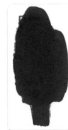

Mechani_____
breathing

D0710641

FEB 13 2015

Mechanics of Breathing

Andrea Aliverti • Antonio Pedotti
Editors

Mechanics of Breathing

New Insights from New Technologies

Second Edition

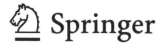 Springer

Editors
Andrea Aliverti
Politecnico di Milano
Milano
Italy

Antonio Pedotti
Politecnico di Milano
Milano
Italy

Videos to this book can be accessed at http://www.springerimages.com/videos/978-88-470-5646-6

ISBN 978-88-470-5646-6   ISBN 978-88-470-5647-3   (eBook)
DOI 10.1007/978-88-470-5647-3
Springer Milan Heidelberg New York Dordrecht London

Library of Congress Control Number: 2014938110

Foreword

Although in the last two decades most of the funds and efforts in respiratory research have been focused on cellular and molecular mechanisms, there are no doubts that a full understanding of the more "classical" respiratory mechanics at organ and system levels is far to be completely reached.

And understanding the mechanics of breathing is important.

As described by Peter Macklem in "A Century of the Mechanics of Breathing" (American Journal of Respiratory and Critical Care Medicine 170:10–15, 2004), the progresses in the knowledge of mechanics of breathing gained in the last century had an enormous impact in the clinical practice and allowed great benefits in terms of prevention, diagnosis and treatment of respiratory diseases.

For instance, the discovery of surfactant role, achieved by studies on alveolar mechanics, resulted in an extraordinary reduction in infant mortality from neonatal respiratory distress syndrome by suggesting treatments based on mechanical ventilation, corticosteroids and replacement of surfactant itself. In respiratory intensive care, the technological progress and intelligent use of mechanical ventilators during anaesthesia, that improved substantially the rate of survival in surgical interventions, would have not been possible without a detailed knowledge of lung and chest wall mechanics. In lung volume reduction surgery for emphysema, suitable mechanical models are of crucial importance for predicting the functional outcome during surgical planning and patient selection. Research in respiratory mechanics has allowed to highlight the abnormalities in obstructive sleep apnea and to propose the successful treatment by nasal continuous positive airway pressure.

We strongly believe that given the complexity of the respiratory system, further insights and improvements in clinical practice can only be obtained by an integrative, multi-scale and multidisciplinary approach based on innovative technologies for measuring and investigating structure and function combined with computational models to process and interpret the available amount of data.

Solving the problem of asthma, the most prevalent respiratory disease in developed countries, will certainly require integration of knowledge from molecular and cellular biology on airway inflammation and from biomechanics on how alteration of airway geometry, load and structure and function of smooth muscles lead to excessive airway narrowing to identify the proper cure. A similar approach is required for better understanding the mechanisms of loss of lung elastic recoil and peripheral airway obstruction in chronic obstructive pulmonary disease (COPD) and identifying proper means to prevent or arrest these processes.

This book was envisioned as a state-of-the-art description of the complexity in normal and pathological respiratory system, mainly observed from the point of view of the mechanics of the airways, lung and chest wall. It is intended as an occasion to spread new insights into the mechanics of breathing obtained by innovative methods of functional imaging of the respiratory system, together with new emerging concepts in physiology and pathophysiology. It is explained how these advances permit the assessment of emerging treatment approaches, including new drugs, innovative surgical techniques and modes of mechanical ventilation and new forms of rehabilitation. In order to ensure a comprehensive coverage of the subject, a multidisciplinary team of authors, comprising basic scientists in respiratory medicine, chest and intensive care physicians and bioengineers involved in both modelling and innovative technologies, was assembled.

The book is structured into four parts. In the first part, eight chapters report last findings on airway, lung and chest wall mechanics during spontaneous breathing at rest and during exercise, and how physiological aspects of mechanics of breathing are altered in presence of diseases, namely asthma, COPD, and acute lung injury (ALI). In the second part, established and emerging methods for assessing respiratory mechanics and, more generally, lung function are illustrated including: spirometry, forced oscillations, optoelectronic plethysmography, gas washout, assessment of respiratory muscle perfusion, and dyspnea.

The third part offers an update on how thoracic functional imaging can provide new insights to the assessment of mechanics of breathing, particularly to study airway distensibility, regional ventilation, diaphragm displacement, and regional perfusion. The fourth part includes six chapters and reports an updated review on how different kinds of intervention (pharmacological treatment, rehabilitation, and invasive and non-invasive mechanical ventilation) affect the mechanics of breathing in selected diseases.

This volume constitutes an updated and significantly revised second edition of the book *Mechanics of Breathing: Pathophysiology, Diagnosis and Treatment*, which was based on a series of lectures delivered during the post-graduate course "What is new in mechanics of breathing: implications for diagnosis and treatment", held in Como, Italy, on April 2001. The present edition contains, in addition, a selection of lectures provided at the ERS Research Seminar "The Limits to Exercise in COPD: New Insights from New Methods", held in Como, Italy, on September 2007. The two chapters authored by Peter Macklem and Solbert Permutt, eminent scientists who have enormously contributed to a better understanding of different aspects of the mechanics of breathing and recently passed away, are reported integrally as in the first edition. This book is dedicated to them.

Milano, Italy   Andrea Aliverti
Milano, Italy   Antonio Pedotti

Contents

Part II   Assessment of Mechanics of Breathing

Part III   Assessment of Mechanics of Breathing: Functional Imaging

Part IV   Different Treatment and Mechanics of Breathing

Part I

Physiological and Pathophysiological Aspects of Mechanics of Breathing

The Act of Breathing

1

Peter T. Macklem[†]

1.1 Introduction

In order to breathe, we must continuously contract and relax our respiratory muscles about 30,000 times a day or a billion times for a lifetime of 90 years. That is quite a marathon that no other skeletal muscles are required to perform. These muscles move the parts of the chest wall that form the boundaries of the thoracic cavity, either enlarging or contracting its volume and thereby displacing air in and out of the lungs. What are the respiratory muscles and how do they accomplish their task?

Ignoring the upper airway muscles that contract to maintain airway patency, the main respiratory muscles are the diaphragm, the abdominal muscles, and the inspiratory and expiratory muscles of the rib cage, including the scalenes, sternocleidomastoids, and triangularis sterni. The compartments they displace are the rib cage and the abdomen. The rib cage can, in turn, be broken down into two compartments, the part that is apposed to the lung, the pulmonary rib cage, and the part apposed to the diaphragm, which forms the cephalad boundary of the abdomen, the abdominal rib cage [1].

1.2 Actions of Individual Respiratory Muscle Groups

Let us consider the actions of the abdominal muscles. Among them, the rectus abdominis does not seem to be important for breathing. The most important is the transversus, while the obliques are probably both postural and respiratory. These

[†]Deceased

P.T. Macklem
Meakins-Christie Laboratories, Montreal Chest Institute of the Royal Victoria Hospital,
McGill University Health Centre, Montreal, QC, Canada

A. Aliverti, A. Pedotti (eds.), *Mechanics of Breathing*,
DOI 10.1007/978-88-470-5647-3_1, © Springer-Verlag Italia 2014

muscles form the anterolateral abdominal wall and insert into the costal margin, and thus can act on the abdominal rib cage [2]. When they contract by themselves, they displace the abdominal wall inward, compress the abdominal contents, increase abdominal pressure (Pab), and passively stretch the relaxed diaphragm. The increase in Pab is transmitted across the diaphragm, but reduced by whatever passive trans-diaphragmatic pressure (Pdi) is present, to increase pleural pressure (Ppl) and thereby inflate the pulmonary rib cage, while deflating the lung [3]. Thus, the volume displaced by the cephalad displacement of the diaphragm, which equals the volume swept by inward displacement of the abdominal wall, is greater than the increase in thoracic volume due to pulmonary rib cage expansion. The actions of the abdominal muscles on both the lungs and abdomen are purely deflationary. They are expiratory muscles.

Their action on the rib cage is considerably more complex. The passively stretched costal diaphragmatic fibers that originate from the costal margin exert an inflationary action on the abdominal rib cage, as does the increase in Pab that is transmitted through the diaphragm to its inner surface. However, any tension transmitted from the abdominal muscles that are also attached at the costal margin would tend to deflate it. The resulting forces acting on the pulmonary and abdominal parts of the rib cage are likely to be different, producing a distortion of the rib cage away from its relaxation configuration. To the extent that the rib cage resists bending, there will be an interaction between the two rib cage compartments tending to minimize distortions [1, 4]. While almost certainly both rib cage compartments expand, the displacements and distortions between the two rib cage compartments have not yet been studied in detail.

Now let us see what happens when the inspiratory muscles of the rib cage contract in isolation. These muscles, of which the most important are the scalenes and parasternal muscles, also include whichever external intercostals that are activated during breathing and the sternocleidomastoids. These muscles insert almost exclusively into the pulmonary rib cage, the caudal border of which is marked by the cephalad extremity of the area of apposition of the diaphragm to the rib cage. This border extends transversely around the rib cage at the level of the xiphisternum. While it is true that the external intercostal muscles extend well into the abdominal rib cage, they do not play much of an inspiratory role, except perhaps when ventilating at maximal breathing capacity. As ventilation increases, these muscles are activated from above downward, so that it is only at very high levels of ventilation that the external intercostals attached to the abdominal rib cage contract [5].

Contracting the inspiratory rib cage muscles therefore has a direct action to expand the rib cage, making Ppl more negative, inflating the lung, and sucking the diaphragm in a cephalad direction, passively stretching it. Because the diaphragm is relaxed, the negative Ppl is transmitted to the abdomen, so that Pab also falls, but not by quite as much as Ppl, because of the passive Pdi resulting from the stretching of the diaphragmatic fibers. The fall in Pab displaces the abdomen inward and thus is expiratory to this compartment. However, the net effect on the whole chest wall is inspiratory; hence, the expiratory displacement of the abdominal wall, which equals the cephalad displacement of the diaphragm, is not as great as the inspiratory displacement of the pulmonary rib cage. Again the effects on the abdominal rib cage and the abdomen are not straightforward. The fall in Pab exerts a deflationary pressure on the abdominal rib cage, while the passive stretching of the diaphragm and the inflation of the pulmonary rib cage both tend to expand it. While the net effect is inflationary, the precise displacements and distortions have not been accurately measured yet. However, the abdominal rib cage and the abdomen move in opposite directions. There is little interaction between these two compartments [6], but under these circumstances the abdomen does not move with a single degree of freedom. The part of the abdominal wall immediately adjacent to the costal margin is "tented" by the abdominal rib cage and moves outward with it, while the rest of the abdominal wall moves inward [7]. This happens to a greater extent than with abdominal muscle contraction when the tensing of these muscles minimizes abdominal wall distortions.

What happens when the diaphragm, often referred to as the most important respiratory muscle, is the only muscle contracting? The diaphragm's connections with the rib cage are all at the costal margin on ribs 7–12 in the abdominal rib cage (except for a tiny slip at the bottom of the sternum). Thus, it has only a minimal action on the pulmonary rib cage. When it contracts, its fibers exert a force on the central tendon, which is displaced caudally compressing the abdominal contents, increasing Pab, and displacing the abdominal wall outward. At the same time the fibers originating from the costal margin exert a cephalad force on the abdominal rib cage through ribs 7–12, and this is augmented by the increase in Pab acting in the area of apposition of diaphragm to the inner surface of the abdominal rib cage. The purpose of diaphragmatic contraction is to develop a pressure difference across the muscle so that as Pab increases, Ppl decreases, thereby inflating the lung. Thus, the action of the diaphragm on the abdomen and the lung is purely inspiratory, but the decrease in Ppl is expiratory to the pulmonary rib cage. If the diaphragm contracts against a closed glottis when to a close approximation chest wall and lung volume remain constant, the pulmonary rib cage is displaced inward as the abdomen is displaced outward. While the increase in Pab and the tension developed in the costal fibers act to expand the abdominal rib cage, this is almost exactly counterbalanced by the expiratory displacement of the pulmonary rib cage and the resistance of the rib cage to bending, so that no net movement of the abdominal rib cage occurs and considerable rib cage distortion takes place [4, 8].

The motions occurring when the diaphragm is the only muscle contracting and air is free to flow into the lung have not been studied yet with precision, but it is likely that significant rib cage distortions would take place. The pulmonary rib cage would be caught between the expiratory force of the fall in Ppl acting over its whole inner surface and the inspiratory action of the expanding abdominal rib cage taking the pulmonary rib cage with it. As most of the force developed by the diaphragm on the rib cage would go into distorting it, and only a small fraction into expanding it [8], this would be an inefficient way to breathe. Rib cage distortions are costly [4, 8], so a good way to breathe is to avoid them altogether.

1.3   Quiet Breathing at Rest

Normally, humans breathe both at rest and during exercise, in a way that the rib cage does not distort [8]. The undistorted configuration of the pulmonary and abdominal rib cage compartments occurs when the pressure acting on both compartments is the same. This occurs during relaxation with all muscles relaxed and Ppl is equal to Pab. During quiet breathing at rest, equal pressures acting on both compartments require that the inspiratory rib cage muscles contract to the extent that the net inflationary pressure acting on the pulmonary rib cage is identical to the net inflationary pressure produced by the agencies acting on the abdominal rib cage. If xPdi is that fraction of Pdi which acts directly on the abdominal rib cage to expand it, and the pressures developed by the inspiratory rib cage muscles is Prcm, then for the pressures to be equal during inspiration on both compartments:

$$\mathrm{Prcm} + \mathrm{Ppl} = x\mathrm{Pdi} + \mathrm{Pab} - y\mathrm{Pabm} \tag{1.1}$$

The left-hand term is the sum of the pressures acting on the pulmonary rib cage, including the deflationary action of Ppl, while the right-hand term is the sum of the pressures acting on the abdominal rib cage, including the action of Pab acting in the area of apposition of the diaphragm to the abdominal rib cage. In the upright position, at least, the abdominal contents passively stretch the abdominal muscles. As they insert into the abdominal rib cage, they have a deflationary action on this compartment represented by $-y\mathrm{Pabm}$, where y is the fraction of the passive pressure developed by the stretched abdominal muscles on the abdominal rib cage. Rearranging,

$$\mathrm{Prcm} = (x+1)\mathrm{Pdi} - y\mathrm{Pabm} \tag{1.2}$$

This assumes that expiratory muscles do not act (except passively) during quiet breathing. This is the case [8]. The inspiratory rib cage muscles must overcome the deflationary action of the fall in Ppl on the pulmonary rib cage and develop an inflationary pressure equal to the combined effects of the direct action of the diaphragm and Pab, minus the deflationary pressure developed by the passively stretched abdominal muscles on the abdominal rib cage. The fact that the measured Prcm is only about half of Pdi during quiet breathing suggests that yPabm is substantial.

1.4   Breathing During Exercise

A quite different pattern of breathing emerges during exercise. As soon as exercise starts, there is an immediate recruitment of expiratory muscles, even at zero workload [9]. The abdominal muscles are the main ones recruited; the expiratory rib cage muscles are recruited to a lesser extent. The expiratory muscles are recruited cyclically, starting at the beginning of expiration, and increasing the pressure that they develop throughout expiration, which reaches its maximal value at end-expiration. Then they do not relax right away, but counterintuitively relax slowly throughout

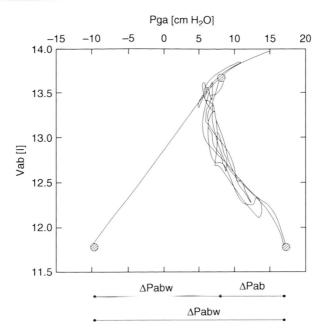

Fig. 1.1 Pressure volume diagram of the abdomen during relaxation, during quiet breathing, and during various levels of exercise [*Vab* volume displaced by the abdominal wall, *Pga* gastric pressure, used as an index of abdominal pressure (*Pab*)]. The *straight* line with a positive slope at lower values of Vab and bending to the right at high Vab is the relaxation pressure volume curve of the abdomen, and *Pabw* is the elastic recoil pressure of the abdomen. The *heavy curve* along the relaxation line ending in the *open circle* is the abdominal pressure volume curve during quiet breathing. The *curved lines* with negative slopes are dynamic abdominal pressure volume curves during various levels of exercise. The *open circle* at the bottom end of the largest of these curves is a zero flow point at end-expiration. The upper *open circle* is a zero flow point at end-inspiration. The pressure generated by the abdominal muscles (*Pabm*) at any Vab is the horizontal distance between the relaxation and dynamic curves at that Vab (From Aliverti et al. [9], modified)

inspiration (Fig. 1.1). This results in a Pab that is high at the beginning of inspiration, but falls progressively throughout inspiration, in striking contrast to breathing at rest when Pab increases throughout inspiration [9].

Evidently as soon as exercise starts, there is an immediate change in the central drive to the respiratory muscles. This drive activates the muscles to produce power, the product of the flow they generate and the pressure they produce. But how this power is partitioned between flow and pressure is not determined by the central drive; it is a unique function of the load the muscle acts against. During breathing at rest, when Pab rises throughout inspiration, this load on the diaphragm increases continuously. Furthermore, Ppl decreases continuously throughout inspiration. The increase in Pab and decrease in Ppl represent the interaction between the activation of the diaphragm produced by the central drive and the elastic loads of the lung and chest wall that the diaphragm is acting against. For a given degree of activation, as these loads increase during inspiration, more of the central drive to the diaphragm is converted into Pdi and less is converted into flow.

Quite the opposite situation is true during exercise. The decrease in Pab during inspiration parallels the decrease in Ppl. If ΔPab equals ΔPpl, then the diaphragm would contract isotonically. It would have to develop a Pdi that equaled Pab-Ppl, either actively or passively, but then merely maintain that Pdi constant during inspiration. The elastic loads disappear.

During exercise the conditions for no rib cage distortion are the same as in Eq. 1.2, except that Pabm is both active and passive. Expressing Eq. 1.2 in terms of changes,

$$\Delta Prcm = (x+1)\Delta Pdi - y\Delta Pabm \qquad (1.3)$$

Prcm now includes both inspiratory and expiratory rib cage muscles. Probably the most important expiratory rib cage muscle is the triangularis sterni, which originates from the lateral border of the sternum and runs axially and laterally in a cephalad direction to insert into the lower border of the ribs of the pulmonary rib cage. The condition for both lack of rib cage distortion and isotonic diaphragm contraction is obtained by setting $\Delta Pdi = 0$ in Eq. 1.3:

$$Prcm = -y Pabm \qquad (1.4)$$

Equation 1.4 states that a simple control system by which the central drive to the combined inspiratory and expiratory rib cage muscles is exactly 180° out of phase with the drive to the abdominal muscles, with a constant of proportionality equal to y, accomplishes two remarkable phenomena: it prevents costly rib cage distortions and removes the elastic load from the diaphragm [9]. Removing the elastic load allows more of the diaphragmatic activation to be converted into flow and less into pressure; that is, during exercise the diaphragm acts as a flow generator, whereas at rest it acts as a pressure generator [9]. The plot of Prcm versus Pabm during exercise is shown in Fig. 1.2 and confirms that the pressures developed by these two muscle groups are, in fact, nearly 180° out of phase.

This explains a puzzling feature of the diaphragm's role in exercise. From breathing at rest to zero load exercise, Pdi actually falls, and at maximal exercise workload Pdi is only about double what it is during breathing at rest, while the pressures developed by the rib cage and abdominal muscles increase, much more than Pdi does [9]. What has happened to the diaphragm's vaunted role as the most important respiratory muscle? It is acting as a flow generator of course. Because it is unloaded, most of its power is expressed as flow and little is expressed as pressure. The increase in diaphragmatic power with exercise workload is just as great as the increase in power of the rib cage and abdominal muscles [9]. Looking at pressures alone gives a very misleading picture.

In addition to preventing rib cage distortions and allowing the diaphragm to act as a flow generator, the abdominal muscles play another important role: end-expiratory lung volume progressively decreases as exercise workload increases. This allows elastic energy to be stored in the system below functional residual capacity, which can be released to perform useful external work during inspiration. Furthermore, the reduction in end-expiratory lung volume is entirely accomplished

Fig. 1.2 Relationship between the pressures developed by the abdominal muscles (*Pabm*) and those developed by the rib cage muscles (*Prcm*) during quiet breathing (*QB*) and at increasing levels of exercise to a maximum of 70 % maximal power output (70 %). During all levels of exercise, these pressures are nearly 180° out of phase (From Aliverti et al. [9])

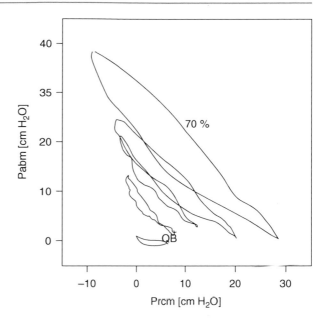

by a reduction in the volume of the abdominal compartment; there is no decrease in the volume of the rib cage at end-expiration [9]. As the volume of the abdomen is the main determinant of diaphragmatic fiber length, its inward displacement lengthens the diaphragm fibers, allowing it to generate more power for a given degree of central activation.

To summarize, there are three sets of respiratory muscles, namely, the diaphragm, the abdominal muscles, and the rib cage muscles. Each has a unique action on the three compartments comprising the chest wall, namely, the pulmonary or lung-apposed rib cage, the abdominal or diaphragm-apposed rib cage, and the abdomen. Although it is possible to breathe with only one or other of these three, isolated contraction of each has unwanted effects on at least one of the compartments. To prevent these effects, coordinated recruitment of two or three sets of muscles is required. During breathing at rest, this is accomplished by the coordinated activity of the diaphragm and inspiratory rib cage muscles. Normally no expiratory muscles are used. During exercise, the abdominal muscles, and to a lesser extent the expiratory rib cage muscles, are immediately recruited. The abdominal muscles in concert with the rib cage muscles play a double role of preventing costly rib cage distortions and unloading the diaphragm, so that it acts as a flow generator while the rib cage and abdominal muscles take on the task of developing the pressures required to move the rib cage and abdomen, respectively. The abdominal muscles play a third role in decreasing end-expiratory lung volume by decreasing the volume of the abdomen. This stores elastic energy in the respiratory system that can be released during inspiration to perform useful external work. It also lengthens diaphragmatic fibers so that they develop more power for a given level of activation.

References

1. Ward ME, Ward JW, Macklem PT (1992) Analysis of human chest wall motion using a two compartment rib cage model. J Appl Physiol 72:1338–1347
2. De Troyer A, Sampson A, Sigrist S, Kelly S (1983) How the abdominal muscles act on the rib cage. J Appl Physiol 54:465–469
3. Goldman MD, Mead J (1973) Mechanical interaction between the diaphragm and rib cage. J Appl Physiol 35:197–204
4. Chihara K, Kenyon CM, Macklem PT (1996) Human rib cage distortability. J Appl Physiol 81: 437–447
5. Whitelaw WA, Feroah T (1989) Patterns of intercostal activity in humans. J Appl Physiol 67: 2087–2094
6. Deschamps C, Rodarte JR, Wilson TA (1988) Coupling between rib cage and abdominal compartments of the relaxed chest wall. J Appl Physiol 65:2265–2269
7. Mead J, Loring SH (1982) Analysis of volume displacement and length changes of the diaphragm during breathing. J Appl Physiol 53:750–755
8. Kenyon CM, Cala SJ, Yan S et al (1997) Rib cage mechanics during quiet breathing and exercise in humans. J Appl Physiol 83:1242–1255
9. Aliverti A, Cala SJ, Duranti R et al (1997) Human respiratory muscle actions and control during exercise. J Appl Physiol 83:1256–1269

Work of Breathing During Exercise: Implications for Performance

Lee M. Romer and Jerome A. Dempsey

2.1 Introduction

This chapter describes the mechanical and metabolic costs of meeting the ventilatory requirements of exercise in healthy humans. We also deal with whether the respiratory muscles fatigue during exercise, what factors contribute to any such respiratory muscle fatigue, what the implications of these factors are for blood flow distribution and endurance exercise performance, and whether it is possible to overcome these potential respiratory limitations.

2.2 What Are the Ventilatory Costs of Exercise?

During whole-body exercise the respiratory control system functions to increase alveolar ventilation to a level sufficient to regulate arterial blood-gas tensions and acid–base balance at or near resting levels while minimizing the mechanical work performed by the respiratory muscles. These ventilatory demands are met by increases in tidal volume and airflow, requiring increases in negative intrapleural pressure. The peak dynamic pressure generated by the inspiratory muscles expressed relative to the subjects' ability to generate pressure at the lung volumes and flow rates adopted during maximal exercise is only 40–60 % in moderately fit

L.M. Romer, PhD (✉)
Centre for Sports Medicine and Human Performance, Brunel University,
Uxbridge, Middlesex UB8 3PH, UK
e-mail: lee.romer@brunel.ac.uk

J.A. Dempsey, PhD
John Rankin Laboratory of Pulmonary Medicine,
Department of Population Health Sciences, University of Wisconsin,
1300 University Ave., Room 4245 MSC, Madison, WI 53706-1532, USA
e-mail: jdempsey@wisc.edu

A. Aliverti, A. Pedotti (eds.), *Mechanics of Breathing*,
DOI 10.1007/978-88-470-5647-3_2, © Springer-Verlag Italia 2014

individuals [1]. In contrast, endurance-trained subjects elevate peak dynamic inspiratory muscle pressure to 90 % of capacity or greater [1].

The O_2 consumption of the respiratory muscles ($\dot{V}rmO_2$) during exercise increases progressively relative to minute ventilation ($\dot{V}_E$). However, the relationship is concave upward, i.e., a greater increment in $\dot{V}rmO_2$ is required to establish a given increase in $\dot{V}_E$ as work rate increases [2]. The $\dot{V}rmO_2$ during near-maximal exercise requires approximately 10 % of $\dot{V}O_{2\,max}$ for moderately fit subjects, whereas in highly fit subjects at higher peak work rates and $\dot{V}_E$, the $\dot{V}rmO_2$ approaches 15 % of $\dot{V}O_{2\,max}$ [3]. Respiratory muscle perfusion naturally plays an important role in determining $\dot{V}rmO_2$. By measuring the reduction in cardiac output achieved via mechanical ventilation, Harms et al. [4] estimated that the respiratory muscle work under normal physiological conditions at maximal exercise in fit subjects requires approximately 16 % of the cardiac output to be directed to the respiratory muscles to support their metabolic requirements (Fig. 2.1). These indirect estimates in humans are in agreement with microsphere studies in the exercising pony, which show large increases in blood flow to both inspiratory and expiratory muscles amounting to approximately 16 % of total cardiac output during maximal exercise [5].

Nevertheless, the quantitation of respiratory muscle blood flow during exercise in the human remains controversial. Recent estimates of "trunk and head" blood flow based on the difference between cardiac output and flow to the arms plus legs (measured with dye dilution via catheterization of the subclavian and femoral veins) suggest that the lumped structure of the head, neck, heart, abdomen viscera, kidney, respiratory muscles, and gluteal muscles receives about 20 % of the cardiac output and 15 % of the $\dot{V}O_2$ during maximal upright cycling exercise [6]. These data would attribute a substantially less than 15 % share of the cardiac output to the respiratory muscles. One problem not yet addressed in any study is the identification of all muscles – in the chest wall, abdomen, upper back, and shoulders – which are actually engaged (both dynamically and as fixators) in producing the hyperpnea accompanying heavy exercise.

2.3   Do the Respiratory Muscles Fatigue with Exercise?

Muscle fatigue has been defined as "a condition in which there is a loss in the capacity for developing force and/or velocity of a muscle, resulting from muscle activity under load and which is reversible by rest" [7]. Respiratory muscle fatigue thus defined and its significance to whole-body exercise performance were poorly documented and had generated little interest before the late 1970s. The seminal paper of Roussos and Macklem [8], however, illustrated that the diaphragm under resistive load exhibits task failure in a fashion similar to that expected of any other skeletal muscle.

More recently, nerve stimulation techniques have been used to provide objective evidence of exercise-induced respiratory muscle fatigue. In subjects with a wide range of fitness performing sustained exercise for more than 8–10 min at intensities greater than 80–85 % of $\dot{V}O_{2\,max}$, reductions of 15–30 % in the transdiaphragmatic

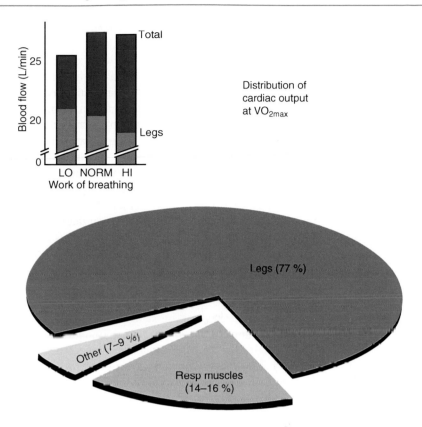

Fig. 2.1 Distribution of cardiac output at $\dot{V}O_{2\,max}$. *Left panel*: distribution of total cardiac output among legs, respiratory muscles, and other metabolically active tissues (skin, heart, brain, kidneys, and liver) at $\dot{V}O_{2\,max}$. Respiratory muscle blood flow at $\dot{V}O_{2\,max}$ was assumed to be equal to the fall in cardiac output obtained with respiratory muscle unloading at $\dot{V}O_{2\,max}$ and extrapolated to zero work of breathing. *Right panel*: total cardiac output and leg blood flow were measured under control conditions (normal work of breathing), with respiratory muscle unloading (low work of breathing) and with respiratory muscle loading (high work of breathing). Total blood flow was significantly lower with unloading and unchanged with loading, whereas leg blood flow and vascular conductance were significantly increased with unloading and decreased with loading (Data from Harms et al. [4, 26])

pressure response to supramaximal stimulation of the phrenic nerves were consistently obtained across a wide range of lung volumes and stimulation frequencies (1–100 Hz), and persisted for 1–2 h after exercise [9, 10]. These findings of diaphragmatic fatigue obtained at end-exercise have been confirmed using phrenic nerve stimulation "during" exercise, showing that significant fatigue occurs early during sustained, heavy exercise [11]. Like the diaphragm, the abdominal muscles are also susceptible to peripheral fatigue after sustained, heavy exercise (>90 % $\dot{V}O_{2\,max}$), as demonstrated by 15–25 % reductions in the gastric pressure response to stimulation of the thoracic nerves [12].

2.4   What Are the Factors Contributing to Respiratory Muscle Fatigue?

There appear to be two general causes of exercise-induced diaphragmatic fatigue, namely, one cause attributable to the force production by the diaphragm itself and a second due to the effects of whole-body exercise, per se. Babcock et al. [13] examined the role that diaphragmatic pressure generation played in the fatigue process independent of the whole-body "exercise effect." Subjects who demonstrated exercise-induced diaphragmatic fatigue were required to mimic at rest the essential mechanical components of breathing during exercise as well as the diaphragmatic pressure production for an identical time period as produced during exercise at 95 % of $\dot{V}O_{2\,max}$. This mimicking protocol caused a less than 10 % decline in evoked diaphragmatic pressure. Furthermore, sustained force outputs of the diaphragm that were 1.5–2 times those normally experienced during exhaustive exercise were required to cause diaphragmatic fatigue when the subject was in the resting state and increased ventilation voluntarily. These data show that the influence of whole-body exercise on diaphragmatic fatigue is substantial. We believe that this whole-body exercise effect is likely due to less blood flow availability to the diaphragm during exercise (vs. hyperpnea during the resting state) in the face of high blood flow demands by the locomotor muscles.

A second study showed that greatly reducing the force output of the diaphragm during exhaustive prolonged exercise prevented exercise-induced diaphragmatic fatigue [14]. Thus, while the force output of the diaphragm experienced during exercise was insufficient to cause fatigue in the absence of locomotor muscle force output, it was critical to the development of diaphragmatic fatigue in the presence of whole-body exercise. These findings were consistent with the additional observation that the effect of exhaustive high-intensity whole-body exercise, per se, did not elicit fatigue in non-exercising muscles of the hand [13].

Based on the evidence summarized above, we postulate that the development of diaphragmatic fatigue during exercise is a function of the relationship between the magnitude of diaphragmatic work and the adequacy of its blood supply: the less blood flow is available, the less diaphragmatic work is required to produce fatigue. In healthy subjects of varying fitness levels [15], an imbalance of muscle force output versus blood flow and/or O_2 transport availability to the diaphragm which favors fatigue appears to occur during exhaustive endurance exercise only when either the relative intensity of the exercise exceeds 85 % of $\dot{V}O_{2\,max}$ [9] or arterial hypoxemia is present [16].

2.5   What Are the Consequences of Respiratory Muscle Fatigue?

2.5.1   Effects on Exercise Performance

Experiments that have deliberately fatigued the respiratory muscles prior to exercise using either voluntary hyperpnea [17, 18] or resistive loading [19, 20] have noted a decrease [17, 18, 20] or no change [19] in time-to-exhaustion during subsequent short-term, heavy exercise; the influence of fatigue upon more prolonged exercise remains untested. On balance, these findings suggest that there is potential for respiratory muscle fatigue to impair short-duration, high-intensity exercise performance. A potential limitation of pre-fatigue studies, however, is that the number and type of motor units recruited during loaded breathing may be substantially different than during subsequent exercise. There may also be an effect of prior fatigue on the breathing pattern during subsequent exercise, such that any changes in exercise performance could be due to changes in exertional dyspnea. Furthermore, it is difficult to determine the contribution of subject expectation because it is impossible to placebo the pre-fatigue condition.

Several studies have noted increases in exercise capacity with partial unloading of the respiratory muscles using either low-density gas mixtures [21] or proportional assist mechanical ventilation [22]. For example, mechanical unloading of the respiratory muscles by over 50 % of their total inspiratory and expiratory work during heavy exercise (>90 % of $\dot{V}O_{2\,max}$) prevented diaphragmatic fatigue [14] and resulted in a statistically significant 14 % increase in exercise time-to-exhaustion in trained male cyclists, with reductions in oxygen uptake and the rate of rise in perceptions of respiratory and limb discomfort [22] (Fig. 2.2). Other studies have not found a significant effect of respiratory muscle unloading on exercise capacity in less fit subjects [23–25], although these studies were conducted at lower relative exercise intensities, and the respiratory muscle unloading did not affect oxygen uptake. Collectively, these findings suggest that the work of breathing normally encountered during heavy sustained exercise has a significant influence on exercise performance.

2.5.2 Cardiorespiratory Interactions

2.5.2.1 Respiratory Muscle Metaboreflex

Perhaps the most likely aspect of respiratory muscle work limiting exercise performance is a reflex effect from fatiguing respiratory muscles which increases sympathetic vasoconstrictor outflow and compromises perfusion of limb muscle during prolonged exercise, thereby limiting its ability to perform work. Harms et al. [26] used a proportional assist ventilator to decrease the work of breathing in endurance-trained cyclists exercising at greater than 80 % of $\dot{V}O_{2\,max}$. An increase in limb blood flow was observed commensurate with a 50–60 % decrease in the work of breathing. Conversely, when the work of breathing was increased by a comparable amount, limb blood flow and vascular conductance fell (Fig. 2.1). It seems likely that the local reductions in vascular conductance were sympathetically mediated because these changes correlated inversely with changes in norepinephrine spillover across the limb. When the study was repeated at an exercise intensity of only 50–75 % of $\dot{V}O_{2\,max}$, changes in limb blood flow, vascular conductance, and norepinephrine spillover did not occur, even though changes in respiratory muscle work were still sufficient to alter oxygen uptake and cardiac output [27].

Fig. 2.2 Effects of respiratory muscle unloading via mechanical ventilation upon endurance exercise capacity at a workload requiring ~90 % of VO_{2max} in trained male cyclists ($n=7$). Group mean data are shown for minutes 1–5 of exercise and at exhaustion. Absolute time-to-exhaustion under control conditions averaged 9.1 ± 2.6 min. Unloading normal work of breathing by 50 % from control increased time-to-exhaustion in 76 % of trials by a mean ± SD of 1.3 ± 0.4 min (14 ± 5 %). Respiratory muscle unloading caused reductions in oxygen uptake and the rate of rise in perceptions of limb and respiratory discomfort throughout the duration of exercise. * Significantly different from control, $p < 0.05$ (Data from Harms et al. [22])

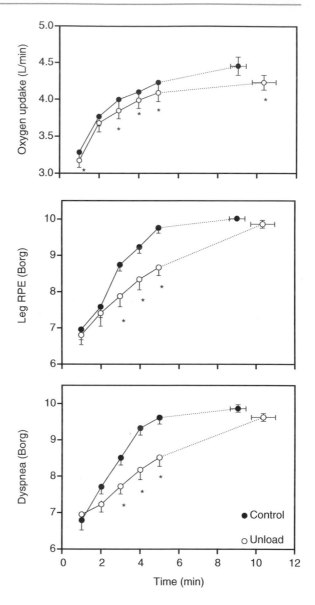

What caused these sympathetically mediated changes in limb vascular conductance when respiratory muscle work was altered during maximal exercise? We postulate that reflex mechanisms of sympathoexcitation are triggered by metaboreceptors in the diaphragm and expiratory muscles that begin to accumulate metabolic end products during heavy exercise when cardiac output is insufficient to adequately meet the high metabolic requirements of both respiratory and limb musculature. Evidence in support of this postulate is fourfold. First, diaphragmatic fatigue caused a time-dependent increase in multiunit activity in small diameter phrenic afferents in anesthetized cats [28, 29] and in single-unit activity in group IV afferents in anesthetized rats [30]. Second, electrical or pharmacological stimulation of thin-fiber phrenic afferents in anesthetized animals using capsaicin, bradykinin or lactic acid injections, or diaphragm muscle ischemia elicited increases in efferent sympathetic nerve activity and/or vascular resistance in several vascular beds, including the limb musculature and renal and coronary vasculature [31–33]. Third, in the resting or mildly exercising canine, infusing lactic acid into the phrenic artery and diaphragm caused vasoconstriction and reduced blood flow in the contracting limb muscle, and this vasoconstrictive effect was prevented via adrenergic blockade [34]. Finally, in a series of studies in humans, high-intensity contractions of the diaphragm [35] or expiratory muscles [36] against airway resistance to the point of task failure and/or fatigue caused a time-dependent increase in muscle sympathetic nerve activity (MSNA) in the resting leg, despite a corresponding increase in systemic blood pressure. This time-dependent increase in MSNA was accompanied by a significant decrease in limb vascular conductance and limb blood flow along with an increase in mean arterial pressure and heart rate [37] (Fig. 2.3). A similar time-dependent increase in ulnar nerve MSNA elicited via voluntary increases in inspiratory muscle work has recently been shown during cycling exercise [38].

To determine the precise mechanisms responsible for these time dependent increases in MSNA and vascular responses, additional experiments were conducted to differentiate the potential effect of diaphragmatic fatigue from associated changes in lung volume, intrathoracic pressure, mechanical deformation of muscle, and central respiratory motor output, all of which accompanied the fatiguing voluntary respiratory efforts carried out to task failure. These potential excitatory effects on MSNA were ruled out by showing no effect of non-fatiguing voluntary increases in central respiratory motor output per se and a vasodilatory effect of increasing tidal volume by itself [35, 36]. Furthermore, the increase in MSNA was gradual and time dependent and was not evident at the initiation of the fatiguing trial despite marked increases in effort, diaphragmatic force production, and negativity of intrathoracic pressure. A more recent study using multiple trials of gradually increasing inspiratory effort showed that limb vasoconstriction only occurred when the rhythmic contractions of the diaphragm were of sufficient force and frequency to cause fatigue [39]. Thus, the apparent threshold for activation of MSNA from rhythmic respiratory muscle contractions was surpassed, not at a specific intensity of muscle force output, but only by respiratory muscle fatigue or at least a regimen of rhythmic muscular contractions that was likely sufficient to cause significant accumulation of muscle metabolites.

Collectively, the MSNA and blood flow data in humans and animals studied at rest and during exercise suggest that significant respiratory muscle metabolite accumulation will evoke a metaboreflex effect, which increases sympathetic vasoconstrictor outflow to limb locomotor muscle (Fig. 2.4), and perhaps explain the observed effects of changes in respiratory muscle work on limb vascular conductance, blood flow, and fatigue during maximal exercise [26, 40].

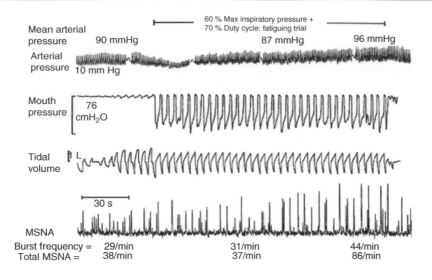

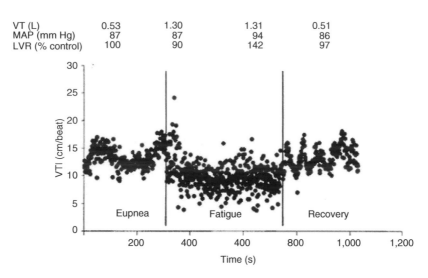

Fig. 2.3 Upper panel (**a**): effects of fatiguing the diaphragm on muscle sympathetic nerve activity (MSNA) in the resting leg in one representative subject during eupnea and diaphragmatic breathing at 60 % of maximum inspiratory mouth pressure (MIP) with a $T_IT_{TOT}=0.7$ and $f_b=15$ breaths/min. Note that the frequency and amplitude of MSNA were unchanged at the onset of increased diaphragmatic force output but increased thereafter in a time-dependent manner. Lower panel (**b**): beat-by-beat velocity of femoral artery blood flow (*VTI* velocity time integral) in the resting leg in one representative subject during eupnea and fatiguing diaphragmatic work at 60 % MIP with a $T_IT_{TOT}=0.7$ and $f_b=15$ breaths/min and during recovery. Femoral artery diameter was unchanged during the experiment; therefore, any changes in measured blood velocity reflected those in blood flow. Note that leg blood flow decreased and leg vascular resistance increased during fatiguing diaphragmatic work, despite an increase in MAP (Data from St. Croix et al. [35] and Sheel et al. [37])

Respiratory muscle metaboreflex

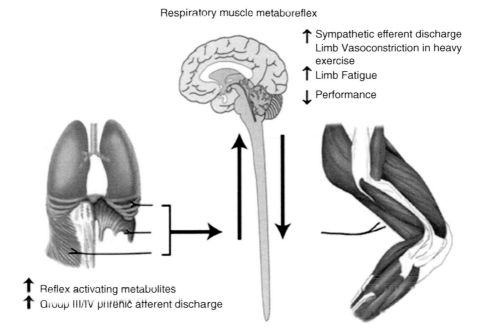

↑ Sympathetic efferent discharge
Limb Vasoconstriction in heavy
exercise
↑ Limb Fatigue
↓ Performance

↑ Reflex activating metabolites
↑ Group III/IV phrenic afferent discharge

Fig. 2.4 Schematic representation of the proposed respiratory muscle metaboreflex from the diaphragm and expiratory muscles activated by fatiguing contractions of these muscles and eliciting increased sympathetic discharge and limb vasoconstriction during heavy exercise with consequences of enhanced rate of development of limb fatigue and reduced exercise performance (see text) (From Dempsey et al. [63])

2.5.2.2 Intrathoracic Pressures and Cardiac Output

In exercising humans and dogs, reducing the negativity of inspiratory intrapleural pressure reduces right ventricular preload and stroke volume in health [4]. On the other hand, increasing expiratory threshold pressure reduces stroke volume – presumably because left ventricular afterload is increased – thereby reducing transventricular pressure differences which would slow the rate of ventricular filling during diastole [41, 42]. Further, increasing abdominal versus intrathoracic pressure with predominantly diaphragm versus ribcage inspirations, respectively, has marked cyclical effects on femoral venous return from the limbs at rest and even during mild-intensity leg exercise [43]. Understanding how the cardiovascular effects of isolated alterations in pressures during various phases of the respiratory cycle translate into the complex effects of breathing during whole-body exercise will be a formidable task – especially in the elite athlete ventilating in excess of 150 l/min who experiences expiratory flow limitation, positive expiratory pressures which often exceed the critical closing pressure of the airways, and hyperinflation with inspiratory pressures that are approaching the limits of the dynamic capacity of the inspiratory muscles [1]. Equally intriguing and clinically relevant is why reducing the magnitude of negative pressure on inspiration increases stroke volume and cardiac output in a dose-dependent manner in heart failure animals [44] and humans [45] during exercise – effects which are in the opposite direction to those in the healthy subject.

2.6   Can These Respiratory Limitations Be Overcome?

Evidence from studies that have specifically trained the respiratory muscles of healthy subjects using strength (resistive/threshold) or endurance (hyperpnea) training suggests it might be possible to overcome the aforementioned respiratory limitations on exercise. Early studies produced contradictory findings, primarily due to poor research designs and inappropriate outcome measures [46]. More recent evidence from adequately controlled studies suggests that there might be small but significant effects on exercise performance during constant load tests, time trials, and intermittent tests [47–50].

The mechanisms by which respiratory muscle training might improve exercise performance are not entirely clear. Increases in respiratory muscle strength, velocity of shortening, and endurance have been consistently observed with respiratory muscle training in healthy subjects [51]. The functional significance of such improvements in respiratory muscle function would presumably be to prevent or delay the respiratory muscle fatigue that is known to occur during heavy sustained exercise (see above). Changes in respiratory muscle fiber size, subtype ratio, and myofiber contractile properties induced by respiratory muscle training may reduce the force contribution from each active myofiber or the number of myofibers at a given submaximal level of ventilation. In conjunction, a stronger type I fiber may allow individuals to delay the recruitment of less efficient type II fibers. Fatigue-resistant respiratory muscles may cause reductions in the rate of carbohydrate breakdown, lactate accumulation, and intracellular pH in these muscles, contributing to an overall improvement in cellular homeostasis. Fewer metabolic stimuli in the respiratory muscles would be expected to attenuate reflex activity from type III/IV receptors of these muscles and thereby reduce sympathetic vasoconstrictor activity in the limbs. The concomitant increase in limb blood flow would increase oxygen delivery to the limbs and potentially reduce both limb muscle fatigue and peripheral effort sensations. There is evidence that respiratory muscle training reduces exercise-induced respiratory muscle fatigue [52], increases the oxidative and/or lactate transport capacity of the inspiratory muscles [53], alleviates calf muscle fatigue during plantar flexion exercise [54], and increases the threshold for activation of the respiratory muscle metaboreflex [55]. However, direct evidence for a benefit of respiratory muscle training on blood flow redistribution during dynamic whole-body exercise is not yet available. In addition to the potential effects of respiratory muscle training on exercise-induced respiratory muscle fatigue and its associated vasoconstrictive effects on the locomotor muscle vasculature, there might also be perceptual benefits. Attenuation of sensory input to the central nervous system may be expected to occur in line with a decrease in inhibitory feedback from fatiguing respiratory muscles, an alteration in breathing pattern (e.g., reduce operating lung volumes), a delay in the recruitment of accessory respiratory muscles, an alteration in the motor recruitment within a given respiratory muscle, or a reduction in the fraction of maximum tension generated with each breath [56, 57].

To what extent should exercise performance be affected by respiratory muscle training? Several studies have noted increases in time-to-exhaustion with partial unloading of the respiratory muscles of healthy subjects [21, 22]. For example, mechanical unloading of the respiratory muscles by over 50 % of their total inspiratory and expiratory work during heavy exercise prevented diaphragmatic fatigue [14] and resulted in at most a 14 % improvement in endurance capacity in trained cyclists (Fig. 2.2) with no change in circulating lactate, a reduction in oxygen uptake and cardiac output, a decrease in the rate of rise of both respiratory and limb discomfort, and variable effects on ventilation [22]. Although some respiratory muscle training studies have reported huge improvements (25–50 %) in exercise capacity [47, 48], it seems inconceivable that the effects could surpass those seen with substantial mechanical unloading – unless respiratory muscle training imparts some additional influences on locomotor muscles that are not realized via substantial respiratory muscle unloading and the prevention of diaphragmatic fatigue. A potential reason why previous studies have found greater improvements in exercise capacity with respiratory muscle training may be due to a large intraindividual variance in exercise performance coupled with a failure to use carefully matched and designed placebo groups.

If respiratory muscle training were to attenuate exercise-induced respiratory muscle fatigue, it is likely that the benefit would only occur in near-maximal exercise conditions. Increases in time-to-exhaustion with respiratory muscle unloading have been noted in healthy, fit subjects only at exercise intensities greater than 85 % of $\dot{V}O_{2\,max}$ [21, 22]. Interestingly, exercise-induced diaphragmatic fatigue also only occurred consistently at exercise intensities greater than 85 % of $\dot{V}O_{2\,max}$ [9], and the effects of respiratory muscle unloading on limb vascular resistance during exercise only occurred when the intensity exceeded 80 % of maximum [26, 27]. On the other hand, there are several examples where respiratory muscle work exerts significant cardiovascular effects, even during submaximal exercise. In patients with congestive heart failure [58] or those with chronic obstructive pulmonary disease [59], sustained exercise at only 50–60 % of maximum caused fatigue of limb locomotor muscles [60]. In rodent models of heart failure (vs. healthy controls), microsphere distribution studies showed a reduced limb blood flow and enhanced diaphragm blood flow during exercise [61]. In human chronic heart failure patients, respiratory muscle unloading [45] was shown to increase limb vascular conductance and limb blood flow and enhance exercise performance. These effects reflect the combination of increased respiratory muscle work with limited cardiac output in chronic heart failure. Finally, even the healthy person exercising submaximally in hypoxic environments undergoes hyperventilation and increased work of breathing; under these conditions, unloading the respiratory muscles significantly reduces the rate of development of limb fatigue and improves endurance performance [62].

References

1. Johnson BD, Saupe KW, Dempsey JA (1992) Mechanical constraints on exercise hyperpnea in endurance athletes. J Appl Physiol 73:874–886
2. Otis AB (1954) The work of breathing. Physiol Rev 34:449–458

3. Aaron EA, Seow KC, Johnson BD et al (1992) Oxygen cost of exercise hyperpnea: implications for performance. J Appl Physiol 72:1818–1825
4. Harms CA, Wetter TJ, McClaran SR et al (1998) Effects of respiratory muscle work on cardiac output and its distribution during maximal exercise. J Appl Physiol 85:609–618
5. Manohar M (1986) Blood flow to the respiratory and limb muscles and to abdominal organs during maximal exertion in ponies. J Physiol 377:25–35
6. Calbet JA, Gonzalez-Alonso J, Helge JW et al (2007) Cardiac output and leg and arm blood flow during incremental exercise to exhaustion on the cycle ergometer. J Appl Physiol 103:969–978
7. NHLBI Workshop summary. Respiratory muscle fatigue. Report of the Respiratory Muscle Fatigue Workshop Group (1990) Am Rev Respir Dis 142:474–480
8. Roussos CS, Macklem PT (1977) Diaphragmatic fatigue in man. J Appl Physiol 43:189–197
9. Johnson BJ, Babcock MA, Suman OE et al (1993) Exercise-induced diaphragmatic fatigue in healthy humans. J Physiol 460:385–405
10. Romer LM, Polkey MI (2008) Exercise-induced respiratory muscle fatigue: implications for performance. J Appl Physiol 104:879–888
11. Walker DJ, Walterspacher S, Schlager D et al (2011) Characteristics of diaphragmatic fatigue during exhaustive exercise until task failure. Respir Physiol Neurobiol 176:14–20
12. Taylor BJ, How SC, Romer LM (2006) Exercise-induced abdominal muscle fatigue in healthy humans. J Appl Physiol 100:1554–1562
13. Babcock MA, Pegelow DF, McClaran SR et al (1995) Contribution of diaphragmatic power output to exercise-induced diaphragm fatigue. J Appl Physiol 78:1710–1719
14. Babcock MA, Pegelow DF, Harms CA et al (2002) Effects of respiratory muscle unloading on exercise-induced diaphragm fatigue. J Appl Physiol 93:201–206
15. Babcock MA, Pegelow DF, Johnson BD et al (1996) Aerobic fitness effects on exercise-induced low-frequency diaphragm fatigue. J Appl Physiol 81:2156–2164
16. Babcock MA, Johnson BD, Pegelow DF et al (1995) Hypoxic effects on exercise-induced diaphragmatic fatigue in normal healthy humans. J Appl Physiol 78:82–92
17. Dodd SL, Powers SK, Thompson D et al (1989) Exercise performance following intense, short-term ventilatory work. Int J Sports Med 10:48–52
18. Martin B, Heintzelman M, Chen HI (1982) Exercise performance after ventilatory work. J Appl Physiol 52:1581–1585
19. Mador MJ, Acevedo FA (1991) Effect of respiratory muscle fatigue on subsequent exercise performance. J Appl Physiol 70:2059–2065
20. Taylor BJ, Romer LM (2008) Effect of expiratory muscle fatigue on exercise tolerance and locomotor muscle fatigue in healthy humans. J Appl Physiol 104:1442–1451
21. Wilson GD, Welch HG (1980) Effects of varying concentrations of N2/O2 and He/O2 on exercise tolerance in man. Med Sci Sports Exerc 12:380–384
22. Harms CA, Wetter TJ, St Croix CM et al (2000) Effects of respiratory muscle work on exercise performance. J Appl Physiol 89:131–138
23. Gallagher CG, Younes M (1989) Effect of pressure assist on ventilation and respiratory mechanics in heavy exercise. J Appl Physiol 66:1824–1837
24. Krishnan B, Zintel T, McParland C et al (1996) Lack of importance of respiratory muscle load in ventilatory regulation during heavy exercise in humans. J Physiol 490(Pt 2):537–550
25. Marciniuk D, McKim D, Sanii R et al (1994) Role of central respiratory muscle fatigue in endurance exercise in normal subjects. J Appl Physiol 76:236–241
26. Harms CA, Babcock MA, McClaran SR et al (1997) Respiratory muscle work compromises leg blood flow during maximal exercise. J Appl Physiol 82:1573–1583
27. Wetter TJ, Harms CA, Nelson WB et al (1999) Influence of respiratory muscle work on VO2 and leg blood flow during submaximal exercise. J Appl Physiol 87:643–651
28. Balzamo E, Lagier-Tessonnier F, Jammes Y (1992) Fatigue-induced changes in diaphragmatic afferents and cortical activity in the cat. Respir Physiol 90:213–226

29. Jammes Y, Balzamo E (1992) Changes in afferent and efferent phrenic activities with electrically induced diaphragmatic fatigue. J Appl Physiol 73:894–902
30. Hill JM (2000) Discharge of group IV phrenic afferent fibers increases during diaphragmatic fatigue. Brain Res 856:240–244
31. Hussain SN, Chatillon A, Comtois A et al (1991) Chemical activation of thin-fiber phrenic afferents. 2. Cardiovascular responses. J Appl Physiol 70:77–86
32. Offner B, Dembowsky K, Czachurski J (1992) Characteristics of sympathetic reflexes evoked by electrical stimulation of phrenic nerve afferents. J Auton Nerv Syst 41:103–111
33. Szulczyk A, Szulczyk P, Zywuszko B (1988) Analysis of reflex activity in cardiac sympathetic nerve induced by myelinated phrenic nerve afferents. Brain Res 447:109–115
34. Rodman JR, Henderson KS, Smith CA et al (2003) Cardiovascular effects of the respiratory muscle metaboreflexes in dogs: rest and exercise. J Appl Physiol 95:1159–1169
35. St Croix CM, Morgan BJ, Wetter TJ et al (2000) Fatiguing inspiratory muscle work causes reflex sympathetic activation in humans. J Physiol 529(Pt 2):493–504
36. Derchak PA, Sheel AW, Morgan BJ et al (2002) Effects of expiratory muscle work on muscle sympathetic nerve activity. J Appl Physiol 92:1539–1552
37. Sheel AW, Derchak PA, Morgan BJ et al (2001) Fatiguing inspiratory muscle work causes reflex reduction in resting leg blood flow in humans. J Physiol 537(Pt 1):277–289
38. Katayama K, Iwamoto E, Ishida K et al (2012) Inspiratory muscle fatigue increases sympathetic vasomotor outflow and blood pressure during submaximal exercise. Am J Physiol Regul Integr Comp Physiol 302:R1167–R1175
39. Sheel AW, Derchak PA, Pegelow DF et al (2002) Threshold effects of respiratory muscle work on limb vascular resistance. Am J Physiol Heart Circ Physiol 282:H1732–H1738
40. Romer LM, Lovering AT, Haverkamp HC et al (2006) Effect of inspiratory muscle work on peripheral fatigue of locomotor muscles in healthy humans. J Physiol 571(Pt 2):425–439
41. Miller JD, Hemauer SJ, Smith CA et al (2006) Expiratory threshold loading impairs cardiovascular function in health and chronic heart failure during submaximal exercise. J Appl Physiol 101:213–227
42. Stark-Leyva KN, Beck KC, Johnson BD (2004) Influence of expiratory loading and hyperinflation on cardiac output during exercise. J Appl Physiol 96:1920–1927
43. Miller JD, Pegelow DF, Jacques AJ et al (2005) Skeletal muscle pump versus respiratory muscle pump: modulation of venous return from the locomotor limb in humans. J Physiol 563(Pt 3):925–943
44. Miller JD, Smith CA, Hemauer SJ et al (2007) The effects of inspiratory intrathoracic pressure production on the cardiovascular response to submaximal exercise in health and chronic heart failure. Am J Physiol Heart Circ Physiol 292:H580–H592
45. Olson TP, Joyner MJ, Dietz NM et al (2010) Effects of respiratory muscle work on blood flow distribution during exercise in heart failure. J Physiol 588:2487–2501
46. McConnell AK, Romer LM (2004) Respiratory muscle training in healthy humans: resolving the controversy. Int J Sports Med 25:284–293
47. HajGhanbari B, Yamabayashi C, Buna T et al (2012) Effects of respiratory muscle training on performance in athletes: a systematic review with meta-analyses. J Strength Cond Res. doi:10.1519/JSC.0b013e318269f73f
48. Illi SK, Held U, Frank I et al (2012) Effect of respiratory muscle training on exercise performance in healthy individuals: a systematic review and meta-analysis. Sports Med 42(8):707–724
49. McConnell AK (2012) CrossTalk opposing view: respiratory muscle training does improve exercise tolerance. J Physiol 590:3397–3398
50. Patel MS, Hart N, Polkey MI (2012) CrossTalk proposal: training the respiratory muscles does not improve exercise tolerance. J Physiol 590:3393–3395
51. Leith DE, Bradley M (1976) Ventilatory muscle strength and endurance training. J Appl Physiol 41:508–516

52. Verges S, Lenherr O, Haner AC (2007) Increased fatigue resistance of respiratory muscles during exercise after respiratory muscle endurance training. Am J Physiol Regul Comp Physiol 292(3):R1246–R1253

53. Brown PI, Sharpe GR, Johnson MA (2012) Inspiratory muscle training abolishes the blood lactate increase associated with volitional hyperpnoea superimposed on exercise and accelerates lactate and oxygen uptake kinetics at the onset of exercise. Eur J Appl Physiol 112:2117–2129

54. McConnell AK, Lomax M (2006) The influence of inspiratory muscle work history and specific inspiratory muscle training upon human limb muscle fatigue. J Physiol 577(Pt 1):445–457

55. Witt JD, Guenette JA, Rupert JL et al (2007) Inspiratory muscle training attenuates the human respiratory muscle metaboreflex. J Physiol 584(Pt 3):1019–1028

56. McConnell AK, Romer LM (2004) Dyspnoea in health and obstructive pulmonary disease: the role of respiratory muscle function and training. Sports Med 34(2):117–132

57. Sheel AW, Foster GE, Romer LM (2004) Exercise and its impact on dyspnea. Curr Opin Pharmacol 11(3):195–203

58. O'Donnell DE, D'Arsigny C, Raj S et al (1999) Ventilatory assistance improves exercise endurance in stable congestive heart failure. Am J Respir Crit Care Med 160:1804–1811

59. Richardson RS, Sheldon J, Poole DC et al (1999) Evidence of skeletal muscle metabolic reserve during whole-body exercise in patients with chronic obstructive pulmonary disease. Am J Respir Crit Care Med 159:881–885

60. Amann M, Regan MS, Kobitary M et al (2010) Impact of pulmonary system limitations on locomotor muscle fatigue in patients with COPD. Am J Physiol Regul Integr Comp Physiol 299:R314–R324

61. Musch TI (1993) Elevated diaphragmatic blood flow during submaximal exercise in rats with chronic heart failure. Am J Physiol 265:H1721–H1726

62. Amann M, Pegelow DF, Jacques AJ et al (2007) Inspiratory muscle work in acute hypoxia influences locomotor muscle fatigue and exercise performance of healthy humans. Am J Physiol Regul Integr Comp Physiol 293:R2036–R2045

63. Dempsey JA, Romer L, Rodman J et al (2006) Consequences of exercise-induced respiratory muscle work. Respir Physiol Neurobiol 151:242–250

Pathology of COPD and Asthma

3

Simonetta Baraldo, Riccardo Cazzuffi, Erica Bazzan,
Fabrizio Luppi, Graziella Turato, and Marina Saetta

3.1   Introduction

Although there is no doubt that the major site of increased resistance in COPD locates in the peripheral airways, the central airways are involved in the disease as well [1–5]. Conversely, in asthma, though the majority of studies focused on the pathophysiology of central airways, there is an increasing appreciation of a critical involvement of the peripheral airways [6]. Distinctive patterns of airway inflammation and structural remodelling are constitutive parts of the pathological picture of the two diseases [7, 8]. These include both cellular and structural changes that may contribute to the clinical manifestations and functional impairment characteristic of each condition.

S. Baraldo • R. Cazzuffi • E. Bazzan • G. Turato
Department of Cardiologic, Thoracic and Vascular Sciences,
Respiratory Diseases Clinic, University of Padova, Padova, Italy

F. Luppi
Department of Oncology Hematology and Respiratory Diseases,
Center for Rare Lung Diseases, University Hospital of Modena,
Modena, Italy

M. Saetta (✉)
Department of Cardiologic, Thoracic and Vascular Sciences,
Respiratory Diseases Clinic, University of Padova, Padova, Italy

Department of Cardiologic, Thoracic and Vascular Sciences,
Section of Respiratory Diseases, University of Padova,
Via Giustiniani 3, 35128 Padova, Italy
e-mail: marina.saetta@unipd.it

A. Aliverti, A. Pedotti (eds.), *Mechanics of Breathing*,
DOI 10.1007/978-88-470-5647-3_3, © Springer-Verlag Italia 2014

3.2   Conducting Airways

3.2.1   Asthma

Much of the current knowledge on the mechanisms of asthma came from studies performed on allergic asthma, where antigen exposure could activate antigen presenting cells and, in turn, T-lymphocytes, thus inducing an immune response characterised by a shift towards a Th2 phenotype, with production (among other cytokines) of IL-4, that sustains increased IgE levels, and of IL-5, that promotes eosinophilia. Accordingly, the characteristic airway inflammatory response involves activated T-lymphocytes, eosinophils and mast cells [7, 9–11]. In particular, mast cells infiltrating the airway muscle layer are believed to have important implications in asthma by affecting the degree of airway reactivity and airway remodelling [11]. Indeed, mast cells can release a variety of mediators, including those that induce airway smooth muscle contraction, resulting in bronchoconstriction, but also those that promote the development of structural changes in the airways, thus airway remodelling. The characteristic components of airway remodelling in asthma are: increased smooth muscle mass, thickening of the reticular basement membrane (RBM), angiogenesis and bronchial epithelial damage [7, 12].

Traditionally, remodelling has been considered the unavoidable consequence of long-term inflammation, but the exact relationship between airway inflammation and remodelling is still poorly understood. Of interest, the first studies that evaluated the pathology of asthma in children showed that both airway eosinophilia and all the structural changes characteristic of asthma were already present even in young children, at the first stages of the disease [13–15]. These observations indicate that the processes leading to remodelling of the airway wall begin early in the course of the disease and most probably occur in parallel with the establishment of chronic inflammation rather than being a consequence of it. Furthermore, recent evidence suggests that the presence of eosinophils and eosinophilic mediators is not required for the development of airway remodelling [16, 17]. Indeed, although eosinophil levels are on average increased in asthmatic patients, up to 50 % of asthmatic subjects do not show evidence of airway eosinophilia despite having all the clinical and functional features of the disease. Of interest, we have demonstrated that the typical aspects of airway remodelling (epithelial damage, basement membrane thickening and angiogenesis) develop in asthmatic children even in the absence of eosinophils or the eosinophil-related cytokines IL-4 and IL-5 [16]. In line with our observations, a recent study provided evidence that bronchoconstriction, independently of inflammation, may induce epithelial stress and initiate a tissue response that leads to structural changes in the airways [17]. These results do not throw into question the importance of eosinophils as effector cells in asthma, but rather suggest that other pathways may be involved in remodelling, thus highlighting the complexity of the disease. Finally, although eosinophils, T-lymphocytes and mast cells are the predominant cell types in asthma, evidence is now emerging that neutrophils may play a key role, at least in a subset of patients. Neutrophils have been traditionally associated with severe asthma [18–20], but subsequent studies showed that this phenotype is rather common even among patients with milder forms of the disease [21, 22]. Several factors can contribute to airway neutrophilia, including respiratory infections, smoking and corticosteroid therapy, which reduces eosinophils but increases neutrophils inhibiting their apoptosis [22, 23].

As highlighted above, most of the studies on the pathogenesis of asthma performed so far traditionally concentrated on environmental stimuli, mainly aeroallergens, and the consequent adaptive immune response with priming of Th2 T-lymphocytes and recruitment of eosinophils. However, this is probably not the only pathway, since airway eosinophilia and remodelling are present not only in children with atopic asthma but even in those with non-atopic asthma, indicating that the airway pathology characteristic of asthma may develop even in the absence of atopy [24]. Of interest, it is becoming increasingly evident that disturbance of innate immune responses could play a key role in the pathogenesis of asthma which has been underappreciated so far. In this context viral infections, and particularly rhinoviruses, probably play a crucial role. Viral upper respiratory tract infections are, directly or indirectly, responsible for vast health-care use worldwide. Viral infections are particularly important in asthmatic patients, in whom rhinovirus is the most frequent cause of exacerbations both in adults and children [25]. Moreover, data from longitudinal studies suggest that wheezing episodes associated with viral infections early in life are a major risk factor for the development of asthma later in life [26, 27]. Impaired immune response to viral infections, with decreased IFN production, has been proposed as a mechanism for increased susceptibility to infections in asthmatic patients. Indeed, previous studies suggested that the immune response to viral infections is deficient in adult atopic asthmatics and that this deficiency correlates with the severity of virus-induced asthma exacerbations and asthma symptoms [28–30]. Whether this abnormal immune response is already present in the airways of young children or whether it develops later on as a consequence of long-term immune deregulation or sustained corticosteroid therapy was not known. To address this issue we have recently studied the epithelial production of IFN-β and IFN-λ in response to rhinovirus and reported a deficient IFN response in children with asthma, not only in those with atopy but also in non-atopic ones [31]. This altered innate response was associated to increased viral replication ex vivo and was correlated with the degree of airway eosinophilia and epithelial damage. These results suggest that disturbance of the airway immunopathological profile early in life, by affecting innate immune responses, could explain the greater susceptibility to viral infections observed in asthmatic patients and, possibly, the persistence of symptoms.

The role of the peripheral airways in asthma is increasingly being recognised as a relevant target for asthma knowledge and adequate control [32]. Evidence accumulating in recent decades indicates that inflammatory changes characteristic of the proximal airways of asthmatics also occur in the distal airways [33]. Of interest, the distribution of the inflammatory cell infiltration within the airway wall varies significantly moving from the central to the peripheral airways [34]. In central airways the preponderance of inflammatory cells has been observed in the airway submucosa (i.e. the inner area which lies between the epithelial basement membrane and the smooth muscle), whereas in peripheral airways the greatest density of eosinophils is in the adventitia (i.e. the external area which lies between the smooth muscle and the alveolar attachments). These regional differences in inflammatory cell density could have important physiologic implications in the relative mechanisms contributing to airflow limitation at these two anatomic sites. In large airways the increased eosinophil density in the "inner" region would promote airway constriction by amplifying the effect of bronchial smooth muscle shortening on the airway calibre. Conversely, in peripheral airways the increased eosinophil density in the "outer" region would promote airway constriction by decreasing the tethering effects of the parenchyma on the airway wall [35].

3.2.2 COPD

The pathological mechanisms leading to airflow limitation in chronic obstructive pulmonary disease have been the focus of several studies that highlighted the concept, now well accepted, that COPD is also characterised by an important airway inflammatory process involving the central and the peripheral airways [4, 5, 36]. Cigarette smoking is the most important risk factor for the development of COPD, and it has long been recognised that smokers show evidence of inflammatory changes in their airways, consisting predominantly of macrophages infiltration in the airway wall and neutrophil accumulation in the airway lumen [2]. This early inflammatory infiltrate probably represents the non-specific response of the innate immunity to the insult of cigarette smoking. In smokers who develop chronic airflow limitation, this inflammatory process is further amplified, due to the activation of an adaptive immune response [37]. Indeed, in smokers who develop COPD, there is an increase in the number of lymphocytes (particularly CD8+ T-lymphocytes and B-lymphocytes) and macrophages [4, 5, 36–39]. High numbers of CD8+ T-lymphocytes are present not only in the peripheral airways of smokers with COPD but also in central airways in the lung parenchyma and in the adventitia of the pulmonary arterioles, suggesting that it is a consistent trait in this disease [4, 5, 40]. The findings of increased numbers of lymphocytes, and especially CD8+ T-cells, only in smokers who develop COPD is intriguing and supports the notion that a T-cell inflammation may be essential for the development of the disease. Traditionally the major activity of CD8 cytotoxic T-lymphocytes has been considered the rapid resolution of acute viral infections, and viral infections are a frequent occurrence in patients with COPD. The observation that people with frequent respiratory infections in childhood are more prone to develop COPD supports the role of viral infections in this disease [41]. It is conceivable that, in response to repeated viral infections, an excessive recruitment of CD8 cytotoxic T-lymphocytes may occur and damage the lung in susceptible smokers, possibly through the release of perforins and TNF-α [42]. On the other hand, it is also possible that CD8 T-lymphocytes are able to damage the lung even in the absence of a stimulus such as a viral infection, as shown by Enelow and coworkers [43] who demonstrated that recognition of a lung "autoantigen" by cytotoxic T-cells may directly produce a marked lung injury. Along with the inflammatory response, several structural changes have been described in the conducting airways of smokers with established COPD that would result in narrowing of the airway lumen and in loss of the tethering function of the lung parenchyma, thus promoting a reduction of expiratory flow. These pathological lesions include thickening of the airway wall, with increased smooth muscle mass and fibrosis, hypertrophy of mucous glands and hyperplasia of goblet cells [36, 44, 45].

A significantly increased number of mucus-secreting goblet cells are seen in the peripheral airway epithelium of smokers with COPD. The increased number of goblet cells correlates with the degree of lung function impairment, as assessed by FEV_1/FVC [45]. This goblet cell metaplasia can have important functional consequences, potentially contributing to the development of smoking-induced airflow obstruction in at least two ways: first, by producing an excess of mucus which could alter the surface tension of the airway lining fluid, rendering the peripheral airways unstable and facilitating their closure and second, by inducing luminal occlusion through the formation of mucous plugs in peripheral airways. Indeed, luminal occlusion by mucous and inflammatory exudates is frequently observed in smokers with COPD [46, 47]. In addition neutrophils, which are not usually found within the airway wall, are increased in the peripheral airway epithelium and in bronchial glands of smokers with COPD [45, 48]. As neutrophil elastase is a remarkably potent secretagogue, it has been proposed that the location of neutrophils in close contact with the mucus-secreting structures of the glands and of the epithelium is crucial for the activation of their secretory function. While the excessive mucus production from goblet cells in peripheral airways may indeed contribute to airway obstruction, whether chronic bronchitis (due to mucus hypersecretion from bronchial glands in the central airways) could promote the development of functional abnormalities has been the matter of an extensive debate, with no definite answer yet. Nevertheless, it is now increasingly being recognised that, when present in patients with COPD, chronic bronchitis has numerous clinical consequences including an increased exacerbation rate, accelerated decline in lung function, worse quality of life and, possibly, increased mortality [49, 50].

Besides their role on mucus hypersecretion, neutrophils may have important effector functions even on airway smooth muscle. Indeed, an enlarged smooth muscle area is an important component of airway wall thickening, which is increased in smokers with COPD compared with those with normal lung function and augments progressively with worsening of airflow limitation [36]. This increase in smooth muscle can be due to several mechanisms, including hypertrophy and hyperplasia of smooth muscle cells and matrix deposition within smooth muscle bundles. Of interest, we reported an increased number of neutrophils infiltrating the smooth muscle of patients with COPD; these cells through the release of inflammatory mediators, cytokines and growth factors, could modulate smooth muscle proliferation and contractility [51]. Indeed, it is well known that the airways of smokers can react to non-specific stimuli by constricting, and this constriction results in airway hyper-reactivity. Whether hyperresponsiveness is a primary event that might contribute to the natural history of COPD or is a consequence of the already decreased airway dimensions is still an open question. In any case, the abnormalities found in the airways of smokers, particularly chronic inflammation, could contribute to the constriction even of a normal airway smooth muscle.

Another important component of remodelling is fibrosis of the airway wall. It has been previously reported that cigarette smoke induces oxidative stress in human lung fibroblasts, which may then initiate a process of repair and collagen deposition [52]. Furthermore, the interaction between fibroblasts and inflammatory cells may also play a role in fibrotic remodelling. On this line is the observation that mast cells, which have important profibrotic and prorepair properties, are increased in the airways of smokers with COPD, particularly in those with centrilobular emphysema [53]. Fibrosis, along with an increased airway smooth muscle and other inflammatory components, ought to increase the airway wall thickness and change the mechanical characteristics of the airway to decrease the luminal diameter. Indeed, the same degree of smooth muscle shortening may cause considerably greater luminal narrowing in airways with a thickened airway wall than in normal airways [54]. In the context of a chronic disease such as COPD, it is well conceivable that the pathological changes observed in small airways are associated to various attempts to repair, which may result in fibrosis, and thickening of the airway wall. On this line it should be noted that thickening of the airway wall is the parameter found to correlate best with airflow limitation in smokers across the different stages of disease severity [46, 55].

3.3   Lung Parenchyma

3.3.1   Asthma

Only a few studies have examined the inflammation of the lung parenchyma in asthma, focusing their analysis on transbronchial biopsies [20, 56, 57]. Patients with nocturnal asthma, when examined at night, have an increase in the number of alveolar tissue eosinophils and CD4 T-lymphocytes as compared with those with non-nocturnal asthma, and these cells correlate with the overnight decrement in lung function [56]. Furthermore, patients with uncontrolled asthma had increased number of mast cells in the alveolar walls, with increased expression of FcεRI and surface-bound IgE, compared to healthy controls [57]. Finally, in the alveolar walls of patients with severe steroid-dependent asthma, the inflammatory response is characterised by a prominent neutrophilia [22] which could represent a marker of severity, but could also be a consequence of corticosteroid therapy.

Taken together, these results point towards the presence of an excessive alveolar inflammation particularly in asthma phenotypes difficult to control. Moreover, they go along with the observation that inflammation in small airways predominates in the outer region of the airway wall that is in the adventitial layer and may spread out to the surrounding alveolar walls that is the site of alveolar attachments. Indeed, it is known that the elastic load provided by the lung parenchyma is transmitted to the airways through the alveolar attachments, resulting in mechanical interdependence between airways and parenchyma [54]. Of note, it has been shown that patients who died of fatal asthma have an increased number of damaged alveolar attachments and decreased elastic fibre content in the adventitial layer of small airways and peribronchial alveoli [58]. These alterations can contribute to the pathogenesis of some of the functional abnormalities observed in patients with the most severe forms of asthma, such as the loss of deep breath bronchodilator effect and enhanced airway closure [59].

3.3.2 COPD

Investigation of the inflammatory changes in the alveolar region of COPD patients is of particular interest, as a localisation of inflammatory cells within the alveolar walls might contribute to the smoking-induced parenchymal destruction that characterises the disease. Emphysema, which is one of the major contributors to airflow limitation in COPD, is defined anatomically as a permanent "destructive" enlargement of airspaces distal to the terminal bronchiole without obvious fibrosis [60]. However, this last statement has been debated since some studies have shown that, in emphysema, the destructive process is accompanied by a net increase in the mass of collagen, suggesting that, contrary to the definition of the disease, there is indeed an active alveolar wall fibrosis in emphysematous lungs [61, 62].

Smokers can develop two main morphological forms of emphysema that can be distinguished according to the region of the acinus which is destroyed. Centriacinar (or centrilobular) emphysema is characterised by focal destruction restricted to respiratory bronchioles and the central portions of the acinus surrounded by areas of grossly normal lung parenchyma. This form of emphysema is usually most severe in the upper lobes of the lung. Panacinar (or panlobular) emphysema is characterised by destruction of the alveolar walls in a fairly uniform manner, i.e. all the air spaces beyond the terminal bronchiole are involved. The panacinar form is characteristic of patients who develop emphysema early in life, usually associated with deficiency of alpha1-antitrypsin, and in contrast to the centriacinar form has a tendency to involve the lower lobes more than the upper ones. Nonetheless, heavy smokers with normal alpha1-antitrypsin levels can develop both the centrilobular and panlobular phenotype [63].

The two forms of emphysema have distinct mechanical properties and distinct peripheral airway involvement [63, 64]. In particular, the lung compliance is greater in panlobular than in centrilobular emphysema, whereas the extent of peripheral airway inflammation is greater in the centrilobular than in the panlobular form. Thus, in panlobular emphysema, airflow limitation seems to be primarily a function of loss of elastic recoil as suggested by the correlation between reduced expiratory flow and increased compliance observed in this form of emphysema [64]. By contrast, in centrilobular emphysema airflow limitation seems primarily a function of peripheral airway inflammation, as supported by the correlation between reduced expiratory flow and increased airway inflammation. In support of a central role of inflammation in this form of emphysema, we recently reported that patients with centrilobular emphysema show a more severe inflammatory infiltrate in both the lung parenchyma and peripheral airways. Mast-cell infiltration was a prominent component of this response and was related to the degree of airway reactivity, suggesting that centrilobular emphysema shares some pathogenetic traits with asthma [53].

Inflammation has been identified as a key component of COPD, and it has been shown that inflammatory cell infiltration in the lung can persist for years after cessation of smoking [65]. The implication of an inflammatory response to the pathogenesis of emphysema is not new, but our knowledge of the mechanisms regulating the activation and persistence of this response in the lung is continuously evolving.

Starting from the hypothesis of elastase-antielastase imbalance, proposed more than 40 years ago, studies first focused on the role of neutrophils and macrophages and their ability to induce lung destruction through the release of protcolytic enzymes. However, the activation of neutrophils and macrophages by itself is not sufficient to explain all the pathogenetic traits of COPD, and more recent evidences suggest a crucial role for acquired immunity, with involvement of dendritic cells and lympho-cytes [37]. This hypothesis was based on the observation that B- and T-lymphocytes, especially of the CD8[+] subset, were the predominant cells infiltrating lung tissue of patients with COPD, and their numbers were strongly related to the apoptosis of structural cells and lung function impairment [36–40]. Adding to this, it has been recently proposed that this adaptive immune response, at least in some patients, could have an autoimmune component due to the recognition of pulmonary self-antigens modified by cigarette smoking and to the failure of mechanisms regulating immunological tolerance. In support of this hypothesis is the observation that, in non-smoking subjects who develop COPD, the disease seems to be associated with organ-specific autoimmunity [66].

3.4   Overlap between Asthma and COPD

As we have seen, asthma and COPD are two distinct obstructive lung diseases with distinctive clinical presentations and different patterns of airway inflamma-tion and remodelling of lung structure. Indeed, the two conditions usually differ in the pattern of inflammatory cells most frequently encountered and the typical structural changes. Asthma is characterised by an increase of eosinophils, CD4[+] T-lymphocytes and mast cells; whereas, in COPD, CD8[+]T-lymphocytes, macro-phages and neutrophils predominate. Furthermore, a typical increase in basement membrane thickness is frequently observed in patients with asthma that is not present in those with COPD.

Nevertheless, despite the distinctive features of the two conditions, some asth-matic patients may experience a fixed airflow obstruction that persists despite opti-mal pharmacologic treatment [67]. Indeed, up to 30 % of subjects with airflow obstruction have a history of asthma rather than COPD, and these are patients usu-ally excluded from clinical trials as they cannot be labelled as having either asthma or COPD. Instead, they would deserve clinical and research attention because their disease is usually misjudged, their prognosis is unknown, and treatment has never been properly explored. Even the pathological traits at bases of asthma with fixed airflow obstruction were not completely understood. In particular, it was unknown whether these patients will maintain the pathological changes typical of asthma or whether, with the development of irreversible airflow obstruction, they will show the features typical of COPD. Of interest, we have shown that, within a group of patients with fixed airflow obstruction, those with a history of asthma have a distinct airway pathology compared with those with a history of smoking-induced COPD. Indeed, patients with a history of asthma and fixed airflow obstruction have the same pathological changes that are present in patients with asthma with variable airflow obstruction in terms of both eosinophilia and increased basement membrane thickness [68]. These findings suggest that the asthmatic airway pathology does not change with the development of fixed airflow obstruction and, thus, does not become similar to the one characteristic of COPD. Furthermore, in a longitudinal follow-up of that study, we have shown that patients with fixed airflow obstruction due to asthma, just as patients with COPD, have accelerated lung function decline and increased frequency of exacerbations compared with asthmatic patients fully reversible to bronchodilators [69]. Yet, the lung function decline in patients with fixed airflow obstruction is associated with the pathogenetic substrates specific for the underlying disease, i.e. asthma vs. COPD. In particular, the fall in FEV_1 correlates with exhaled nitric oxide levels and sputum eosinophils in asthmatic patients, while it correlates with neutrophil counts and emphysema score in patients with COPD [69]. In conclusion, while fixed airflow obstruction is associated with accelerated lung function decline both in asthma and in COPD, the rate of functional decline depends on the distinctive pathological and clinical features of the underlying diseases. These observations have important clinical implications since therapeutic strategies should be addressed to the different pathogenetic traits in the two diseases, and patients with fixed airflow obstruction due to asthma should not be grouped under the general heading of COPD.

References

1. Saetta M, Turato G, Maestrelli P et al (2001) Cellular and structural bases of chronic obstructive pulmonary disease. Am J Respir Crit Care Med 163(6):1304–1309
2. Baraldo S, Turato G, Saetta M (2012) Pathophysiology of the small airways in chronic obstructive pulmonary disease. Respiration 84(2):89–97
3. Hogg JC, Macklem PT, Thurlbeck WM (1968) Site and nature of airway obstruction in chronic obstructive lung disease. N Engl J Med 278(25):1355–1360
4. O'Shaughnessy TC, Ansari TW, Barnes NC et al (1997) Inflammation in bronchial biopsies of subjects with chronic bronchitis: inverse relationship of CD8+ T lymphocytes with FEV1. Am J Respir Crit Care Med 155(3):852–857
5. Saetta M, Di Stefano A, Maestrelli P et al (1993) Activated T-lymphocytes and macrophages in bronchial mucosa of subjects with chronic bronchitis. Am Rev Respir Dis 147(2):301–306
6. Contoli M, Bousquet J, Fabbri LM et al (2010) The small airways and distal lung compartment in asthma and COPD: a time for reappraisal. Allergy 65(2):141–151
7. Bousquet J, Jeffery PK, Busse WW et al (2000) Asthma. From bronchoconstriction to airways inflammation and remodeling. Am J Respir Crit Care Med 161(5):1720–1745
8. Cosio M, Ghezzo H, Hogg JC et al (1978) The relations between structural changes in small airways and pulmonary- function tests. N Engl J Med 298(23):1277–1281
9. Azzawi M, Bradley B, Jeffery PK et al (1990) Identification of activated T lymphocytes and eosinophils in bronchial biopsies in stable atopic asthma. Am Rev Respir Dis 142 (6 Pt 1):1407–1413
10. Bentley AM, Maestrelli P, Saetta M et al (1992) Activated T-lymphocytes and eosinophils in the bronchial mucosa in isocyanate-induced asthma. J Allergy Clin Immunol 89(4):821–829
11. Brightling CE, Bradding P, Symon FA et al (2002) Mast-cell infiltration of airway smooth muscle in asthma. N Engl J Med 346(22):1699–1705
12. Xiao C, Puddicombe SM, Field S et al (2011) Defective epithelial barrier function in asthma. J Allergy Clin Immunol 128(3):549–556

13. Barbato A, Turato G, Baraldo S et al (2006) Epithelial damage and angiogenesis in the airways of children with asthma. Am J Respir Crit Care Med 174(9):975–981
14. Barbato A, Turato G, Baraldo S et al (2003) Airway inflammation in childhood asthma. Am J Respir Crit Care Med 168(7):798–803
15. Snijders D, Agostini S, Bertuola F et al (2010) Markers of eosinophilic and neutrophilic inflammation in bronchoalveolar lavage of asthmatic and atopic children. Allergy 65(8):978–985
16. Baraldo S, Turato G, Bazzan E et al (2011) Noneosinophilic asthma in children: relation with airway remodelling. Eur Respir J 38(3):575–583
17. Grainge CL, Lau LC, Ward JA et al (2011) Effect of bronchoconstriction on airway remodeling in asthma. N Engl J Med 364(21):2006–2015
18. Lamblin C, Gosset P, Tillie-Leblond I et al (1998) Bronchial neutrophilia in patients with noninfectious status asthmaticus. Am J Respir Crit Care Med 157(2):394–402
19. Sur S, Crotty TB, Kephart GM et al (1993) Sudden-onset fatal asthma. A distinct entity with few eosinophils and relatively more neutrophils in the airway submucosa? Am Rev Respir Dis 148(3):713–719
20. Wenzel SE, Szefler SJ, Leung DY et al (1997) Bronchoscopic evaluation of severe asthma. Persistent inflammation associated with high dose glucocorticoids. Am J Respir Crit Care Med 156:737–743
21. Green RH, Brightling CE, Woltmann G et al (2002) Analysis of induced sputum in adults with asthma: identification of subgroup with isolated sputum neutrophilia and poor response to inhaled corticosteroids. Thorax 57:875–879
22. Cowan DC, Cowan JO, Palmay R et al (2010) Effects of steroid therapy on inflammatory cell subtypes in asthma. Thorax 65:384–390
23. Cox G (1995) Glucocorticoid treatment inhibits apoptosis in human neutrophils. Separation of survival and activation outcomes. J Immunol 154(9):4719–4725
24. Turato G, Barbato A, Baraldo S et al (2008) Non-atopic children with multitrigger wheezing have airway pathology comparable to atopic asthma. Am J Respir Crit Care Med 178(5):476–482
25. Corne JM, Marshall C, Smith S et al (2002) Frequency, severity, and duration of rhinovirus infections in asthmatic and non-asthmatic individuals: a longitudinal cohort study. Lancet 359:831–834
26. Kusel MM, de Klerk NH, Kebadze T et al (2007) Early-life respiratory viral infections, atopic sensitization, and risk of subsequent development of persistent asthma. J Allergy Clin Immunol 119(5):1105–1110
27. Lemanske RF Jr, Jackson DJ, Gangnon RE et al (2005) Rhinovirus illnesses during infancy predict subsequent childhood wheezing. J Allergy Clin Immunol 116:571–577
28. Papadopoulos N, Stanciu L, Papi A et al (2002) A defective type 1 response to rhinovirus in atopic asthma. Thorax 57:328–332
29. Wark PAB, Johnston SL, Bucchieri F et al (2005) Asthmatic bronchial epithelial cells have a deficient innate immune response to infection with rhinovirus. J Exp Med 201:937–947
30. Contoli M, Message SD, Laza-Stanca V et al (2006) Role of deficient type III interferon-lambda production in asthma exacerbations. Nat Med 12:1023–1029
31. Baraldo S, Contoli M, Bazzan E et al (2012) Deficient antiviral immune responses in childhood: distinct roles of atopy and asthma. J Allergy Clin Immunol 130:1307–1314
32. Contoli M, Kraft M, Hamid Q et al (2012) Do small airway abnormalities characterize asthma phenotypes? In search of proof. Clin Exp Allergy 42:1150–1160
33. Balzar S, Wenzel SE, Chu HW (2002) Transbronchial biopsy as a tool to evaluate small airways in asthma. Eur Respir J 20:254–259
34. Haley KJ, Sunday ME, Wiggs BR et al (1998) Inflammatory cell distribution within and along asthmatic airways. Am J Respir Crit Care Med 158(2):565–572
35. James AL, Pare PD, Hogg JC (1989) The mechanics of airway narrowing in asthma. Am Rev Respir Dis 139(1):242–246
36. Saetta M, Di Stefano A, Turato G et al (1998) CD8+ T-lymphocytes in peripheral airways of smokers with chronic obstructive pulmonary disease. Am J Respir Crit Care Med 157:822–826

37. Cosio MG, Saetta M, Agusti A (2009) Immunologic aspects of chronic obstructive pulmonary disease. N Engl J Med 360(23):2445–2454
38. van der Strate BW, Postma DS, Brandsma CA et al (2006) Cigarette smoke-induced emphysema: a role for the B cell? Am J Respir Crit Care Med 173:751–758
39. Polverino F, Baraldo S, Bazzan E et al (2010) A novel insight into adaptive immunity in chronic obstructive pulmonary disease: B cell activating factor belonging to the tumor necrosis factor family. Am J Respir Crit Care Med 182(8):1011–1019
40. Saetta M, Baraldo S, Corbino L et al (1999) CD8+ve cells in the lungs of smokers with chronic obstructive pulmonary disease. Am J Respir Crit Care Med 160(2):711–717
41. Paoletti P, Prediletto R, Carrozzi L et al (1989) Effects of childhood and adolescence-adulthood respiratory infections in a general population. Eur Respir J 2(5):428–436
42. Liu AN, Mohammed AZ, Rice WR et al (1999) Perforin-independent CD8(+) T-cell-mediated cytotoxicity of alveolar epithelial cells is preferentially mediated by tumor necrosis factor-alpha: relative insensitivity to Fas ligand. Am J Respir Cell Mol Biol 20(5):849–858
43. Enelow RI, Mohammed AZ, Stoler MH et al (1998) Structural and functional consequences of alveolar cell recognition by CD8(+) T lymphocytes in experimental lung disease. J Clin Invest 102(9):1653–1661
44. Reid L (1960) Measurement of the bronchial mucous gland layer: a diagnostic yardstick in chronic bronchitis. Thorax 15:132–141
45. Saetta M, Turato G, Baraldo S et al (2000) Goblet cell hyperplasia and epithelial inflammation in peripheral airways of smokers with both symptoms of chronic bronchitis and chronic airflow limitation. Am J Respir Crit Care Med 161:1016–1021
46. Hogg JC, Chu F, Utokaparch S et al (2004) The nature of small airway obstruction in chronic obstructive pulmonary disease. N Engl J Med 350(26):2645–2653
47. Caramori G, Casolari P, Di Gregorio C et al (2009) MUC5AC expression is increased in bronchial submucosal glands of stable COPD patients. Histopathology 55(3):321–331
48. Saetta M, Turato G, Facchini FM et al (1997) Inflammatory cells in the bronchial glands of smokers with chronic bronchitis. Am J Respir Crit Care Med 156(5):1633–1639
49. Vestbo J, Prescott E, Lange P (1996) Association of chronic mucus hypersecretion with FEV1 decline and chronic obstructive pulmonary disease morbidity. Copenhagen City Heart Study Group. Am J Respir Crit Care Med 153(5):1530–1535
50. Montes de Oca M, Halbert RJ, Lopez MV et al (2012) The chronic bronchitis phenotype in subjects with and without COPD: the PLATINO study. Eur Respir J 40:28–36
51. Baraldo S, Turato G, Badin C et al (2004) Neutrophilic infiltration within the airway smooth muscle in patients with COPD. Thorax 59(4):308–312
52. Carnevali S, Luppi F, D'Arca D et al (2006) Clusterin decreases oxidative stress in lung fibroblasts exposed to cigarette smoke. Am J Respir Crit Care Med 174(4):393–399
53. Ballarin A, Bazzan E, Zenteno RH et al (2012) Mast cell infiltration discriminates between histopathological phenotypes of chronic obstructive pulmonary disease. Am J Respir Crit Care Med 186(3):233–239
54. Macklem PT (1998) The physiology of small airways. Am J Respir Crit Care Med 157:S181–S183
55. Corsico A, Milanese M, Baraldo S et al (2003) Small airway morphology and lung function in the transition from normality to chronic airway obstruction. J Appl Physiol 95(1):441–447
56. Kraft M, Martin RJ, Wilson S et al (1999) Lymphocyte and eosinophil influx into alveolar tissue in nocturnal asthma. Am J Respir Crit Care Med 159(1):228–234
57. Andersson CK, Bergqvist A, Mori M et al (2011) Mast cell–associated alveolar inflammation in patients with atopic uncontrolled asthma. J Allergy Clin Immunol 127(4):905–912
58. Mauad T, Silva LF, Santos MA et al (2004) Abnormal alveolar attachments with decreased elastic fiber content in distal lung in fatal asthma. Am J Respir Crit Care Med 170(8):857–862
59. Allen ND, Davis BE, Cockcroft DW (2008) Correlation between airway inflammation and loss of deep-inhalation bronchoprotection in asthma. Ann Allergy Asthma Immunol 101(4):413–418

60. Standards for the diagnosis and care of patients with chronic obstructive pulmonary disease. American Thoracic Society (1995) Am J Respir Crit Care Med 152(5 Pt 2):S77–S121
61. Lang MR, Fiaux GW, Gillooly M et al (1994) Collagen content of alveolar wall tissue in emphysematous and non- emphysematous lungs. Thorax 49(4):319–326
62. Vlahovic G, Russell ML, Mercer RR et al (1999) Cellular and connective tissue changes in alveolar septal walls in emphysema. Am J Respir Crit Care Med 160(6):2086–2092
63. Kim WD, Eidelman DH, Izquierdo JL et al (1991) Centrilobular and panlobular emphysema in smokers. Two distinct morphologic and functional entities. Am Rev Respir Dis 144(6): 1385–1390
64. Saetta M, Kim WD, Izquierdo JL et al (1994) Extent of centrilobular and panacinar emphysema in smokers' lungs: pathological and mechanical implications. Eur Respir J 7(4):664–671
65. Turato G, Di Stefano A, Maestrelli P et al (1995) Effect of smoking cessation on airway inflammation in chronic bronchitis. Am J Respir Crit Care Med 152(4 Pt 1):1262–1267
66. Birring SS, Brightling CE, Bradding P et al (2002) Clinical, radiologic, and induced sputum features of chronic obstructive pulmonary disease in nonsmokers: a descriptive study. Am J Respir Crit Care Med 166:1078–1083
67. ten Brinke A (2008) Risk factors associated with irreversible airflow limitation in asthma. Curr Opin Allergy Clin Immunol 8:63–69
68. Fabbri LM, Romagnoli M, Corbetta L et al (2003) Differences in airway inflammation in patients with fixed airflow obstruction due to asthma or chronic obstructive pulmonary disease. Am J Respir Crit Care Med 167(3):418–424
69. Contoli M, Baraldo S, Marku B et al (2010) Fixed airflow obstruction due to asthma or chronic obstructive pulmonary disease: 5-year follow-up. J Allergy Clin Immunol 125(4):830–837

Pathophysiology of Airflow Obstruction

4

Vito Brusasco

4.1 Introduction

Airflow obstruction is a hallmark of asthma and chronic obstructive pulmonary disease (COPD), though it may be present in other, less frequent, pulmonary disorders. After the pioneering work of Tiffeneau and Pinelli in 1947 [1], airflow obstruction has been usually defined as a reduced ratio of forced expiratory volume in the first second (FEV_1) to vital capacity (VC) or forced vital capacity (FVC). However, several studies have suggested that this ratio may remain within the range of normality in the early stages of disease [2] and may be reduced in healthy subjects having a lung volume that is disproportionately large compared with the airway cross-sectional area, a condition that has been called "dysanaptic growth" [3]. Therefore, the diagnosis of airflow obstruction in clinical settings is not always straightforward. The functional complexity of intrathoracic airways in vivo originates from the interaction of several factors, including geometry of tracheobronchial tree, fluid dynamics, and mechanical interdependence between airways and lung parenchyma. In this chapter, the factors governing fluid dynamics in the airways will be first summarized, then the changes in lung mechanics responsible for airflow obstruction in asthma and COPD will be reviewed.

V. Brusasco
Department of Internal Medicine, University of Genoa,
Viale Benedetto XV, 6, Genoa, 16132, Italy
e-mail: vito.brusasco@unige.it

A. Aliverti, A. Pedotti (eds.), *Mechanics of Breathing*,
DOI 10.1007/978-88-470-5647-3_4, © Springer-Verlag Italia 2014

4.2   Fluid Dynamics in the Airways

4.2.1   Pressure-Flow Relationships

Airflow through the bronchial tree is dependent on the pressure difference between alveoli and airway opening. At a given lung volume, the alveolar pressure is the sum of the lung recoil pressure and the pressure generated by respiratory muscles. The pressure-flow relationship of the lung during tidal breathing can be analyzed by applying the general equation of motion

$$P_{tp} = P_{FRC} + EV + R\dot{V}$$

where P_{tp} is transpulmonary pressure, i.e., the difference between pleural and airway opening pressures, P_{FRC} is pressure at functional residual capacity, E is elastance, V is volume relative to functional residual capacity, R is resistance, and $\dot{V}$ is flow. Thus, the terms EV and $R\dot{V}$ represent the pressures required to expand the lung and overcome flow resistance, respectively. In this simple model, the P-V relationship is assumed to be linear and independent of V amplitude and breathing frequency. However, even in healthy subjects, EV is volume dependent, because of the exponential relationship between pressure and volume [4], and $R\dot{V}$ is frequency dependent, because of the viscoelastic behavior of lung tissue [5, 6]. Moreover, in severely obstructed subjects, the estimates of pulmonary E and R are affected by expiratory flow limitation, which causes varying nonlinear pressure-flow relationships [7].

During expiration, pressure differences along the airways are caused by frictional pressure losses and convective acceleration. Frictional losses are due to laminar flow in small airways and turbulent flow in large airways, the former being directly proportional to $\dot{V}$ and gas viscosity, the latter to $\dot{V}^2$ and gas density ρ. Pressure losses due to convective acceleration represent the energy dissipated in order to increase fluid velocity, according to the Bernoulli equation

$$P = \frac{1}{2}\rho \cdot \left(\dot{V} / A\right)^2$$

where P is elastic pressure and A is the local cross-sectional area. Because the denominator is A^2, the convective pressure drop is inversely proportional to the 4th power of airway radius. During forced expiration, convective acceleration is the major determinant of pressure loss because the velocity of gas molecules is greatly increased as flow moves from the large (peripheral) to a small (central) cross-sectional area of bronchial tree [8].

4.2.2   Maximal Expiratory Flow

Even in healthy subjects, the lungs exhibit the phenomenon of expiratory flow limitation. That is, once a threshold value of P_{tp} is achieved, $\dot{V}$ does not increase with further increases of effort. In rigid tubes, the relationship between $\dot{V}$ and P can be

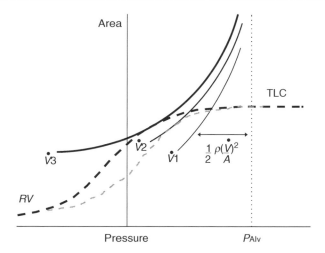

Fig. 4.1 Diagrammatic relationships between cross-sectional area, pressure, and flow ($\dot{V}$). Continuous lines are plots of the Bernoulli equation for $\dot{V}$ of 1, 2, and 3 L/s; interrupted lines are transmural pressure (P_{tm}) area curves of two hypothetical airways from total lung capacity (*TLC*) to residual volume (*RV*). For a given $\dot{V}$, the pressure drop due to convective acceleration is the distance between the alveolar pressure (P_{Alv}) and the corresponding plot of the Bernoulli equation. To pass through a given airway, $\dot{V}$ must meet simultaneously the pressure-area and the P_{tm}-area relationships of that airway. Note that V_{max} is less in a more compliant (*thin interrupted line*) than a less compliant (*thick interrupted line*) airway (Modified from Ref. [91]. With permission from Comprehensive Physiology)

simply described by the Bernoulli equation. In collapsible tubes like the airways, the maximum flow ($\dot{V}_{max}$) is limited at the point of intersection between Bernoulli equation plots and the *P-V* relationship of each given airway (Fig. 4.1), as described by the following equation:

$$\dot{V}_{max} / A = \left(A / \rho \cdot \Delta P / \Delta A \right)^{1/2}$$

where $\Delta P/\Delta A$ is airway *E*. This equation is also called "wave-speed equation" because $\dot{V}_{max} / A$ corresponds to the velocity at which a pressure disturbance can be transmitted in a tube the compliance of which exceeds the compliance of gas [9]. The point at which $\dot{V}_{max}$ is achieved along the bronchial tree is called "choke point," and its location is determined by the pressure-area relationship of the entire bronchial tree at a given recoil pressure. Because the latter is a function of lung volume, the choke point moves from central to peripheral airways as the lung empties during expiration. From the above analysis it follows that if *P* is reduced because of frictional losses upstream from the limiting segment are increased or alveolar pressure is decreased due to loss of elastic recoil, then the plots of Bernoulli equations are displaced to the left and $\dot{V}_{max}$ is reduced (Fig. 4.2). This unique relationship between $\dot{V}$, *V*, and *P* [10] makes it impossible to separate the determinants of expiratory flow limitation by simple spirometry.

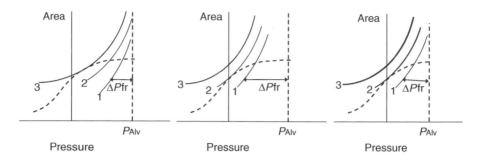

Fig. 4.2 Effect of frictional pressure (*Pfr*) losses and reduced elastic pressure on maximal $\dot{V}$. *Left panel*: $\dot{V}$ cannot exceed 3 L/s, because the Bernoulli plot for greater $\dot{V}$ would not meet the airway P_{tm}-area curve. *Middle panel*: the Bernoulli plots are displaced to the left, because of increased Pfr losses in peripheral airways, then the point of tangency with the P_{tm}-area curve is at lower $\dot{V}$, and maximal $\dot{V}$ will be less. *Right panel*: A reduction of P_{Alv} due to loss of lung elastic recoil would have the same effect of displacing the Bernoulli plots to the left, thus also reducing maximal $\dot{V}$ (Modified from Ref. [91]. With permission from Comprehensive Physiology)

4.3 Physiologic Determinants of Airway Caliber

4.3.1 Airway Smooth Muscle (ASM)

Unquestionably, the ASM tone is a major determinant of airway caliber even in healthy subjects. The mechanical behavior of ASM has been described by length-tension and force-velocity relationships [11]. In vitro, the ASM exhibits length-tension characteristics that are not very dissimilar from those of skeletal muscle, but there are quantitative differences that may have an impact on airway narrowing in vivo. First, unloaded ASM can shorten to ~10 % of initial length, as compared to ~65 % of striated muscle [11]. Second, the ASM exhibits a length-adaptation phenomenon [12], i.e., a leftward shift of the length-tension curve (Fig. 4.3), that can occur within minutes after length changes [13], as compared to weeks in the diaphragm [14, 15] or other skeletal muscles [16]. Third, although ASM is much slower than striated muscle in achieving maximum shortening, 90 % of such a shortening occurs within 3 s [17].

4.3.2 Effect of Lung Volume

The intrapulmonary airways are coupled to lung parenchyma by a connective tissue network. Therefore, for purely geometric reasons, the airways are expected to change their diameter proportionally to the cube root of changes in lung volume. A primary consequence of this interdependence between airways and lung parenchyma is that, being the resistance of a given airway inversely proportional to the fourth power of its radius, a hyperbolic inverse relationship exists between airway resistance and lung volume. In healthy subjects of different body size, the products

Fig. 4.3 Length adaptation of airway smooth muscle. The force-length curve of airway smooth muscle is displaced to the left after shortening. Thus, the force-generation capacity is reduced immediately after shortening (from point *A* to point *B*) but then is recovered (from point *B* to point *C*) (From Ref. [92] by permission)

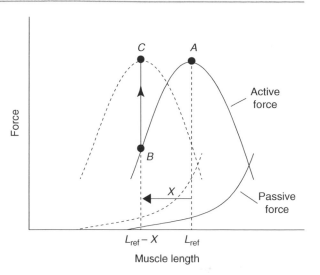

of airway resistance and lung volume (*specific airway resistance*) and its inverse (*specific airway conductance*) are relatively constant. But this relationship may be altered if the transmission of the lung elastic force to airway walls is impeded or ASM tone is increased. Indeed, agreement between measured and predicted changes of airway resistance with lung volume was observed when ASM tone was abolished by atropine [18]. The effects of changes in lung volume on airway caliber also depend on the airway wall compliance; this, in turn, depends on ASM tone, airway wall stiffness, and the structural support of a given airway.

4.3.3   Mechanical Factors Limiting Airway Narrowing

When ASM shortens, all incompressible tissues internal to its perimeter must be accommodated within a reduced space. For geometric reasons, it can be calculated that maximal linear shortening of ASM in vivo would result in complete closure of airways, even if their wall thickness is normal [19]. In healthy subjects, however, the response to maximal doses of different bronchoconstrictor agents given alone or in combination is limited to a degree that is much less than expected from the ASM shortening capacity [20–22]. Modeling studies [23–25] based on morphometric observations have led to the concept that the extent to which airways can narrow depends on the balance between the force developed by ASM and the load it works against (Fig. 4.4). Sources of mechanical load on ASM are both internal and external to the airway walls.

4.3.3.1   Internal Load
The airway wall is provided with noncontractile elastic elements in parallel to ASM and also within the ASM itself. Altogether, these represent the so-called internal load, which the ASM must overcome before it can shorten. It has also been proposed

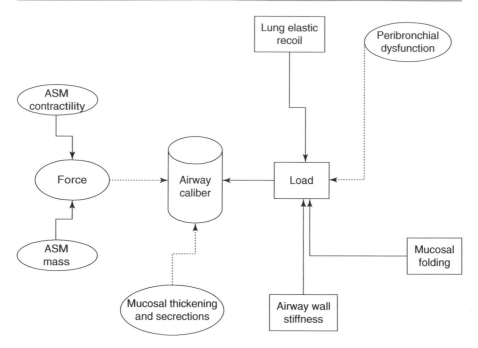

Fig. 4.4 Schematic representation of factors favoring (*within ovals*) and factors opposing (*within rectangles*) airway narrowing. Continuous and interrupted *arrows* denote positive and negative effects, respectively. The effect of airway smooth muscle (*ASM*) shortening is amplified by mucosal thickening and presence of bronchial secretions. Airway wall stiffness, mucosal folding, and lung elastic recoil provide the load limiting ASM shortening, thus opposing airway narrowing (From Ref. [93]. With permission from Comprehensive Physiology)

that mucosal folding could provide an additional load on ASM [26–28]. Theoretical analyses by Lambert and coworkers showed that the greater the number of folds, the greater the pressure difference across the folding membrane [29], and the number of folds increases with the degree of airway narrowing [26]. Furthermore, the pressure required to produce a given number of folds is shown to depend on the rigidity of the folding membrane and its thickness [30].

Compared with those of other species, human bronchi are stiffer and also develop less active force [31], features that seem to be due to relatively larger content of connective tissue and less ASM. In large airways, an important preload on airway smooth muscle is also provided by cartilage rings.

4.3.3.2 External Load

In a seminal study, Ding and coworkers showed that maximal bronchoconstriction in healthy subjects was increased by breathing at reduced lung volume and decreased at increased volume [32]. This observation led to the concept that the elastic elements of lung parenchyma surrounding the airways represent a major source of load on ASM. Because airways and lung parenchyma are interdependent systems [33], when the ASM contracts the surrounding parenchyma is stretched, thus generating a tethering force on ASM. The external load on the contracting ASM approximates lung elastic recoil plus the pressure necessary to overcome the tension generated when the outer wall perimeter decreases [26]. Therefore, the magnitude of external load on ASM is expected to depend on lung volume, lung elastic recoil, and the anatomical integrity of bronchial adventitia, where the force of interdependence is applied.

4.3.4   Relationships Between ASM Force, Velocity, and Load

When ASM shortens, the overall load increases with the decrease of airway caliber. This is due to the stretching of the surrounding lung parenchyma and mucosal folding, despite a decrease in the load represented by transmural pressure (Fig. 4.5, upper panel). For years it was believed that ASM force-generation capacity decreases during length changes either above or below the so-called optimal length. Thus, airway narrowing would be limited at the point where ASM force is balanced by the increase in load (Fig. 4.5, lower panel). However, recent studies have shown that ASM can rapidly adapt to length changes [12, 13], so it can recover its maximal force-generation capacity soon after shortening. Thus, repeated or sustained stimulation may lead to excessive airway narrowing.

Under normal conditions, ASM stretching during inspiration causes a transient reduction in ASM tone [34]. The repeated cyclic stretching of tidal breathing may be sufficient to maintain the ASM in a relaxed state if the time required to recover contractile force is longer than expiratory time. Because ASM shortening is near maximal in 3 s, which approximately corresponds to a tidal expiratory time, it has been suggested that even small increments of shortening may decrease or abolish the relaxant effect of tidal stretching, thus possibly resulting in a progressive increase of ASM tone and excessive airway narrowing [35, 36].

4.4   Pathological Changes

4.4.1   Asthma

Morphological studies on postmortem and surgical specimens have shown important structural changes in the asthmatic airways [37, 38]. The precise consequences of these changes are difficult to establish, as they depend on where they occur within the airway wall, the nature and the mechanical characteristics of the material deposited, and the degree of interdependence between airways and lung parenchyma.

A characteristic feature of asthma is an increased thickness of ASM, resulting more likely from hyperplasia than hypertrophy [39]. An increased ASM mass can result in an enhanced force-generation capacity, thus possibly accounting for the increased airway narrowing in response to bronchoconstrictor stimuli [24], even if this concept is based on the unproven assumption that hyper-proliferating myocytes have the same contractile properties as the normal ones. A key question that is still unanswered is whether asthmatic ASM has abnormal contractile properties. Studies comparing the force-generation capacity of ASM from asthmatic and non-asthmatic

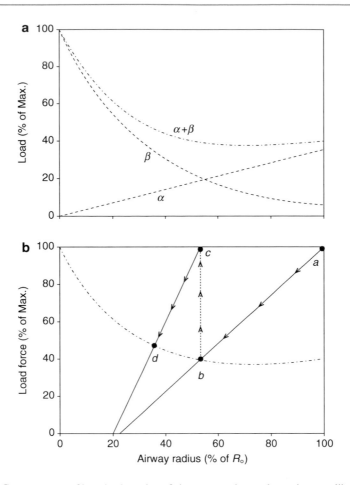

Fig. 4.5 Consequences of length adaptation of airway smooth muscle on airway caliber. (**a**) When airway radius decreases the load due to P_{tm} (α) decreases according to the LaPlace law, while the load represented by parenchymal tethering and mucosal folding (β) increases more, thus total load ($\alpha + \beta$) increases. (**b**) When the muscle is stimulated, the airway radius decreases from point a to point b, where the load equals the force, and force-generation capacity decreases. If the muscle is allowed to adapt at the shortened length, then its force-generation capacity can increase and may fully recover (point c). If the muscle is stimulated again, it will shorten and airway radius may be further reduced to point d, where a new balance between force and load is achieved (Reprinted with permission of the American Thoracic Society. Copyright © 2013 American Thoracic Society. Bossé et al. [12])

subjects gave inconsistent results [40–48]. But other studies have consistently reported an increase of shortening velocity in ASM cells from asthmatic subjects [49], human bronchial ASM passively sensitized with IgE-containing serum [50], and ASM from animal models of allergic [51–53] or innate airway hyperresponsiveness [54–56]. Consistent with these findings, in vivo studies have shown that airway renarrowing after a deep inspiration is faster in asthmatic than healthy subjects [57–59].

Another morphological feature of asthmatic airways is an increased thickness of the adventitial layer. It has been proposed that peribronchial inflammation or edema may enhance airway responsiveness, independent of ASM contractility, by uncoupling the airways from lung parenchyma [25]. However, fluid loading in healthy subjects enhanced the bronchoconstrictor response to methacholine without reducing the bronchodilator effect of deep breaths [60], suggesting that airway wall edema may not be sufficient to effectively uncouple airways and lung parenchyma.

The airways of asthmatic subjects have been shown to be less distensible than the normal ones [61–63]. One of the most consistent pathological findings in asthma is an increased thickness of the subepithelial layer, resulting from deposition of type IV and type V collagen, proteoglycans, and fibronectin below the normal basement membrane made of type III collagen [64–66]. The overall thickness of subepithelial layer observed in asthmatic airways was 10–15 μm, compared to 5–8 μm in non-asthmatic airways, which makes it unlikely that it directly contributes to reduce airway caliber. Rather, there are reasons to predict that an increased stiffness of airways in asthma may be protective against bronchoconstriction. First, a reduced airway wall compliance at choke point tends to increase $\dot{V}_{max}$, thus partially counteracting the effect of reduced airway caliber [8, 9]. Second, deposition of collagen fibers running parallel to the ASM would increase elastic afterload, thus attenuating ASM shortening and airway responsiveness [67]. Third, part of the increase in ASM layer is represented by an increase in the amount of connective tissue surrounding individual myocytes due to increased deposition of extracellular matrix [68]. This may provide an additional constraint to shortening by limiting radial expansion, in order to maintain the same volume [69]. In vitro, treatment with collagenase increased ASM cell shortening [70]. In vivo, an inverse relationship between subepithelial fibrosis and response to methacholine was observed in subjects with asthma [71].

For geometric reasons, an increased thickness of the airway wall layer internal to ASM would be expected to result in a greater reduction of caliber for a given ASM shortening [19]. However, pathological observations have suggested that the airways do not narrow concentrically but the mucosal layer is folded. This distortion process absorbs part of ASM energy, thus representing an additional elastic load opposing its shortening [27–30]. The bending stiffness of a layer increases with its thickness cubed, thus thickening of the whole airway wall could represent an efficient protective mechanism independent of tissue properties.

Studies using computed tomography have consistently shown that airway wall thickening is associated with a decrease in airway function [72, 73]. Two studies [74, 75] found a direct relationship between airway wall thickening and hyperresponsiveness to methacholine. However, in a study in which the two components of airway responsiveness, i.e., airway sensitivity and airway reactivity, were separately evaluated, the latter resulted to be inversely correlated with airway wall thickness [76]. Notwithstanding, a decreased airway distensibility may be also responsible for a reduced response to bronchodilators, thus possibly leading to fixed obstruction in asthmatic subjects [62].

4.4.2 COPD

In subjects with COPD, airway wall remodeling due to inflammation is variably associated with parenchymal destruction due to emphysema. Therefore, excessive airflow limitation may result from airway narrowing, loss of lung elastic recoil, or both.

Thickening of airway wall has been consistently reported in COPD, and modeling studies have suggested that it may represent a major mechanism for increased airflow resistance in COPD [19, 23]. Morphological observations in surgical samples have shown that thickening of the wall layer internal to ASM in COPD correlated with bronchoconstrictor and bronchodilator responses [77, 78]. Changes in the adventitial layer have been hypothesized to contribute to airway narrowing in COPD by uncoupling airways and lung parenchyma but no relationships were observed between airway hyperresponsiveness and thickness of adventitial layer either in penlobular or centrilobular emphysema [78]. Therefore, adventitial thickening by itself may not be sufficient to effectively impede force transmission from lung parenchyma to the airways.

Parenchymal destruction and reduction of lung elastic recoil, which are characteristic features of emphysema, may contribute to airflow obstruction in different ways. First, a reduction in number and integrity of alveolar attachments to small airways together with a reduction of P_{tp} may decrease the distending force on airway walls [79]. Second, a reduction in alveolar pressure shifts the Bernoulli equation plots to the left, thus limiting $\dot{V}_{max}$ at a level lower than normal (Fig. 4.2). During forced expiration, airways downstream from the choke point are dynamically compressed because the intraluminal pressure is reduced below the pleural pressure at the same lung volume. This phenomenon is enhanced in COPD because airway distending pressure and driving pressure are decreased due to loss of lung recoil pressure [80], increased frictional losses in peripheral airways, or reduced tethering force on airway walls [81]. An increased collapsibility of central airways was initially reported in patients with chronic airflow obstruction [82, 83] but not confirmed in a larger and more recent study [84].

The ASM layer has also been found to be thicker than normal in COPD due to hyperplasia [85], though not as much as in asthma. Modeling studies based on morphometric data have suggested that the amount of ASM is unlikely to play a major role in COPD airway narrowing [24]. Studies comparing preoperative lung function with morphometric observations on surgical samples found that airflow obstruction [77] and response to constrictor stimuli [79, 86] were related to total airway wall thickness whereas a relationship with ASM mass was not consistently reported [24, 87–89]. In one study, a weak correlation was found between the isometric force developed in vitro by ASM and airflow obstruction determined preoperatively [90], suggesting a possible role for an increased ASM contractility in COPD. Indeed, several studies have reported significant bronchodilator responses in COPD patients, which would suggest that ASM does contribute to airflow obstruction in this disease. This, however, does not prove that ASM is abnormal in COPD because, even in the presence of a normal ASM tone, the response to bronchodilators may appear greater than in normal subjects because of the amplifying effect of airway wall thickening.

Conclusions

Airway caliber in vivo is regulated by a complex interaction between morphological and mechanical factors. In asthma, airflow obstruction seems to be mainly dependent on airway wall remodeling, with ASM playing a key role, though some morphological changes may be even protective against excessive airway narrowing. In COPD, airflow obstruction may result from changes in airway wall geometry, lung parenchymal properties, or both.

References

1. Tiffeneau R, Pinelli A (1947) Air circulant et air captif dans l'exploration de la fonction venti-latoire pulmonaire. Paris Med 133:624–631
2. Bates DV, Woolf CR, Paul GI (1962) A report on the first two stages of the co-ordinated study of chronic bronchitis in the Department of Veterans Affairs, Canada. Med Serv J Can 18:211–303
3. Mead J (1980) Dysanapsis in normal lungs assessed by the relationship between maximal flow, static recoil, and vital capacity. Am Rev Respir Dis 121.339–342
4. Hoppin FG Jr, Stothert JC Jr, Greaves IA, Lai Y-L, Hildebrandt J (1986) Lung recoil: elastic and rheological properties. In: Macklem PT, Mead J (eds) Handbook of physiology. The respiratory system. Mechanics of breathing, Section 3, vol III, part 1 American Physiological Society, Bethesda, pp 195–215
5. Bailyss LE, Robertson GW (1939) The visco-elastic properties of the lungs. Q J Exp Physiol 29:27–47
6. Hildebrandt J (1969) Dynamic properties of air-filled excised cat lung determined by liquid plethysmograph. J Appl Physiol 27:246–250
7. Officer TM, Pellegrino R, Brusasco V, Rodarte JR (1998) Measurement of pulmonary resistance and dynamic compliance with airway obstruction. J Appl Physiol 85:1982–1988
8. Lambert RK, Wilson TA (1973) A model for the elastic properties of the lung and their effect on expiratory flow. J Appl Physiol 34:34–48
9. Dawson SV, Elliott EA (1977) Wave-speed limitation on expiratory flow – a unifying concept. J Appl Physiol 43:498–515
10. Fry DL, Hyatt RE (1960) Pulmonary mechanics. A unified analysis of the relationship between pressure, volume and gas flow in the lungs of normal and diseased human subjects. Am J Med 29:672–689
11. Stephens NL, Hoppin FG (1986) Mechanical properties of airway smooth muscle. In: Macklem PT, Mead J (eds) Handbook of physiology, Section 3, vol III, part 1. The respiratory system. Mechanics of breathing. American Physiological Society, Bethesda, pp 263–276
12. Bossé Y, Sobieszek A, Paré PD, Seow CY (2008) Length adaptation of airway smooth muscle. Proc Am Thorac Soc 5(1):62–67
13. Kuo KH, Wang L, Pare PD, Ford LE, Seow CY (2001) Myosin thick filament lability induced by mechanical strain in airway smooth muscle. J Appl Physiol 90:1811–1816
14. Supinski GS, Kelsen SG (1982) Effect of elastase-induced emphysema on the force-generating ability of the diaphragm. J Clin Invest 70:978–988
15. Farkas GA, Roussos C (1983) Diaphragm in emphysematous hamsters: sarcomere adaptability. J Appl Physiol 54:1635–1640
16. Williams PE, Goldspink G (1978) Changes in sarcomere length and physiological properties in immobilized muscle. J Anat 127:459–468

17. Li W, Stephens NL (1994) Auxotonic loading and airway smooth muscle shortening. Can J Physiol Pharmacol 72:1458–1463
18. Pedley TJ, Schroeter RC, Sudlow MF (1977) Gas flow and mixing in the airways. In: West JB (ed) Bioengineering aspects of the lung. Marcel Dekker, New York, pp 163–265
19. Moreno RH, Hogg JC, Paré PD (1986) Mechanics of airway narrowing. Am Rev Respir Dis 133:1171–1180
20. Sterk PJ, Timmers MC, Bel EH, Dijkman JH (1988) The combined effects of histamine and methacholine on maximal airway narrowing in normal humans in vivo. Eur Respir J 1:34–40
21. Bel EH, Van der Veen H, Kramps JA, Dijkman JH, Sterk PJ (1987) Maximal airway narrowing to inhaled leukotriene D_4 in normal subjects: comparison and interaction with methacholine. Am Rev Respir Dis 136:979–984
22. Pellegrino R, Violante B, Crimi E, Brusasco V (1993) Effects of aerosol methacholine and histamine on airways and lung parenchyma in healthy humans. J Appl Physiol 74:2681–2686
23. Wiggs BR, Bosken C, Paré PD, James A, Hogg JC (1992) A model of airway narrowing in asthma and in chronic obstructive pulmonary disease. Am Rev Respir Dis 145:1251–1258
24. Lambert RK, Wiggs BR, Kuwano K, Hogg JC, Paré PD (1993) Functional significance of increase airway smooth muscle in asthma and COPD. J Appl Physiol 74:2771–2781
25. Macklem PT (1996) A theoretical analysis of the effect of airway smooth muscle load on airway narrowing. Am J Respir Crit Care Med 153:83–89
26. Lambert RK, Codd SL, Alley MR, Pack RJ (1994) Physical determinants of bronchial mucosal folding. J Appl Physiol 77:1206–1216
27. Wiggs BR, Hroussis CA, Drazen JM, Kamm RD (1997) On the mechanism of mucosal folding in normal and asthmatic airways. J Appl Physiol 83:1814–1821
28. Seow CY, Wang L, Paré PD (2000) Airway narrowing and internal structural constraints. J Appl Physiol 88:527–533
29. Lambert RK (1991) Role of bronchial basement membrane in airway collapse. J Appl Physiol 71:666–673
30. Lambert RK, Paré PD, Okazawa M (2001) Stiffness of peripheral airway folding membrane in rabbits. J Appl Physiol 90:2041–2047
31. Ishida K, Paré PD, Hards J, Schellemberg RR (1992) Mechanical properties of human bronchial smooth muscle in vitro. J Appl Physiol 73:1481–1485
32. Ding DJ, Martin JG, Macklem PT (1987) Effects of lung volume on maximal methacholine-induced bronchoconstriction in normal humans. J Appl Physiol 62:1324–1330
33. Mead J, Takishima T, Leith D (1970) Stress distribution in lungs: a model of pulmonary elasticity. J Appl Physiol 28:596–608
34. Fredberg JJ, Jones KA, Nathan M, Raboudi S, Prakash YS, Shore SA, Butler JP, Sieck GC (1996) Friction in airway smooth muscle mechanisms: latch and implications in asthma. J Appl Physiol 81:2703–2712
35. Solway J, Fredberg JJ (1997) Perhaps airway smooth muscle dysfunction contributes to asthmatic bronchial hyperresponsiveness after all. Am J Respir Cell Mol Biol 17:144–146
36. Bullimore SR, Siddiqui S, Donovan GM, Martin JG, Sneyd J, Bates JH, Lauzon AM (2011) Could an increase in airway smooth muscle shortening velocity cause airway hyperresponsiveness? Am J Physiol Lung Cell Mol Physiol 300:L121–L131
37. Dunnill MS (1960) The pathology of asthma with special reference to change in the bronchial mucosa. J Clin Pathol 13:27–33
38. Kuwano K, Bosken C, Paré PD, Wiggs B, Hogg JC (1993) Small airways dimensions in asthma and chronic obstructive pulmonary disease. Am Rev Respir Dis 148:1220–1225
39. Woodruff PG, Dolganov GM, Ferrando RE, Donnelly S, Hays SR, Solberg OD, Carter R, Wong HH, Cadbury PS, Fahy JV (2004) Hyperplasia of smooth muscle in mild to moderate asthma without changes in cell size or gene expression. Am J Respir Crit Care Med 169:1001–1006
40. Bai TR (1990) Abnormalities in airway smooth muscle in fatal asthma. Am Rev Respir Dis 141:552–557

41. Bai TR (1991) Abnormalities in airway smooth muscle in fatal asthma. A comparison between trachea and bronchus. Am Rev Respir Dis 143:441–443
42. Cerrina J, Labat C, Haye-Legrande I, Raffestin B, Benveniste J, Brink C (1989) Human isolated bronchial muscle preparations from asthmatic patients: effects of indomethacin and contractile agonists. Prostaglandins 37:457–469
43. Cerrina J, Le Roy Ladurie M, Labat C, Raffestin B, Bayol A, Brink C (1986) Comparison of human bronchial muscle responses to histamine in vivo with histamine and isoproterenol agonists in vitro. Am Rev Respir Dis 134:57–61
44. Chan V, Burgess JK, Ratoff JC, O'Connor BJ, Greenough A, Lee TH, Hirst SJ (2006) Extracellular matrix regulates enhanced eotaxin expression in asthmatic airway smooth muscle cells. Am J Respir Crit Care Med 174:379–385
45. Chin LY, Bossé Y, Jiao Y, Solomon D, Hackett TL, Paré PD, Seow CY (2010) Human airway smooth muscle is structurally and mechanically similar to that of other species. Eur Respir J 36:170–177
46. de Jongste JC, Mons H, Bonta IL et al (1987) In vitro responses of airways from an asthmatic patient. Eur J Respir Dis 71:23–29
47. Schellenberg RR, Foster A (1984) In vitro responses of human asthmatic airway and pulmonary vascular smooth muscle. Int Arch Allergy Appl Immunol 75:237–241
48. Thomson RJ, Bramley AM, Schellenberg RR (1996) Airway muscle stereology: implications for increased shortening in asthma. Am J Respir Crit Care Med 154:749–757
49. Ma X, Cheng Z, Kong H, Wang Y, Unruh H, Stephens NL, Laviolette M (2002) Changes in biophysical and biochemical properties of single bronchial smooth muscle cells from asthmatic subjects. Am J Physiol Lung Cell Mol Physiol 283:L1181–L1189
50. Mitchell RW, Rühlmann E, Magnussen H, Leff AR, Rabe KF (1994) Passive sensitization of human bronchi augments smooth muscle shortening velocity and capacity. Am J Physiol 267:L218–L222
51. Antonissen LA, Mitchell RW, Kroeger EA, Kepron W, Tse KS, Stephens NL (1979) Mechanical alterations of airway smooth muscle in a canine asthmatic model. J Appl Physiol 46:681–687
52. Fan T, Yang M, Halayko A, Mohapatra SS, Stephens NL (1997) Airway responsiveness in two inbred strains of mouse disparate in IgE and IL-4 production. Am J Respir Cell Mol Biol 17:156–163
53. Mitchell RW, Ndukwu IM, Arbetter K, Solway J, Leff AR (1993) Effect of airway inflammation on smooth muscle shortening and contractility in guinea-pig trachealis. Am J Physiol Lung Cell Mol Physiol 265:L549–L554
54. Blanc FX, Coirault C, Salmeron S, Chemla D, Lecarpentier Y (2003) Mechanics and cross-bridge kinetics of tracheal smooth muscle in two inbred rat strains. Eur Respir J 22:227–234
55. Duguet A, Biyah K, Minshall E, Gomes R, Wang CG, Taoudi-Benchekroun M, Bates JHT, Eidelman DH (2000) Bronchial responsiveness among inbred mouse strains: role of airway smooth-muscle shortening velocity. Am J Respir Crit Care Med 161:839–848
56. Wang CG, Almirall JJ, Dolman CS, Dandurand RJ, Eidelman DH (1997) In vitro bronchial responsiveness in two highly inbred rat strains. J Appl Physiol 82:1445–1452
57. Jackson AC, Murphy MM, Rassulo J, Celli BR, Ingram RH (2004) Deep breath reversal and exponential return of methacholine-induced obstruction in asthmatic and nonasthmatic subjects. J Appl Physiol 96:137–142
58. Jensen A, Atileh H, Suki B, Ingenito EP, Lutchen KR (2001) Airway caliber in healthy and asthmatic subjects: effects of bronchial challenge and deep inspirations. J Appl Physiol 91:506–515
59. Pellegrino R, Wilson O, Jenouri G, Rodarte JR (1996) Lung mechanics during induced bronchoconstriction. J Appl Physiol 81:964–975
60. Pellegrino R, Dellacà R, Macklem PT, Aliverti A, Bertini S, Lotti P, Agostoni PG, Locatelli A, Brusasco V (2003) Effects of rapid saline infusion on lung mechanics and airway responsiveness in humans. J Appl Physiol 95:728–734

61. Wilson JW, Li X, Pain MCF (1993) The lack of distensibility of asthmatic airways. Am Rev Respir Dis 148:806–809
62. Ward C, Johns DP, Bish R, Pais M, Reid DW, Ingram C, Feltis B, Walters EH (2001) Reduced airway distensibility, fixed airflow limitation, and airway wall remodeling in asthma. Am J Respir Crit Care Med 164:1718–1721
63. Brackel HJL, Pedersen OF, Mulder PGH, Overbeek SE, Kerrebijn KF, Bogaard JM (2000) Central airways behave more stiffly during forced expiration in patients with asthma. Am J Respir Crit Care Med 162:896–904
64. Roche WR, Beasley R, Williams JH, Holgate ST (1989) Subepithelial fibrosis in the bronchi of asthmatics. Lancet 1:520–524
65. Wilson JW, Li X (1997) The measurement of reticular basement membrane and submucosal collagen in the asthmatic airway. Clin Exper Allergy 27:363–371
66. Huang J, Olivenstein R, Taha R, Hamid Q, Ludwig M (1999) Enhanced proteoglycan deposition in the airway wall of atopic asthmatics. Am J Respir Crit Care Med 160:725–729
67. Palmans E, Kips JC, Pauwels RA (2000) Prolonged allergen exposure induces structural airway changes in sensitized rats. Am J Respir Crit Care Med 161:627–635
68. Bai TR, Cooper J, Koelmeyer T, Paré PD, Weir T (2000) The effect of age and duration of disease on airway structure in fatal asthma. Am J Respir Crit Care Med 162:663–669
69. Meiss RA (1999) Influence of intercellular tissue connections on airway muscle mechanics. J Appl Physiol 86:5–15
70. Bramley AM, Roberts CR, Schellenberg RR (1995) Collagenase increases shortening of human bronchial smooth muscle in vitro. Am J Respir Crit Care Med 152:1513–1517
71. Milanese M, Crimi E, Scordamaglia A, Riccio A, Pellegrino R, Canonica GW, Brusasco V (2001) On the functional consequences of bronchial basement membrane thickening. J Appl Physiol 91:1035–1040
72. Niimi A, Matsumoto H, Amitani R, Nakano Y, Mishima M, Minakuchi M, Nishimura K, Itoh H, Izumu T (2000) Airway wall thickness in asthma assessed by computed tomography: relation to clinical indices. Am J Respir Crit Care Med 162:1518–1523
73. Siddiqui S, Gupta S, Cruse G, Haldar P, Entwisle J, Mcdonald S, Whithers PJ, Hainsworth SV, Coxson HO, Brightling C (2009) Airway wall geometry in asthma and nonasthmatic eosinophilic bronchitis. Allergy 64:951–958
74. Boulet L-P, Belanger M, Carrier G (1995) Airway responsiveness and bronchial-wall thickness in asthma with or without fixed airflow obstruction. Am J Respir Crit Care Med 152:865–871
75. Little SA, Sproule MW, Cowan MD, Macleod KJ, Robertson M, Love JG, Chalmers GW, McSharry CP, Thomson NC (2002) High resolution computed tomographic assessment of airway wall thickness in chronic asthma: reproducibility and relationship with lung function and severity. Thorax 57:247–253
76. Niimi A, Matsumoto H, Takemura M, Ueda T, Chin K, Mishima M (2003) Relationship of airway wall thickness to airway sensitivity and airway reactivity in asthma. Am J Respir Crit Care Med 168:983–988
77. Tiddens HAWM, Paré PD, Hogg JC, Hop WCJ, Lambert R, De Jongste JC (1995) Cartilagineous airway dimensions and airflow obstruction in human lungs. Am J Respir Crit Care Med 152:260–266
78. Finkelstein R, Hong-Da MA, Ghezzo H, Whittaker K, Fraser RS, Cosio MG (1995) Morphometry of small airways in smokers and its relationship to emphysema type and hyperresponsiveness. Am J Respir Crit Care Med 152:267–276
79. Corsico A, Milanese M, Baraldo S, Casoni GL, Papi A, Riccio AM, Cerveri I, Saetta M, Brusasco V (2003) Small airway morphology and lung function in the transition from normality to chronic airway obstruction. J Appl Physiol 95:441–447
80. Funicane KE, Colebatch HJ (1969) Elastic behavior of the lung in patients with airway obstruction. J Appl Physiol 26:330–338
81. Saetta M, Ghezzo H, Kim WD, King M, Angus GE, Wang NS, Cosio MG (1985) Loss of alveolar attachments in smokers. A morphometric correlate of lung function impairment. Am Rev Respir Dis 132:894–900

82. Macklem PT, Fraser RG, Bates DV (1963) Bronchial pressures and dimensions in health and obstructive airway disease. J Appl Physiol 18:699–706

83. Leaver DG, Tattersfield AE, Pride NB (1973) Contributions of loss of lung recoil and of enhanced airway collapsibility to the airflow obstruction of chronic bronchitis and emphysema. J Clin Invest 52:2117–2128

84. Tiddens HAWM, Bogaard JM, de Jongste JC, Hop WCJ, Coxson HO, Paré PD (1996) Physiological and morphological determinants of maximal expiratory flow in chronic obstructive lung disease. Eur Respir J 9:1785–1794

85. Hossain S, Heard BE (1970) Hyperplasia of bronchial muscle in chronic bronchitis. J Pathol 101:171–184

86. Riess A, Wiggs B, Verburgt L, Wright JL, Hogg JC, Paré PD (1996) Morphologic determinants of airway responsiveness in chronic smokers. Am J Respir Crit Care Med 154:1444–1449

87. Taylor SM, Paré PD, Armour CL, Hogg JC, Schellenberg RR (1985) Airway reactivity in chronic obstructive pulmonary disease: failure of in vivo methacholine responsiveness to correlate with cholinergic, adrenergic, or nonadrenergic responses in vitro. Am Rev Respir Dis 132:30–35

88. Vincenc KS, Black JL, Yan K, Armour CL, Donnelly PD, Woolcock AJ (1983) Comparison of in vivo and in vitro responses to histamine in human airways. Am Rev Respir Dis 128:875–879

89. Armour CL, Lazar NM, Schellenberg RR, Taylor SM, Chan N, Hogg JC, Paré PD (1984) A comparison on in vivo and in vitro human airway reactivity to histamine. Am Rev Respir Dis 129:907–910

90. Opazo Saez AM, Seow CY, Paré PD (2000) Peripheral airway smooth muscle mechanics in obstructive airways disease. Am J Respir Crit Care Med 161:910–917

91. Brusasco V, Martinez FJ (2014) Chronic obstructive pulmonary disease. Compr Physiol 4:1–31

92. An SS, Bai TR, Bates JHT, Black JL, Brown RH, Brusasco V, Chitano P, Deng L, Dowell M, Eidelman DH, Fabry B, Fairbank NJ, Ford LE, Fredberg JJ, Gerthoffer WT, Gilbert SH, Gosens R, Gunst SJ, Halayko AJ, Ingram RH, Irvin CG, James AL, Janssen LJ, King GG, Knight DA, Lauzon AM, Lakser OJ, Ludwig MS, Lutchen KR, Maksym GN, Martin JG, Mauad T, McParland BE, Mijailovich SM, Mitchell HW, Mitchell RW, Mitzner W, Murphy TM, Paré PD, Pellegrino R, Sanderson MJ, Schellenberg RR, Seow CY, Silveira PSP, Smith PG, Solway J, Stephens NL, Sterk PJ, Stewart AG, Tang DD, Tepper RS, Tran T, Wang L (2007) Airway smooth muscle dynamics: a common pathway of airway obstruction in asthma. Eur Respir J 29:834–860

93. Brusasco V, Pellegrino R. (2003) Complexity of factors modulating airway narrowing in vivo: Relavance to assessment of airway hyperresponsiveness. J Appl Physiol 95:1305–1313

Role of Airway Smooth Muscle Mechanical Properties in the Regulation of Airway Caliber

5

Susan J. Gunst

5.1 Introduction

The mechanical properties of airway smooth muscle play an important role in regulating the caliber of the airways during breathing. During breathing, the smooth muscle in the airway wall is subjected to stretch and contraction as the lung expands and contracts during changes in lung volume. These cycles of stretch and retraction of the muscle are important in maintaining a normal low level of airway tone and in reducing airway responsiveness to bronchoconstrictor stimuli. The effects of stretch on airway smooth muscle also account for the well-known dilatory effects of deep inspiration on the airways. Deep inspiration following bronchoconstriction causes a reduction in airway resistance in normal human subjects, whereas many asthmatic subjects demonstrate either no change or a slight decrease in airway resistance after deep inspiration [1–5]. Conversely, the prevention of deep inspiration during methacholine challenge of normal subjects results in an increase in airway reactivity that can reach levels comparable to those observed in asthmatics [6–8]. The fundamental mechanical properties of the airway smooth muscle cells play an important role in regulating the effects of lung volume changes on airway tone and responsiveness.

5.2 Mechanical Plasticity of Airway Smooth Muscle

Airway smooth muscle exhibits the property of "mechanical plasticity," which refers to the ability of the muscle to modulate its properties in response to changes in its external mechanical environment. The mechanical plasticity of airway smooth muscle appears to underlie many of the effects of changes in lung volume

S.J. Gunst, PhD
Department of Cellular and Integrative Physiology, Indiana University
School of Medicine, 635 Barnhill Dr., Indianapolis, IN 46202-5120, USA
e-mail: sgunst@iupui.edu

A. Aliverti, A. Pedotti (eds.), *Mechanics of Breathing*,
DOI 10.1007/978-88-470-5647-3_5, © Springer-Verlag Italia 2014

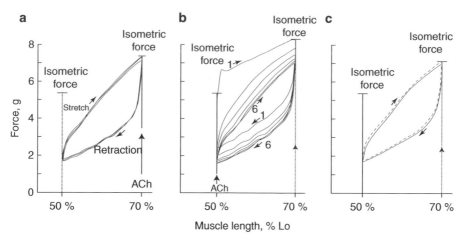

Fig. 5.1 *Mechanical plasticity of airway smooth muscle*. Changes in force during cyclical length oscillations of canine tracheal smooth muscle strip after isometric contraction with acetylcholine (*ACh*) in vitro. (**a**) After isometric contraction at a long muscle length (70 % Lo), successive length-force loops obtained during repeated oscillations to a short length (50 % Lo) are immediately reproducible. (**b**) After isometric contraction at a short length (50 %) Lo, the muscle is initially very stiff as it is stretched from 50 to 70 % Lo. The length-force loop changes during six successive oscillations to a long length (70 %) Lo until a stable loop is finally achieved. This demonstrates plastic adaptation of the muscle caused by stretch beyond its initial length of contraction. (**c**) The final loop obtained after isometric contraction at either length followed by repeated oscillations between 50 and 70 % Lo is the same (Adapted from Gunst [9])

on airway caliber and airway responsiveness that are observed in vivo. An example of the property of mechanical plasticity of tracheal smooth muscle is illustrated in Fig. 5.1 [9]. In Fig. 5.1a, a trachealis muscle strip is stimulated with acetylcholine (ACh) to contract isometrically at a length of 70 % of its "optimal" length, Lo. Lo is the length of the muscle at which isometric force is maximal. Muscle length is held constant until a stable isometric force is achieved. The contracted muscle is then subjected to repeated cycles of length oscillation between lengths of 70 % Lo and a shorter length of 50 % Lo. As the muscle strip is retracted to a shorter length, its force declines dramatically. When the muscle strip is stretched back to 70 % Lo, force increases to the original level of isometric force. The muscle force over most of the length range during the oscillation cycle is much lower than that sustained by the muscle when it is contracted under static isometric conditions at any length within the oscillation cycle, and it remains reproducible and stable with each successive length cycle. In Fig. 5.1b, the same muscle strip is stimulated to contract isometrically at the shortest length within the oscillation cycle, 50 % Lo, and then again subjected to repeated cycles of length oscillation between 50 and 70 % Lo. This time a very different behavior is observed. The muscle is initially very stiff when it is stretched, and it exhibits a high level of tension during the first full cycle of stretch and retraction. The force gradually declines with each successive cycle of length oscillation, and until after 5–6 cycles, it stabilizes and exhibits the same length-force loop that it maintained

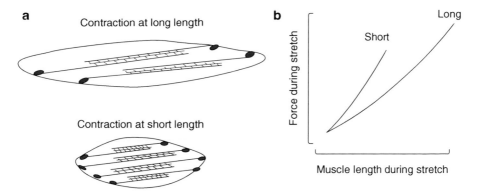

Fig. 5.2 *Mechanism for mechanical plasticity of airway smooth muscle.* (**a**) Contractile activation at a short muscle length results in organization of the contractile apparatus into a short thick filament array, whereas contraction at a long length results in the organization of the contractile apparatus into a long thin filament array. (**b**) As a result of structural differences, the muscle is predicted to be stiffer after contraction at a short length than after contraction at a long length (Adapted from Gunst et al. [10])

when it was oscillated after isometric contraction at the longer length of 70 % Lo (Fig. 5.1b, c). Clearly, after contraction at the shorter length (50 % Lo), the muscle must undergo a transitional process in order to reach the same mechanical state that is obtained when the contraction is initiated at the longer length (70 % Lo). This transition in mechanical behavior characterizes the property of "mechanical plasticity." It represents an adaptive response of the muscle to accommodate to the mechanical forces that are imposed on it.

Evidence suggests that mechanical plasticity results from an ability of the smooth muscle cell to modulate the organization of its contractile/cytoskeletal apparatus in order to accommodate to changes in cell shape imposed by the mechanical forces imposed on it by its external environment [10–13]. Activation of the muscle at a short length results in the contractile apparatus organizing into a shorter, thicker filament array that conforms to the shorter, thicker morphology of the muscle cell; whereas activation of the muscle at a long length results in a longer thinner array of contractile filaments that is adapted to the longer, narrower shape of the elongated muscle cell [12] (Fig. 5.2a). Thus, the muscle is stiffer and less extensible after contractile activation at a short length than after it is activated at a long length (Fig. 5.2b). Stretch of the muscle after activation at a short length causes reorganization of the cytoskeleton and contractile apparatus to accommodate to the change in shape of the muscle cell caused by the stretch (Fig. 5.1b). The stiffness of the muscle thus decreases when the contracted muscle is stretched from a short length to a long length [10, 12].

The effect of muscle length on the stiffness of isolated tracheal smooth muscle strips after contractile activation was evaluated by stimulating each tissue strip to contract isometrically at three different muscle lengths (Fig. 5.3a): Lo, 0.75 Lo, and 0.50 Lo [12]. After 5 min of isometric contraction, the muscle was rapidly shortened to a minimal length and then stretched slowly back to the length at which it was originally contracted isometrically. The force during each stretch maneuver was plotted

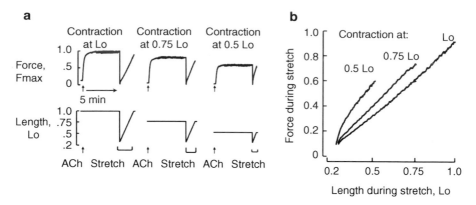

Fig. 5.3 *Effect of muscle length during contractile activation on muscle force and stiffness.* (**a**) tra-chealis muscle strip is contracted isometrically with acetylcholine (*ACh*) at Lo, 0.75 Lo, and 0.50 Lo in successive contractions. After the force stabilizes, the muscle is rapidly shortened to a minimal length and then stretched slowly in order to assess stiffness. (**b**) *Force during stretch* in A is plotted versus *length during stretch* to assess muscle stiffness after isometric contraction at each length. Stiffness is highest after contraction at the shortest length, 0.50 Lo, lower after contraction at 0.75 Lo, and lowest after contraction at the longest length, Lo (Adapted from Gunst and Wu [12])

against muscle length during stretch to evaluate muscle stiffness (Fig, 5.3b). After isometric contraction at a short muscle length (0.5 Lo), the muscle was stiffer and generated more force during stretch than after it was contracted at the medium or long muscle lengths, as indicated by the steeper slope of the force-length plot during stretch (Fig. 5.3b). Thus, as would be predicted from our model of mechanically induced contractile filament reorganization (Fig. 5.2b), the stiffness of the airway muscle tissue was inversely related to the length at which the muscle was stimulated to contract: the muscle was stiffer after contraction at a short length than after contraction at a long length with the same stimulus. Experiments also demonstrated that stretching the muscle beyond the length to which it adapts during static isometric contraction results in a sustained reduction in stiffness, similar to that shown in Fig. 5.1b [12]. These observations support the hypothesis that the structural arrangement of the contractile apparatus of airway smooth muscle cells is modified during contractile stimulation at different muscle lengths, and that stretch of a contracted muscle beyond the length to which it is adapted triggers a realignment of the cytoskeletal system and contractile apparatus [10]. Mechanical properties such as these are difficult to account for solely on the basis of traditional sliding filament models that predict a unique arrangement of contractile filaments based on muscle length [14].

5.3   Role of Mechanical Plasticity in the Regulation of Airway Tone

There is substantial evidence that the "plastic" or length-adaptive properties of airway smooth muscle are important in the normal regulation of airway tone [11, 15–19]. Bronchial segments subjected to physiologic conditions of volume oscillation after

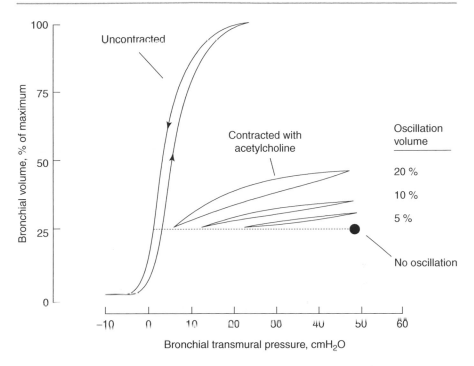

Fig. 5.4 *Effect of cyclical volume oscillations on the transmural pressure of an isolated canine intraparenchymal bronchus contracted with acetylcholine in vitro.* Volume oscillation reduces the magnitude of the airway transmural pressure in proportion to the amplitude of the oscillation volume. Peak pressure during volume oscillation is close to the static isovolume pressure, but pressure at the low end of the volume cycle is reduced well below the static pressure at that volume (Adapted from Gunst et al. [17])

contraction with acetylcholine exhibit plastic properties that are analogous to those observed in trachealis smooth muscle strips [17]. Isolated canine intraparenchymal bronchi were subjected to volume oscillations at amplitudes chosen to approximate the size of volume oscillations that bronchi are subjected to in vivo during tidal breathing (Fig. 5.4) [17]. Under static isovolumetric conditions, bronchial transmural pressure reached a pressure of over 50 cmH₂O during stimulation with acetylcholine. Even a very small magnitude, volume oscillation (5 %) caused a marked reduction in the transmural pressure of the contracted bronchus below the static pressure. As the size of the volume oscillation was increased, the transmural pressure at any particular airway volume declined. The lowest transmural pressures were observed when the magnitude of the volume oscillation was the largest. These observations in isolated bronchi in vitro subjected to small oscillations in volume suggest that oscillation of the airways during tidal breathing would inhibit airway contraction and increase airway compliance.

Tidal breathing has been shown to have a profound effect on airway tone and airway responsiveness in experimental animals. The increase in airway resistance that occurs in response to bronchial challenge is significantly lower during tidal breathing than under static conditions in both dogs and rabbits [20–22]. In ventilated rabbits, tidal breathing inhibits the increase in airway resistance in response to methacholine: the degree of

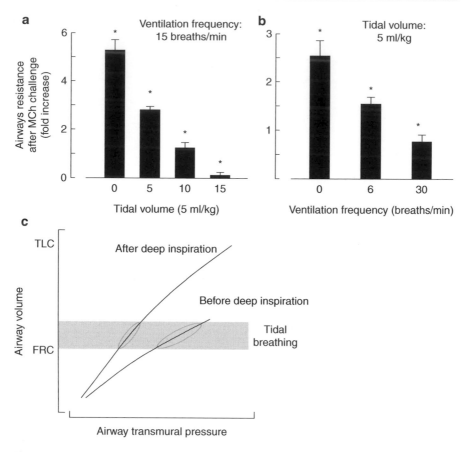

Fig. 5.5 *Effect of tidal breathing and deep inspiration on airway responsiveness.* (**a**) Airway reactivity to methacholine decreases as the magnitude or frequency of tidal volume oscillation increases (Adapted from Shen et al. [22]). (**b**) Predicted effect of deep breath on airway transmural pressures during tidal volume oscillations after bronchoconstriction before and after a deep breath. (**c**) Stretch of the airway caused by a deep breath reduces airway stiffness and contraction, resulting in lower transmural pressures during tidal volume oscillations. *Significantly different from each other ($P < 0.05$)

inhibition of the airway response to methacholine increases as the volume of the tidal breath is increased [19] (Fig. 5.5a). Increases in the frequency of tidal breathing at constant volume also cause a reduction in airway resistance in response to methacholine (Fig. 5.5b). The effects of volume oscillation on the airway responsiveness of experimental animals in vivo are analogous to the effects of volume oscillation on isolated bronchi, which suggests that the mechanisms that underlie the behavior of isolated bronchi may also account for many of the properties of the airways in vivo during breathing [17, 19].

In healthy human subjects with induced bronchoconstriction, a single deep inspiration attenuates the degree of airway narrowing [1–4]. The plastic properties of airway smooth muscle may also contribute to the effects of deep inspiration on airway responsiveness. The tension and stiffness of a contracted tracheal muscle strip can be reduced by stretching the muscle beyond the length to which it adapted during its initial contraction [9, 10, 12]: these experimental observations in the trachealis muscle are extrapolated to account for the expected effect of deep inspiration on airway transmural pressures during tidal breathing after bronchoconstriction (Fig. 5.5c). During tidal breathing at functional residual capacity (FRC) before deep inspiration, airway smooth muscle is subjected to minimal stretch; therefore, the muscle stiffens, leading to a decrease in airway compliance and an increase in airway narrowing. Deep inspiration stretches the airway smooth muscle, reducing the stiffness and contractile tension of the muscle. When tidal breathing is resumed following deep inspiration, airway compliance is increased and airway narrowing is reduced.

We measured the effect of deep inspiration (DI) on airway caliber in ventilated rabbits using forced oscillation at 6 Hz to assess changes in airway resistance (Raw) in response to methacholine (MCh) challenge [23]. A single deep inspiration performed immediately after MCh challenge reduced the magnitude of the increase in Raw in response to MCh, confirming that even a single brief stretch of the airways early in the response to a bronchoconstrictor results in a significant reduction in airway narrowing. A deep inspiration performed prior to MCh challenge also inhibited the increase in airways resistance, but to a lesser degree than when it was performed after bronchoconstriction. This observation is consistent with the results of in vitro studies of airway smooth muscle in which stretch of trachealis smooth muscle strips prior to contractile stimulation inhibited force development in response to cholinergic stimulation, suggesting that unstimulated airway smooth muscle also manifests plastic properties [24–27].

5.4   Molecular Mechanisms for the Mechanical Plasticity of Airway Smooth Muscle

The mechanical plasticity of airway smooth muscle cells has been proposed to result from the reorganization of the cytoskeletal system to adapt to changes in the shape of the smooth muscle cell that occur in response to changes in external mechanical conditions [10–13, 19, 27] (Fig. 5.6). This includes both the contractile and noncontractile cytoskeletal filaments, which are closely interconnected. The contractile apparatus of smooth muscle consists of interdigitating actin and myosin filaments that regulate shortening and tension development in smooth muscle by sliding across each other [14]. Although a majority of the actin filaments associate with myosin filaments to form the contractile apparatus, other actin filaments do not have myosin filaments associated with them and form a labile pool of actin at the cortex of the airway smooth muscle cell that undergoes polymerization and depolymerization during contraction and relaxation [28]. Actin filaments anchor at α-actinin-rich complexes within the cytoplasm of the smooth muscle cell. Cortical and cytoplasmic actin filaments also anchor to multiprotein integrin adhesion junction sites along the plasma membrane via a series of linker proteins (e.g., talin and α-actinin) that bind directly to both integrin proteins and filamentous actin, thus linking extracellular matrix proteins outside the cell to the cytoskeleton and thereby

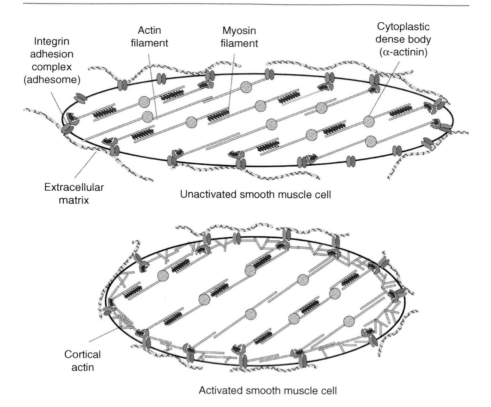

Fig. 5.6 *Cytoskeletal reorganization during contractile activation of the airway smooth muscle cell.* Contractile stimulation of the airway smooth muscle cell triggers the recruitment of adhesome proteins to integrin-associated signaling complexes (adhesomes), cortical actin polymerization, and reorganization of the actin cytoskeleton. The reorganization of actin filaments occurs with the polymerization and depolymerization of cortical actin filaments that regulate the tethering of the cytoskeleton to membrane adhesomes. Because myosin binds to the actin filament lattice, this results in reorganization of the contractile apparatus (Modified from Gunst and Zhang [28])

enabling the transmission of force between the contractile apparatus and the extra-cellular matrix (Fig. 5.6). Integrin proteins also function as mechanotransducers and transduce signals to the cytoskeleton and the nucleus via macromolecular protein complexes associated with integrin adhesion junctions (adhesomes). In addition to linker proteins, these complexes contain dozens of signaling and adaptor proteins that mediate cytoskeletal and nuclear signaling pathways that regulate the organization and activation of cytoskeletal proteins as well as the phenotype and function of the smooth muscle cell [29–32]. Because actin filaments provide a template for myosin filament binding, the arrangement of actin filaments within the cell determines the organization of the contractile apparatus. In airway smooth muscle, modulation of the length and attachment sites of actin filaments in response to environmental conditions would enable the cytoskeletal and contractile filaments to adapt to changes in the shape of the smooth muscle cell (Fig. 5.6).

A wealth of evidence has accumulated to demonstrate that actin polymerization and adhesion junction signaling proteins play critical roles in the regulation of airway

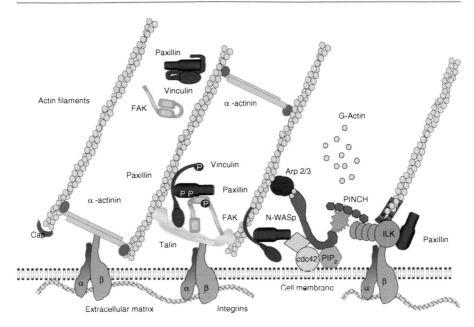

Fig. 5.7 *Molecular organization of membrane adhesion junction (adhesome).* Transmembrane integrins link the extracellular matrix to the cytoskeleton by binding to adhesome linker proteins such as talin and α-actinin. Adhesome complex proteins also bind to actin filaments and catalyze actin remodelling when activated by contractile stimulation. Adhesome proteins transduce mechanical signals to the cytoskeleton and to the nucleus to modulate protein synthesis

smooth muscle contraction, as well as in the regulation of other cellular functions. Agents and molecular interventions that inhibit actin polymerization inhibit force development in tracheal smooth muscle tissues without affecting the activation of contractile proteins, indicating that actin polymerization per se is required for contraction [28, 33, 34]. Contractile stimulation triggers the recruitment of cytoskeletal proteins to integrin-associated plasma membrane adhesion complexes and their assembly into signaling units [35–38]. Many of them, such as focal adhesion kinase (FAK), paxillin, and vinculin, undergo phosphorylation and conformational shifts in structure during the contractile activation of tracheal smooth muscle [29, 32, 36–39]. Thus, it is clear that proteins within adhesion complexes are activated by contractile stimuli to participate in regulating the functions of the airway smooth muscle cells. Both FAK and paxillin phosphorylation are mechanosensitive in tracheal smooth muscle, and both proteins exhibit higher levels of tyrosine phosphorylation when airway muscle is stimulated to contract at a higher level of mechanical strain or load [29]. Other adhesome proteins are also sensitive to mechanical forces and regulate alterations in response to inflammatory and contractile stimuli in response to changes in mechanical load [31]. The length sensitivity of the phosphorylation of both of these proteins is retained even when the muscle strips are stimulated in the absence of Ca^{2+}, under which condition no myosin light chain phosphorylation or force development occurs [29, 40]. These proteins are clearly involved in the regulation of cytoskeletal organization in this tissue and are likely to be critical mediators of the mechanotransduction process that modulates contractility in response to mechanical load (Figs. 5.6, 5.7, and 5.8).

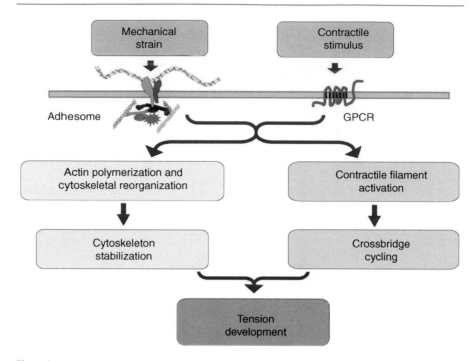

Fig. 5.8 *Mechanism for effects of mechanical strain on contractile tension.* Transmembrane integrins sense mechanical stimuli and initiate mechanosensitive signaling pathways via membrane adhesome signaling complexes that regulate actin dynamics and cytoskeletal organization. These signals collaborate with G protein receptor-mediated signals to regulate the activation of contractile proteins and crossbridge cycling. Both processes are required for the generation of tension development

In summary, the plastic properties of airway smooth muscle most likely underlie many of the physiologic effects of lung volume changes on airway caliber and airway responsiveness in vivo in normal humans and experimental animals. These properties have their basis in dynamic cytoskeletal processes that are being defined at the molecular level. The chronic mechanical and chemical stressors caused by airway inflammation in asthma affect actin filament dynamics and cytoskeletal signaling pathways that may contribute to cell stiffening and airway hyperreactivity as well as modulate the phenotypic properties of the muscle. Further definition of the molecular mechanisms that regulate airway smooth muscle plasticity and cytoskeletal dynamics may lead to new insights in the pathophysiology of asthma and potential new avenues for therapeutic intervention.

Acknowledgments Supported by the USPHS NIH grants HL29289, HL74099, and HL48522.

References

1. Jensen A, Atileh H, Suki B, Ingenito EP, Lutchen KR (2001) Selected contribution: airway caliber in healthy and asthmatic subjects: effects of bronchial challenge and deep inspirations. J Appl Physiol 91:506–515

2. Nadel JA, Tierney DF (1961) Effect of a previous deep inspiration on airway resistance in man. J Appl Physiol 16:717–719
3. Brusasco V, Crimi E, Barisione G, Spanevello A, Rodarte JR, Pellegrino R (1999) Airway responsiveness to methacholine: effects of deep inhalations and airway inflammation. J Appl Physiol 87:567–573
4. Fish JE, Ankin MG, Kelly JF, Peterman VI (1981) Regulation of bronchomotor tone by lung inflation in asthmatic and nonasthmatic subjects. J Appl Physiol 50:1079–1086
5. Wheatley JR, Pare PD, Engel LA (1989) Reversibility of induced bronchoconstriction by deep inspiration in asthmatic and normal subjects. Eur Respir J 2:331–339
6. King GG, Moore BJ, Seow CY, Pare PD (1999) Time course of increased airway narrowing caused by inhibition of deep inspiration during methacholine challenge. Am J Respir Crit Care Med 160:454–457
7. Skloot G, Permutt S, Togias A (1995) Airway hyperresponsiveness in asthma: a problem of limited smooth muscle relaxation with inspiration. J Clin Invest 96:2393–2403
8. Kapsali T, Permutt S, Laube B, Scichilone N, Togias A (2000) Potent bronchoprotective effect of deep inspiration and its absence in asthma. J Appl Physiol 89:711–720
9. Gunst SJ (1983) Contractile force of canine airway smooth muscle during cyclical length changes. J Appl Physiol Respir Environ Exerc Physiol 55:759–769
10. Gunst SJ, Meiss RA, Wu MF, Rowe M (1995) Mechanisms for the mechanical plasticity of tracheal smooth muscle. Am J Physiol 268:C1267–C1276
11. Gunst SJ, Tang DD, Opazo SA (2003) Cytoskeletal remodeling of the airway smooth muscle cell: a mechanism for adaptation to mechanical forces in the lung. Respir Physiol Neurobiol 137:151–168
12. Gunst SJ, Wu MF (2001) Plasticity of airway smooth muscle stiffness and extensibility: role of length-adaptive mechanisms. J Appl Physiol 90:741–749
13. Pratusevich VR, Seow CY, Ford LE (1995) Plasticity in canine airway smooth muscle. J Gen Physiol 105:73–94
14. Gunst SJ (1999) Applicability of the sliding filament/crossbridge paradigm to smooth muscle. Rev Physiol Biochem Pharmacol 134:7–61
15. Xue Z, Zhang L, Liu Y, Gunst SJ, Tepper RS (2008) Chronic inflation of ferret lungs with CPAP reduces airway smooth muscle contractility in vivo and in vitro. J Appl Physiol 104:610–615
16. Xue Z, Zhang W, Desai LP, Gao H, Gunst SJ, Tepper RS. (2013) Increased mechanical strain imposed on murine lungs during ventilation in vivo depresses airway responsiveness and activation of protein kinase Akt. J Appl Physiol 114:1506–1510
17. Gunst SJ, Stropp JQ, Service J (1990) Mechanical modulation of pressure-volume characteristics of contracted canine airways in vitro. J Appl Physiol 68:2223–2229
18. An SS, Bai TR, Bates JH, Black JL, Brown RH, Brusasco V, Chitano P, Deng L, Dowell M, Eidelman DH, Fabry B, Fairbank NJ, Ford LE, Fredberg JJ, Gerthoffer WT, Gilbert SH, Gosens R, Gunst SJ, Halayko AJ, Ingram RH, Irvin CG, James AL, Janssen LJ, King GG, Knight DA, Lauzon AM, Lakser OJ, Ludwig MS, Lutchen KR, Maksym GN, Martin JG, Mauad T, McParland BE, Mijailovich SM, Mitchell HW, Mitchell RW, Mitzner W, Murphy TM, Pare PD, Pellegrino R, Sanderson MJ, Schellenberg RR, Seow CY, Silveira PS, Smith PG, Solway J, Stephens NL, Sterk PJ, Stewart AG, Tang DD, Tepper RS, Tran T, Wang L (2007) Airway smooth muscle dynamics: a common pathway of airway obstruction in asthma. Eur Respir J 29:834–860
19. Shen X, Wu MF, Tepper RS, Gunst SJ (1997) Mechanisms for the mechanical response of airway smooth muscle to length oscillation. J Appl Physiol 83:731–738
20. Tepper RS, Shen X, Bakan E, Gunst SJ (1995) Maximal airway response in mature and immature rabbits during tidal ventilation. J Appl Physiol 79:1190–1198
21. Warner DO, Gunst SJ (1992) Limitation of maximal bronchoconstriction in living dogs. Am Rev Respir Dis 145:553–560
22. Shen X, Gunst SJ, Tepper RS (1997) Effect of tidal volume and frequency on airway responsiveness in mechanically ventilated rabbits. J Appl Physiol 83:1202–1208
23. Gunst SJ, Shen X, Ramchandani R, Tepper RS (2001) Bronchoprotective and bronchodilatory effects of deep inspiration in rabbits subjected to bronchial challenge. J Appl Physiol 91:2511–2516

24. Gunst SJ (1986) Effect of length history on contractile behavior of canine tracheal smooth muscle. Am J Physiol 250:C146–C154
25. Mehta D, Wu MF, Gunst SJ (1996) Role of contractile protein activation in the length-dependent modulation of tracheal smooth muscle force. Am J Physiol 270:C243–C252
26. Wang L, Pare PD, Seow CY (2000) Effects of length oscillation on the subsequent force development in swine tracheal smooth muscle. J Appl Physiol 88:2246–2250
27. Gunst SJ, Wu MF, Smith DD (1993) Contraction history modulates isotonic shortening velocity in smooth muscle. Am J Physiol 265:C467–C476
28. Gunst SJ, Zhang W (2008) Actin cytoskeletal dynamics in smooth muscle: a new paradigm for the regulation of smooth muscle contraction. Am J Physiol Cell Physiol 295:C576–C587
29. Tang DD, Mehta D, Gunst SJ (1999) Mechanosensitive tyrosine phosphorylation of paxillin and focal adhesion kinase in tracheal smooth muscle. Am J Physiol 276:C250–C258
30. Wu Y, Huang Y, Herring BP, Gunst SJ (2008) Integrin-linked kinase regulates smooth muscle differentiation marker gene expression in airway tissue. Am J Physiol Lung Cell Mol Physiol 295:L988–L997
31. Desai LP, Wu Y, Tepper RS, Gunst SJ (2011) Mechanical stimuli and IL-13 interact at integrin adhesion complexes to regulate expression of smooth muscle myosin heavy chain in airway smooth muscle tissue. Am J Physiol Lung Cell Mol Physiol 301:L275–L284
32. Zhang W, Gunst SJ (2008) Interactions of airway smooth muscle cells with their tissue matrix: implications for contraction. Proc Am Thorac Soc 5:32–39
33. Zhang W, Wu Y, Du L, Tang DD, Gunst SJ (2005) Activation of the Arp2/3 complex by N-WASp is required for actin polymerization and contraction in smooth muscle. Am J Physiol Cell Physiol 288:C1145–C1160
34. Mehta D, Gunst SJ (1999) Actin polymerization stimulated by contractile activation regulates force development in canine tracheal smooth muscle. J Physiol 519(Pt 3):829–840
35. Opazo SA, Zhang W, Wu Y, Turner CE, Tang DD, Gunst SJ (2004) Tension development during contractile stimulation of smooth muscle requires recruitment of paxillin and vinculin to the membrane. Am J Physiol Cell Physiol 286:C433–C447
36. Huang Y, Zhang W, Gunst SJ (2010) Activation of vinculin induced by cholinergic stimulation regulates contraction of tracheal smooth muscle tissue. J Biol Chem 286(5):3630–3644
37. Zhang W, Wu Y, Wu C, Gunst SJ (2007) Integrin-linked kinase (ILK) regulates N-WASp-mediated actin polymerization and tension development in tracheal smooth muscle. J Biol Chem 282:34568–34580
38. Zhang W, Huang Y, Gunst SJ (2012) The small GTPase RhoA regulates the contraction of smooth muscle tissues by catalyzing the assembly of cytoskeletal signaling complexes at membrane adhesion sites. J Biol Chem 287:33996–34008
39. Wang Z, Pavalko FM, Gunst SJ (1996) Tyrosine phosphorylation of the dense plaque protein paxillin is regulated during smooth muscle contraction. Am J Physiol 271:C1594–C1602
40. Tang DD, Gunst SJ (2001) Roles of focal adhesion kinase and paxillin in the mechanosensitive regulation of myosin phosphorylation in smooth muscle. J Appl Physiol 91:1452–1459

Nitric Oxide in Asthma Is Like Insulin in Type II Diabetes

Solbert Permutt[†]

6.1   Introduction

The title of this chapter is intentionally provocative, but an accurate characterization of what this chapter is about: a theory of the mechanism of the airway hyperresponsiveness (AHR) in asthma. In non-insulin-dependent diabetes mellitus (type II diabetes), there is compelling evidence that the fundamental cause of the glucose intolerance results from decreased sensitivity to insulin [1]. The theory presented in this chapter is that the fundamental cause of the AHR in asthma results from a decreased sensitivity to endogenous nitric oxide (NO).

6.2   The Role of Deep Inspiration in the Pathogenesis of the AHR of Asthma

While comparing the differences between expiratory flow during forced expirations from total lung capacity (TLC) (full-forced expiration) with those from forced expirations initiated from normal end-tidal volume (partial forced expiration), we became impressed with the increased responsiveness of healthy subjects to inhaled methacholine (MCh) when the partial forced expiration was used [2]. Indeed, with increasing concentrations of Mch in the absence of any deep inspirations (DIs), we found that healthy subjects showed nearly identical responses to mildly asthmatic patients when only partial forced expirations were used. What was exceedingly

[†]Deceased

S. Permutt
Division of Pulmonary and Critical Care Medicine, Department of Medicine,
The Johns Hopkins University School of Medicine, Baltimore, MD, USA

A. Aliverti, A. Pedotti (eds.), *Mechanics of Breathing*,
DOI 10.1007/978-88-470-5647-3_6, © Springer-Verlag Italia 2014

surprising and provocative was the marked decrease in forced expiratory volume in 1 s (FEV_1) and FVC that was present in the healthy subjects after the DIs that were required for the performance of conventional spirometry. Of the ten healthy subjects, six had greater than a 20 % reduction in FEV_1 at doses of Mch less than 8 mg/ml (in the asthmatic range of responsiveness), whereas there was less than a 15 % reduction with 75 mg/ml during routine challenge. These studies indicated that healthy subjects could develop asthmatic responses to low doses of Mch if DIs were suppressed during the challenge. For the asthmatic subjects, there was no effect of suppression of DIs on the response to Mch. We subsequently showed that suppression of DIs for 20 min before challenge with a single dose of Mch markedly increased the response to that single dose as assessed by changes in FEV_1 and FVC [3, 4]. With only five DIs following the 20-min suppression, the increased sensitivity to Mch in the healthy subjects was markedly attenuated. Neither the suppression of DIs nor the five DIs before challenge had an effect on the response to the single dose of Mch in asthmatic patients. Thus, DIs prior to Mch challenge had a protective effect (bronchoprotection) on the response of the airways in healthy subjects, but this protective effect was markedly attenuated in the asthmatic patients. These studies suggest that a major cause of the AHR in asthma could be the loss of the normal protective effect of DIs.

There has been considerable speculation as to the mechanism of the protective effect of DI in healthy subjects and why such an effect is attenuated in asthma [5]. We initially thought that the protective effect of DI in healthy subjects results from the stretch of the airway smooth muscle (ASM) accompanying DI, with the stretch less in asthma because of a decrease in the effectiveness of the tethering forces of the lung parenchyma on the airways. If these tethering forces are decreased in asthma from uncoupling of the interdependence between airways and parenchyma from inflammatory changes within the airways, the load against which the ASM contracts would be decreased, and the degree of shortening increased for the same degree of activation of the ASM [6]. The uncoupling of the forces between the lung parenchyma and airways could account for the increased response to spasmogens in asthma, but this mechanism could not explain why healthy subjects have an asthmatic response to Mch merely because DIs are suppressed prior to the challenge, since the measurement of FEV_1 requires a DI to TLC. There must have been some change in the airways of the normal subjects that occurred during the time that the DIs were suppressed before the Mch challenge.

Fredberg [5] has suggested that if ASM is not cyclically stretched and relaxed, the mechanical properties are changed to a state where ASM becomes much more responsive to spasmogens. He characterized this state of increased responsiveness as a "frozen contractile state." With prolonged suppression of DIs, the magnitude of the stretch during normal tidal breathing might be too small to prevent the frozen state from occurring. The increased responsiveness to spasmogens in asthma could be the result of the ineffectiveness even of DIs to produce the protective effect that occurs in healthy subjects. Fredberg's concepts could account for the findings that suppression of DIs before the spasmogen is given increases the response in healthy subjects if the frozen state is not prevented by tidal breathing alone, but is prevented by a few DIs prior to the challenge in normal subjects. This explanation assumes that the frozen contractile state can develop in healthy subjects when DIs are suppressed, but the frozen contractile state is present at all times in asthma, whether or not DIs are carried out, because the DIs are ineffective in preventing the frozen state in asthma. Fredberg's concepts would apply if DIs are less effective in asthmatic patients because they produce less stretch of the ASM. Recent work, however, does not support this inference: the airways of both groups increase similarly, but in healthy subjects, the diameter remains increased after the DI, while in asthma, the diameter is less than it was prior to the DI [7].

6.3   Hypothesis: DIs Provide Protection Against the Constrictive Effect of Spasmogens by the Release of a Protective Chemical; AHR Occurs When There Is a Decreased Effectiveness of the Putative Protective Chemical

We infer that a protective chemical is released during DIs from stretch of the airways. If the challenge is performed after a prolonged absence of DIs, the protective chemical will not have been released in a quantity sufficient to be effective, and there will be a much greater reduction in FEV_1 and FVC. As few as five DIs can attenuate the constrictive effect of the spasmogen, but once constriction occurs in the absence of DIs, the constriction is not overcome with the DI that precedes the measurement of FEV_1 and FVC. Healthy subjects show asthmatic responses to spasmogens when the challenge occurs following a prolonged absence of DIs, because the protective chemical is not present in an amount that is effective. We believe that DIs are ineffective in asthma, not because of a decrease in the amount released, but rather a lack of effectiveness of the putative protective chemical.

The increased diameter in the normal subject following a DI [7] would be explained by some prolongation of the time of relaxation after a DI releases the chemical. The decreased airway diameter in mildly asthmatic patients following the DI can be explained by a myogenic response from stretch, a characteristic of vascular smooth muscle, but whose role in ASM is less certain [8]. If the myogenic response to stretch (DI) is prevented by the protective chemical, it would only become manifest when the chemical is either not present or is ineffective. A myogenic response from DI that is suppressed only in healthy subjects could explain the frequent constrictive effect of DI in asthma.

6.4   Hypothesis: The Relaxing Chemical That Provides Bronchoprotection Is NO

Exhaled NO is increased in asthma [9]. The NO diffusing capacity of the airways (Dno) is the quantity of NO diffusing per unit time from the airway walls into exhaled gas divided by the difference between the concentration of NO in the airway wall

(Cw) and the lumen [10]. An elevation in the exhaled concentration of NO at a given expiratory flow can be due either to an increase in Cw, largely determined by NO synthase (NOS) activity within the airway walls, or an increase in Dno, a function of the surface area of the airways where NO is being produced. We were surprised to find that the increased concentration of NO that is often found in the exhaled gas of asthmatic patients is largely due to an increase in Dno, not an increase in Cw [10]. We inferred that the increased Dno in asthma is due to an extension of NOS activity toward smaller airways, thus increasing the surface area of the airways where NO is being produced, whereas the Dno of normal subjects is confined to the smaller surface area of the larger airways. We suggested that the increased Dno measured in asthmatic patients may reflect upregulation of non-adrenergic, non-cholinergic NO-producing nerves extending toward the smaller airways in compensation for decreased sensitivity of ASM to the relaxant effects of endogenous NO.

The quantity of diffusible NO was significantly correlated with the degree of airway responsiveness, as determined by the concentration of inhaled Mch required to reduce the FEV_1 by 20 % (PC_{20}) and the baseline pulmonary function (FEV_1), but the correlation was such that the higher the Dno, the greater the PC_{20} and FEV_1. For the mean Dno to be elevated in asthma, with the highest levels in the patients closer to normal subjects than more severe asthmatic patients, makes Dno analogous to insulin in type II diabetes, being usually elevated, but highest in those patients who are the least severe [1]. The explanation for this in type II diabetes is that the fundamental cause of the disease is a decrease in effectiveness of insulin (insulin resistance), and the higher the insulin level, the greater the fasting glucose level and intolerance to a glucose load in early diabetes. As the disease progresses, the high insulin levels cannot be maintained, and then glucose intolerance will increase as insulin levels fall. Thus, there is an inverted U-shaped curve of the relationship between blood glucose or glucose intolerance and insulin level [11].

If the hypothesis is correct, there should be a positive correlation between Dno and PC_{20} in the earliest stages of asthma, that is., an ascending limb of an inverted U-shaped curve. Indeed, we found that Dno was elevated in allergic rhinitis, whether or not AHR was present, and there was a highly significant positive correlation between Dno and PC_{20} within normal subjects, patients with rhinitis, and patients with mild asthma, in contrast to the negative correlation in severe asthmatics [10, 12]. Bronchoprotection from five DIs prior to a single-dose Mch challenge was present in the normal subjects and patients with allergic rhinitis without AHR, but was essentially absent in the allergic rhinitis patients with AHR and the mild asthmatic patients [4].

6.5   Is There Evidence for Diminished Effectiveness of NO in Asthma?

There is good evidence that the modulation of airway tone by NO is less effective in animals with allergic inflammation or genetic predisposition to AHR [10]. The decreased effectiveness in sensitized animals following antigenic challenge might be from decreased expression of type 1 NOS, the neural synthase (nNOS) [13].

Samb et al. [13] found that nNOS was reduced in the lung 6 h following challenge, but not type 2 or type 3 NOS (the inducible and endothelial NOS, respectively). The decreased nNOS expression was accompanied by a decrease in the amount of exhaled NO and an increase in AHR to histamine. The role of the decrease in nNOS is possibly of great importance, because nNOS has now been demonstrated in human ASM cells and has been shown to inhibit ASM cell proliferation that is likely involved in the airway wall remodeling of asthma [14].

Perhaps of greater importance than the association between allergic inflammation and the downregulation of nNOS activity is the effect of the proinflammatory cytokines, interleukin (IL)-1β and tumor necrosis factor (TNF)-α, and type 2 or iNOS, the inducible NOS, on the downregulation of soluble guanylate cyclase (sGC) [15]. The mechanism of the smooth muscle-relaxing effect of NO is through the combination of NO with a heme protein on the enzyme sGC that stimulates the conversion of GTP to cGMP, the intracellular second messenger that mediates smooth muscle relaxation and a number of other effects of NO, including the inhibition of smooth muscle cell proliferation. IL-1β and TNF-α are mediators of the innate immune system that are released from inflamed sites to organize the inflammatory response. They are elevated in asthma and acute severe asthma [16]. Exposure of smooth muscle cells to IL-1β and TNF-α led to NO production by iNOS that stimulated cGMP synthesis through sGS. Prolonged exposure decreased sGC mRNA and protein levels and decreased the ability of the smooth muscle cells to synthesize cGMP when stimulated by NO [15]. The downregulation of sGC was partly through a negative feedback on sGC from the production of NO and cGMP produced by the iNOS, but the cytokines also decreased sGC levels through an independent pathway, since the decrease occurred in iNOS-deficient mice [15]. If a similar process occurs in the ASM of humans, we would expect that the elevated levels of proinflammatory cytokines and iNOS would lead to a decreased ability of NO to relax the ASM. The negative feedback from iNOS on sGC probably plays an important role in protecting the blood pressure in sepsis [17], allowing the antimicrobial effects of iNOS, which do not involve sGC, to occur with less vasodilatation, but the negative feedback is detrimental to the control of ASM tone. Some of the decrease in AHR from corticosteroids might be due to an increase in sGC from the reduction in iNOS and proinflammatory cytokines.

6.6   Is There Evidence That the Effectiveness of NO Is Related to the Degree of AHR in Asthma?

Inhaled NO at 100 ppm caused a significant increase in the FEV_1 in asthmatic patients whose FEV_1 was reduced by 20 % or greater by Mch, but only in the asthmatic patients with $PC_{20} > 1$ mg/ml. In those patients whose $PC_{20} < 1$ mg/ml, there was no improvement in FEV_1 [18]. The authors suggested that the lack of improvement in those patients with a PC_{20} between 0.1 and 1.0 mg/ml might have been due to greater obstruction of small airways, with the ASM-relaxing effect of NO being principally in large airways. There is evidence that NO production in the airways of normal subjects is principally from large airways [10]. There is no support, however, for the constriction in the patients who responded being more confined to larger airway on the basis of the changes in vital capacity (VC). Indeed, there was a greater fall in VC in the responders for the same change in FEV_1. A fall in VC requires virtual closure of airways at residual volume; thus, changes in VC are not significantly affected by changes in the large airways. The lack of responsiveness to the inhaled NO in the more severe reactive asthmatic patients could be explained, however, by less sGC from a greater level of proinflammatory cytokines and a higher level of iNOS.

6.7   Is There Evidence That ASM Sees an Increased Concentration of NO from DIs?

There is considerable evidence that an increase in lung volume causes a reflex decrease in ASM tone through activation of sensory nerves that respond to stretch [19]. It is reasonable to consider how the decreased tone is partitioned between a decrease in cholinergic output and an increase in the output of the inhibitory NANC system (iNANC). There is evidence that baseline tone is a function of the opposing effects of acetylcholine and NO [20], but there is no convincing evidence that reflexes mediated by lung stretch cause an increase in output of NO from the iNANC system. In the guinea pig, an increase in exhaled NO was produced by lung inflation, and at least part of this increased output could have been caused by activity of the vagus nerve, since there was a considerable decrease in output following vagotomy [21]. Later studies from the same laboratory did not support a reflex increase in exhaled NO, because there was no effect of a potent ganglionic blocker (trimetaphan), but the increased NO from lung inflation was essentially abolished by gadolinium, a potent inhibitor of many mechanically sensitive ion channels [22]. The authors suggested that the increased NO from lung stretch could have been caused by "stretch-induced cellular calcium influx." This is known to occur in endothelial cells through activation of type 3 NOS [23] and in striated muscle through activation of nNOS [24]. This raises the possibility that the nNOS, known to be present in human ASM [14], can be activated directly by stretch, so that an increase in NO in ASM need not come from an increased output of the iNANC system.

Conclusions

The theory we propose to account for the AHR of asthma is that the smooth muscle relaxant effects of NO are suppressed by a decrease in sGC and NOS activity within ASM of asthmatics. The decreased sGC and NOS activity within the ASH are the result of inflammatory cytokines, such as IL-1β and TNF-α, which are elevated in asthma. These cytokines decrease the amount and activity of sGC, the enzyme that is required for the production of the second messenger, cGMP, necessary for the smooth muscle relaxant effects of NO. The cytokines also increase the activity of the inducible NO synthase, iNOS, which also decreases the amount and activity of sGC through negative feedback. Stretch of the airways increases the production of NO in ASM through activation of constitutive type 1 NOS, either through activation of the iNANC system or a direct effect of stretch of the ASM itself. The release of NO from the stretch that occurs with DI provides protection against the constrictive effects of spasmogens in normal subjects, but the release of NO is ineffective in asthma because of the downregulation of sGC. The AHR of asthma is, therefore, not due to any increased sensitivity of the ASM to spasmogens, but rather the lack of a protection against the normal constrictive response. The decreased sGC from the inflammatory cytokines is compensated by an increase in constitutive NO production, reflected by an increase in Dno in allergic rhinitis and mild asthma, but this compensation cannot be maintained as the asthma progresses in severity, reflected by a decreasing Dno. The decrease in both sGC and the constitutive NOS in severe asthma could be responsible, at least in part, for the airway remodeling, since a decrease in cGMP has been implicated in the hyperplasia and hypertrophy of ASM.

Acknowledgments I have been very significantly helped in the formation of the ideas expressed by the following people, but in no way should they be held responsible for those ideas: Christina Anderline, Robert Brown, Trisevgeni Kapsali, Mark Liu, George Pyrogos, Nicola Scichilone, Philip Silkoff, Gwen Skloot, Timmie Sylvester, Alkis Togias, and Noe Zamel.

References

1. Reaven GM (1995) Pathophysiology of insulin resistance in human disease. Physiol Rev 75:473–486
2. Skloot G, Permutt S, Togias A (1995) Airway hyperresponsiveness in asthma: a problem of limited smooth muscle relaxation with inspiration. J Clin Invest 96:2393–2403
3. Kapsali T, Permutt S, Laube B et al (2000) Potent bronchoprotective effect of deep inspiration and its absence in asthma. J Appl Physiol 89:711–720
4. Scichilone N, Permutt S, Togias A (2001) The lack of the bronchoprotective and not the bronchodilatory ability of deep inspiration is associated with airway hyperresponsiveness. Am J Respir Crit Care Med 163:413–419
5. Fredberg J (2001) Airway obstruction in asthma: does the response to a deep inspiration matter? Respir Res 2:273–275
6. Macklem PT (1996) A theoretical analysis of the effect of airway smooth muscle load on airway narrowing. Am J Respir Crit Care Med 153:83–89
7. Brown RH, Scichilone N, Mudge B et al (2001) High-resolution computed tomographic evaluation of airway distensibility and the effects of lung inflation on airway caliber in healthy subjects and individuals with asthma. Am J Respir Crit Care Med 163:994–1001
8. Marthan R, Woolcock AJ (1989) Is a myogenic response involved in deep inspiration-induced bronchoconstriction in asthmatics? Am Rev Respir Dis 140:1354–1358
9. Kharitonov SA, Yates D, Robbins RA et al (1994) Increased nitric oxide in exhaled air of asthmatic patients. Lancet 343:133–135
10. Silkoff PE, Sylvester JT, Zamel N, Permutt S (2000) Airway nitric oxide diffusion in asthma. Am J Respir Crit Care Med 161:1218–1228
11. DeFronzo RA (1988) Lilly lecture 1987. The triumvirate: beta-cell, muscle, liver. A collusion responsible for NIDDM. Diabetes 37:667–687
12. Scichilone N, Liu M, Pyrgos G et al (2000) Role of airway NO diffusion in the pathogenesis of asthma. Am J Respir Crit Care Med 163:A757

13. Samb A, Pretolani M, Dinh-Xuan A et al (2001) Decreased pulmonary and tracheal smooth muscle expression and activity of type 1 nitric oxide synthase (nNOS) after ovalbumin immunization and multiple aerosol challenge in guinea pigs. Am J Respir Crit Care Med 164: 149–154

14. Pate HJ, Belvisi MG, Donnelly LE et al (1999) Constitutive expressions of type I NOS in human airway smooth muscle cells: evidence for an antiproliferative role. FASEB J 13: 1810–1816

15. Takata M, Filippov G, Liu H et al (2001) Cytokines decrease sGC in pulmonary artery smooth muscle cells via NO-dependent and NO-independent mechanisms. Am J Physiol Lung Cell Mol Physiol 280:L272–L278

16. Martin C, Wohlsen A, Uhlig S (2001) Changes in airway resistance by simultaneous exposure to TNF-α and IL-1β in perfused rat lungs. Am J Physiol Lung Cell Mol Physiol 280:L595–L601

17. Nathan C (1997) Inducible nitric oxide synthase: what difference does it make? J Clin Invest 100:2417–2423

18. Kacmarek RM, Ripple R, Cockrill BA et al (1996) Inhaled nitric oxide: a bronchodilator in mild asthmatics with methacholine-induced bronchospasm. Am J Respir Crit Care Med 153: 128–135

19. Kesler BS, Canning BJ (1999) Regulation of baseline cholinergic tone in guinea-pig airway smooth muscle. J Physiol 518:843–855

20. Kesler BS, Mazzone SB, Canning BJ (2002) Nitric oxide-dependent modulation of smooth-muscle tone by airway parasympathetic nerves. Am J Respir Crit Care Med 165:481–488

21. Persson MG, Lonnqvist PA, Gustafsson LE (1995) Positive end-expiratory pressure ventilation elicits increases in endogenously formed nitric oxide as detected in air exhaled by rabbits. Anesthesiology 82:969–974

22. Bannenberg GL, Gustafsson LE (1997) Stretch-induced stimulation of lower airway nitric oxide formation in the guinea-pig: inhibition by gadolinium chloride. Pharmacol Toxicol 81:13–18

23. Awolesi MA, Sessa WC, Sumpio BE (1995) Cyclic strain upregulates nitric oxide synthase in cultured bovine aortic endothelial cells. J Clin Invest 96:1449–1454

24. Tidball JG, Lavergne E, Lau KS et al (1998) Mechanical loading regulates NOS expression and activity in developing and adult skeletal muscle. Am J Physiol 275:C260–C266

Static and Dynamic Hyperinflation in Chronic Obstructive Pulmonary Disease

7

Pierantonio Laveneziana, Katherine A. Webb, and Denis E. O'Donnell

7.1 Introduction

Chronic obstructive pulmonary disease (COPD) is a common respiratory condition that is characterized by inflammation of both the large and small (<2 mm) peripheral airways, the alveoli and adjacent capillary networks [1–4]. Expiratory flow limitation (EFL) is generally regarded as the pathophysiological hallmark of COPD. Lung hyperinflation is another important and related physiological manifestation of COPD that has major clinical consequences. In COPD populations, indices of lung hyperinflation have been shown to be predictive of respiratory and all-cause mortality [5–7] and morbidity [6–8]. The progressive decline in resting inspiratory capacity (IC), which mirrors the rise in lung hyperinflation as the disease advances, has major implications for dyspnoea and activity restriction in COPD [9]. For these reasons, there is increasing interest in therapeutic manipulation of lung hyperinflation to improve clinical outcomes in COPD. In this chapter we will attempt to clarify definitions of lung hyperinflation, review causative mechanisms, consider the natural progression of hyperinflation from mild to very severe COPD, outline the negative consequences of lung hyperinflation as it relates to physical activity, and examine the physiological rationale for selective "lung deflating" interventions.

P. Laveneziana
Sorbonne Universités, Neurophysiologie Respiratoire Expérimentale et Clinique,
UPMC Université Paris 06, UMR_S 1158, Paris, France

Neurophysiologie Respiratoire Expérimentale et Clinique,
INSERM, UMR_S 1158, Paris, France

AP-HP, Groupe Hospitalier Pitié-Salpêtrière Charles Foix, Service des Explorations
Fonctionnelles de la Respiration, de l'Exercice et de la Dyspnée, Paris, France
e-mail: pier_lav@yahoo.it

K.A. Webb, MS, MSc • D.E. O'Donnell (✉)
Department of Medicine, Queen's University and Kingston General Hospital,
Kingston, ON, Canada
e-mail: kathy.webb@queensu.ca; odonnell@queensu.ca

A. Aliverti, A. Pedotti (eds.), *Mechanics of Breathing*,
DOI 10.1007/978-88-470-5647-3_7, © Springer-Verlag Italia 2014

7.2   Static and Dynamic Hyperinflation: Definitions and Determinants

The lack of precise definitions of lung hyperinflation and the confusion that abounds over terms such as "static" and "dynamic" hyperinflation have hampered knowledge translation in this area of research. "Static" refers to the determination of lung volume components from the static pressure–volume relaxation curve of the respiratory system. "Dynamic" refers to the influence of dynamic events, such as expiratory timing, during maximal forced or spontaneous tidal breathing, on lung volume measurements. In the absence of any consensus on the definition or severity of lung hyperinflation, it is recommended, when using this term, to specify the volume compartment and express it as percent of predicted normal [10]. Lung hyperinflation is said to be present if measurements of lung volumes such as functional residual capacity (FRC), residual volume (RV) or total lung capacity (TLC) are abnormally increased above the upper limits of natural variability [10]. For the purpose of this chapter, increase in TLC (preferably measured by body plethysmography) exceeding either the upper limit of normal (ULN) (i.e. the upper 95 % confidence limit of a normally distributed reference population) or an empiric 120 % of predicted is consistent with the presence of *lung overinflation*. An increase in plethysmographic FRC above either ULN or 120 % of predicted is termed *lung hyperinflation*. An increase in plethysmographic RV exceeding either ULN or 120 % of predicted is termed *pulmonary gas trapping*, also signified by an increased RV/TLC ratio. In practice, values of these volume components exceeding 120–130 % predicted are deemed to be potentially clinically important, but these "cutoffs" remain arbitrary.

7.2.1   Functional Residual Capacity

FRC or the lung volume at the end of quiet expiration during tidal breathing [i.e. end-expiratory lung volume (EELV)] is increased in COPD subjects compared with healthy subjects [11]. EELV is used interchangeably with FRC in the current chapter. FRC is not always synonymous with the relaxation volume (V_r), which is the static equilibrium volume of the relaxed respiratory system, i.e. the volume at which the elastic recoil pressures of lung and relaxed chest wall are equal and opposite in sign [12] (Fig. 7.1). Active or passive mechanisms often operate to make FRC different from V_r both in healthy and in COPD subjects. For example, in healthy younger subjects during exercise, activation of expiratory muscles commonly drives FRC below the V_r [13].

Increase in FRC has static and dynamic determinants in COPD. Traditionally, increase in FRC is termed "static" lung hyperinflation and is attributed to an increase in the static V_r due to loss of lung recoil [11]. Thus, a change in the elastic properties of the lungs due to emphysema (i.e. increased lung compliance) resets the balance of forces between the lung and chest wall so that the reduced lung recoil pressure requires a greater volume to balance the chest wall recoil [11] (Fig. 7.2). The net

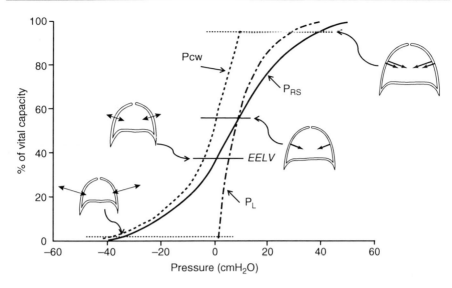

Fig. 7.1 Quasistatic V–P curves of lung (P_L), chest wall (P_{cw}) and total respiratory system (P_{rs}) during relaxation in a sitting position. The static forces of lung and chest wall are indicated by the arrows in the drawings. Please note that the P_L increases its curvature with increasing lung volume, whereas the opposite is true for the P_{cw}. The fall in the compliance of the respiratory system at high lung volumes is therefore mainly due to the decrease in compliance of the lung, whereas at low lung volume it reflects the decreased compliance of the chest wall. In the tidal volume range, the V–P relationships of both the lung and chest wall are nearly linear, and compliance of the lung and chest wall are about the same. In the sitting posture, they amount to 4 % vital capacity per 1 cmH$_2$O or 0.2 L/cmH$_2$O. The volume corresponding to each drawing is indicated by the *horizontal broken lines*

consequence is that the static V_r is higher than that of predicted normal [11] and FRC (or EELV) is increased in COPD compared with health [11] (Fig. 7.2). In this circumstance, resetting of the balance of forces between lung and chest wall at the higher V_r means that the alveolar pressure at end expiration remains atmospheric, i.e. is still zero [11]. Of note, "static" does not necessarily mean "at rest".

A major consequence of the increased compliance and resistance of heterogeneously distributed alveolar units in COPD is ineffective gas emptying on expiration: the mechanical time constant (i.e. the product of compliance and resistance (τ)) for lung emptying is therefore prolonged. The net result is that inhalation begins before full exhalation has been completed because the respiratory system has not yet returned to its V_r. Under this condition, the alveolar pressure at end expiration becomes higher (i.e. positive) than the atmospheric pressure. Consequently, the inspiratory muscles have to offset a threshold load termed auto or intrinsic positive end-expiratory pressure (PEEPi) before inspiratory flow can begin [14]. Lung hyperinflation in this circumstance is "dynamically" determined: EELV no longer occurs at the passive point of equilibrium between chest wall and lung recoil but is abnormally increased above the V_r of the respiratory system due to the presence of inescapable PEEPi [11, 14].

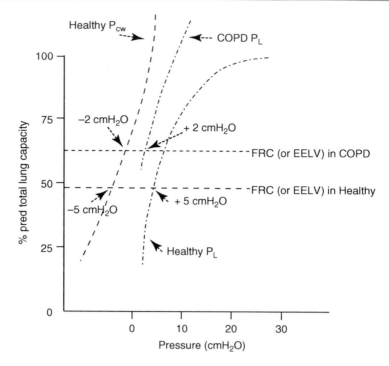

Fig. 7.2 Effect of reduced lung recoil pressure on functional residual capacity (*FRC*). FRC or end-expiratory lung volume (*EELV*) in normal lung represents the volume at which the elastic recoil pressures of lung and relaxed chest wall are equal and opposite in sign (meaning that the net elastic recoil pressure of the total respiratory system equals zero (*long-dashed lines*). Loss of lung elasticity due to emphysema in COPD reduces the lung recoil pressure. Consequently, FRC occurs at a higher lung volume, which defines static hyperinflation (*short-dashed lines*). Please note that under this circumstance, the elastic recoil pressures of lung and relaxed chest wall are equal and opposite in sign, meaning that the alveolar pressure is still atmospheric

The extent of lung hyperinflation is influenced by the prevailing breathing pattern for a given ventilation and the degree of time-constant abnormalities as expressed by the following equation [15]:

$$\text{EELV} - V_r = \frac{V_T}{e^{\frac{T_e}{\tau_{rs}}} - 1}$$

where T_e = expiratory time, τ_{rs} = time constant for emptying of the respiratory system, V_T = tidal volume and base e = 2.718282. In more severe COPD, these factors contribute to lung hyperinflation even at rest. Lung hyperinflation is also influenced by body position and by body mass, for example, EELV decreases when adopting a supine position [16] or with obesity [17]. Variable increases in EELV can also occur when minute ventilation (V'_E) is abruptly increased (e.g. voluntarily, during anxiety/panic attacks, hypoxaemia or physical activity) or when EFL is suddenly worsened (e.g. during exacerbation or increased bronchospasm).

7.2.2   Residual Volume

RV refers to the volume of gas remaining in the lungs after maximal exhalation, regardless of the lung volume at which exhalation is started [10]. In young healthy adults, RV is determined by the balance between expiratory muscle force and the outward elastic recoil of the chest wall [12]. It is the chest wall, and not the lung, that normally contributes the most to the elastic recoil forces of the respiratory system at RV [12] (Fig. 7.1). At RV, these forces are equal and opposite in sign [12]. In older healthy adults, dynamic mechanisms are important in setting RV: the normal loss of lung elasticity with age and associated decreases in maximum expiratory flow rate (premature airway closure and flow limitation) are associated with increased RV, compared to youth [18]. Similarly, RV in COPD is determined by dynamic mechanisms [11]. When expiratory flow rates are very low near RV, the ability to expire maximally may be affected by limited breath-holding ability or subject discomfort before expiration is "complete" (i.e. while expiratory flow is still present) [11]. The consequence is that RV may be greater than the lung volume at which a static balance would have been achieved between expiratory muscle and elastic recoil forces [11].

7.2.3   Inspiratory Capacity

Inspiratory capacity (IC) is defined as the maximal volume of air that can be inspired after a quiet expiration to EELV [10]. The resting IC [9] (or IC/TLC ratio [5, 19]) is also used as indirect measure of lung hyperinflation. Resting IC progressively declines as airway obstruction worsens in COPD [9, 20]. Measurement of IC is motivation dependent and is influenced by static strength of the inspiratory muscles and EELV [21]. The IC represents the operating limits for tidal volume (V_T) expansion in patients with EFL and influences breathing pattern and peak ventilatory capacity during exercise [9, 22] (see below). The IC is diminished in the presence of inspiratory muscle weakness or lung hyperinflation.

7.2.4   Total Lung Capacity

TLC is the greatest volume of gas in the lungs achieved after maximal voluntary inspiration [10]. It depends on the static balance between the outward forces generated by inspiratory muscles during a maximal inspiratory effort and the inward elastic forces of the chest wall and lung [12]. It is the lung that normally contributes the most to the elastic recoil forces of the respiratory system at TLC [12] (Fig. 7.1). At TLC, these two sets of forces are equal and opposite in sign [12]. The increase in TLC in COPD usually reflects the increased lung compliance due to emphysema [12].

7.3 The Natural History of Lung Hyperinflation: From Mild to Advanced COPD

The natural history of the development of lung hyperinflation in COPD patients is unknown, but clinical experience indicates that this is an insidious process that occurs over decades. It is likely that the time course of change in the various volume compartments is highly variable among patients and, in this respect, genetic susceptibility, burden of tobacco smoke and the impact of the frequency and severity of exacerbations may all be important. Until recently, no longitudinal studies have tracked the temporal progression of physiological derangements beyond the decline in forced expiratory volume in 1 s (FEV_1) in a large population of patients with COPD [23]. The 4-year UPLIFT® trial documented a mean rate of decline in pre-bronchodilator IC of 34–50 mL/year in patients with moderate to very severe COPD [7]; patients with the lowest baseline IC were also those with the greatest rates of exacerbations and death [7]. A recent cross-sectional study in 2,265 patients found progressive increases in pulmonary gas trapping and lung hyperinflation (measured by RV and FRC) and corresponding decline of IC across the continuum of COPD severity [20]. Lung volume increases were shown to occur even in the earliest stages of COPD (i.e. GOLD grade I) and increased exponentially with severity of airway obstruction [9, 20] (Fig. 7.3). The magnitude of lung volume components derived from body plethysmography (i.e. expiratory reserve volume, RV and FRC) in both healthy and COPD subjects is strongly influenced by body mass: increased body

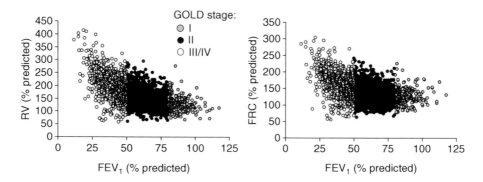

Fig. 7.3 Residual volume (*RV*) and functional residual capacity (*FRC*) versus forced expiratory volume in 1 s (*FEV1*) across GOLD stages (I, II, III/IV). The majority of patients (including many patients with GOLD stage I) were >120 % predicted suggesting evidence of static lung hyperinflation. There was an exponential relationship between static lung volumes and disease severity. GOLD, Global Initiative for Chronic Obstructive Lung Disease (Data from Ref. [20], with permission (pending))

mass index is associated with lower static lung volume components, regardless of the severity of airway obstruction [24].

7.3.1   Mild Symptomatic COPD

It is well established that the presence of apparently minor airflow obstruction (as measured by spirometry) may obscure widespread inflammatory damage to the peripheral airways (<2 mm diameter), lung parenchyma and pulmonary vasculature [2, 25]. Previous studies have shown evidence of active airway inflammation and loss or obliteration of peripheral airways even in those with mild COPD [2, 3, 25]. Loss of peripheral airways may precede the development of centrilobular emphysema. Mucus hypersecretion as a result of chronic bronchitis can result in extensive peripheral airway dysfunction in mild COPD [26, 27]. Alveolar inflammation with destruction of alveolar walls and attachments to airways are integral to the pathogenesis of lung hyperinflation [28]. Previous studies in mild COPD have reported increased static lung compliance [29], and quantitative computed tomography (CT scans) show emphysema and gas trapping [30–32]. Gas trapping, as assessed by expiratory CT scans, can exist in the absence of structural emphysema and is believed to indirectly reflect small airway dysfunction in mild COPD [3]. The presence of lung hyperinflation assessed by quantitative CT scans was found to predict a rapid annual decline in FEV_1 in smokers with a normal FEV_1 [30]. Corbin and coworkers in a 4-year longitudinal study of smokers with chronic bronchitis reported a progressive increase in lung compliance [29]. Interestingly, these investigators reported that increases in TLC in milder COPD served to preserve SVC and IC in the setting of increased RV and FRC, respectively.

7.3.2   Moderate to Severe COPD

There is considerable heterogeneity in FRC and RV across GOLD grades, but many patients in each GOLD category have values that are above the predicted normal values [9, 20] (Fig. 7.3). From cross-sectional studies, it would appear that RV and FRC increase exponentially as airway obstruction worsens [9, 20].

7.4   Consequences of Resting Lung Hyperinflation in Moderate to Severe COPD

The impact of lung hyperinflation on respiratory mechanics and muscle function is highly variable in COPD and varies from minor diaphragmatic dysfunction to overt hypercapnic respiratory failure. Resting lung hyperinflation significantly diminishes ventilatory reserve which can become critically eroded during exacerbations [33–35] and the stress of exercise (see below). Increases in lung volumes in healthy individuals [36] or resting lung hyperinflation in moderate to severe COPD places the inspiratory muscles, especially the diaphragm, at a significant mechanical disadvantage by shortening its fibres, thereby compromising its force-generating capacity by 30–55 % [37, 38]. Lung hyperinflation undoubtedly affects the capacity of the parasternal intercostals and scalenes to shorten, but the extent to which the mechanical effectiveness of intercostals and scalene is compromised is still debated (reviewed in [39]). Potential mechanisms of compromised diaphragmatic function include (1) worsening of the length–tension relationship, (2) decrease in the zone of apposition, (3) decrease in the curvature of the diaphragm, (4) change in the mechanical arrangement of costal and crural components of the diaphragm and (5) increase in the elastic recoil of the thoracic cage.

Lung hyperinflation decreases the resting length of the diaphragm [40, 41] and, less so, of the rib cage muscles [42], although this is controversial [43]. The shortening of the diaphragm is due to a decrease in the length of its zone of apposition, which causes a decrease in its pressure-generating capacity [41]. Lung hyperinflation has traditionally been thought to cause flattening of the diaphragm and to increase its radius of curvature which, in turn, would increase its passive tension and decrease its efficiency in generating transdiaphragmatic pressure, according to Laplace's law. However, this does not seem to be the case because it has been clearly shown that, at resting EELV, the curvature of the diaphragm is only 3.5 % smaller in severe COPD patients than in healthy subjects [44]. The radius of curvature also changes little over the range of IC in both severe COPD patients [44] and healthy subjects [45]. It follows that a change in the curvature of the diaphragm is likely to be less important than a change in length of diaphragmatic fibres in determining contractile force at either EELV or over the range of IC. Lung hyperinflation changes the orientation of the costal and crural fibres of the diaphragm from parallel to series arrangement, as demonstrated in dogs by Zocchi and collaborators [46]. The change in fibre orientation decreases the ability of the diaphragm to generate force, and the diaphragm has an expiratory rather than inspiratory action on the rib cage [46].

When EELV becomes positioned above 70 % of predicted TLC, thoracic elastic recoil is directed inward (i.e. increased) [12] so that the inspiratory muscles have to work, not only against PEEPi and the elastic recoil of the lungs but also against the elastic recoil of the thoracic cage [47] (Fig. 7.1). The net effect is that lung hyperinflation contributes to an increased work and oxygen (O_2) cost of breathing at rest in patients with severe COPD (recently reviewed in [48]).

7.4.1 Lung Hyperinflation and the Heart

Barr et al. [49] reported that in a large population-based sample made up of both smokers and non-smokers, a 10 % increase in the percentage of emphysema (measured by CT) correlated inversely with reductions in left ventricular (LV) diastolic volume, stroke volume and cardiac output, as estimated by magnetic resonance imaging (MRI). Lung hyperinflation has the potential to impair cardiac function by increasing pulmonary vascular resistance [50]. The increased intrathoracic pressure swings linked to increased resistive and increased elastic loading of hyperinflation may result in increased LV afterload as a result of the increased LV transmural pressure gradient. Reduced venous return and reduced right and left ventricular volumes and LV stroke volume are additional consequences of the altered intrathoracic pressure gradients. Severe hyperinflation, as defined as an IC/TLC ratio <25 %, has been shown to be associated with increased all-cause (including cardiovascular) mortality [5], impaired LV filling determined by echocardiography [51] and reduced exercise tolerance [5, 19, 52]. Severe lung hyperinflation has recently been linked to reduced intrathoracic blood volume and reduced LV end-diastolic volume as assessed by MRI [53].

7.4.2 Physiological Adaptations to Chronic Lung Hyperinflation

In the presence of lung hyperinflation, functional muscle weakness (outlined above) is mitigated, to some extent, by long-term adaptations such as shortening of diaphragmatic sarcomeres [54] and a decrease in sarcomere number [55] which causes a leftward shift of the length–tension relationship, thus improving the ability of the muscles to generate force at higher lung volumes. In patients with chronic lung hyperinflation, adaptive alterations in muscle fibre composition (an increase in the relative proportion of slow-twitch, fatigue resistant, type I fibres) [56, 57] and oxidative capacity (an increase in mitochondrial concentration and efficiency of the electron transport chain) [54] are believed to preserve the functional strength of the overburdened diaphragm [37] and make it more resistant to fatigue [54, 56, 58]. In this regard, Similowski and colleagues demonstrated that the reduction in the pressure-generating capacity of the inspiratory muscles of stable COPD patients was related to lung hyperinflation, but that diaphragmatic function in such patients was comparable to normal subjects when measurements were compared at the same lung volume [37]. Despite these impressive temporal adaptations, the presence of severe lung hyperinflation means that ventilatory reserve in COPD is diminished, and the ability to increase V'_E when the demand arises is greatly limited [9].

7.5 Lung Hyperinflation and Exercise

Dynamic lung hyperinflation (DH) has been defined as the temporary and variable increase of EELV above the resting value. Changes in EELV during exercise can be estimated from serial IC measurements [59–61] on the assumption that TLC remains constant [62–64]. When measurements of IC are coupled with those of dynamic inspiratory reserve volume (IRV, calculated as $IC - V_T$) and breathing pattern, further valuable information is provided about the prevailing mechanical constraints on V'_E during exercise [9, 22, 65, 66]. In addition, comparing changes in IC and IRV within and between patients at a standardized V'_E (iso $- V'_E$) during exercise gives us important information on the mechanical constraints on V_T expansion that are independent of the level of ventilatory demand. Small physiological studies and multicentre clinical trials have confirmed high reproducibility and responsiveness of serial IC measurements in moderate to severe COPD [59, 60]. It should be noted that the IC measurement gives only indirect information about changes in absolute lung volumes but, nevertheless, provides important mechanical information, irrespective of possible minor shifts in absolute TLC that may occur [59, 60].

In symptomatic patients with even mild COPD, significant dynamic increases in EELV (or reciprocal decreases in IC) by ~0.5 L have been measured during incremental cycle exercise as a result of the combined effects of increased ventilatory demand (reflecting ventilation–perfusion mismatch) and worsening EFL [9, 67, 68]. Similar changes in EELV (i.e. average decreases in IC of ~0.3–0.5 L) have been reported during exercise in the majority (85 %) of patients with moderate to severe COPD [9, 22, 59–61, 65]. It is unclear why a minority of patients with COPD do not dynamically hyperinflate during exercise, but it may be related, at least in part, to having a smaller resting IC with greater mechanical constraints [22, 61]. Smaller studies using optoelectronic plethysmography have identified more varied behaviours of end-expiratory chest wall motion during exercise and have designated subgroups of COPD as non-hyperinflators ("euvolumics") [69] and "early" and "late" hyperinflators [64]. Differences in IC measured by pneumotachograph and optoelectronic plethysmography during exercise reflect the fact that the latter, measurement of chest wall motion, is influenced by gas compression effects and intrathoracic blood shifts, particularly in the presence of vigorous expiratory muscle recruitment [70].

7.5.1 Benefits of Dynamic Lung Hyperinflation During Exercise

Increases in EELV at low exercise intensities help attenuate expiratory flow limitation and possibly improve ventilation–perfusion relations and pulmonary gas exchange by reducing airway resistance, thus improving gas distribution during inspiration [65, 66]. We have argued that DH, early in exercise, helps to preserve the normally harmonious relationship between central neural drive and the mechanical/muscular response of the respiratory system (i.e. neuromechanical coupling), thus attenuating the rise in dyspnoea [65, 66]. However, when end-inspiratory lung volume (EILV) approaches its maximum value (at approximately 95 % TLC), the benefits of DH are negated by the effects of increased elastic/threshold loading of the respiratory muscles [65, 66, 71].

7.5.2 Negative Effects of Dynamic Lung Hyperinflation

Important consequences of dynamic hyperinflation include (1) V_T constraints resulting in early mechanical ventilatory limitation [9, 22, 61, 65, 66, 72], (2) increased elastic and threshold loading on the inspiratory muscles resulting in an increased work and O_2 cost of breathing [66, 71, 73], (3) functional inspiratory muscle weakness and possible fatigue [66, 71], (4) carbon dioxide (CO_2) retention [74] and (5) adverse effects on cardiac function [51, 52, 75–79].

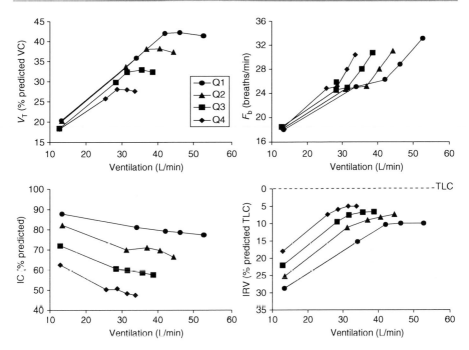

Fig. 7.4 Tidal volume (V_T), breathing frequency (F_b), dynamic inspiratory capacity (IC) and inspiratory reserve volume (IRV) are shown plotted against minute ventilation (V'_E) during constant work rate exercise for each forced expiratory volume in 1 s (FEV_1, expressed as % predicted) quartile (Q). The upper through to lower quartiles (Q1–Q4) represent the mildest to most severe groups, respectively. Note the clear inflection (plateau) in the V_T/V'_E relationship which coincides with a simultaneous inflection in the IRV. After this point, further increases in V'_E are accomplished by accelerating F_b. Data plotted are mean values at steady-state rest, isotime (i.e. 2, 4 min), V_T/V'_E inflection point and peak exercise (Data from Ref. [9], with permission (pending))

7.5.3   Lung Hyperinflation and Tidal Volume Constraints

As airway obstruction increases in severity, there is a progressive decline in the resting IC such that the respiratory system prematurely reaches its physiological limits at a progressively lower peak V'_E during exercise [9]. Resting IC dictates the limits of V_T expansion during exercise in patients with COPD who have EFL [9, 22, 60, 61, 65, 66, 72]. The lower the resting IC, because of lung hyperinflation, the lower peak V_T and peak V'_E achieved during exercise [9, 22, 60, 61, 65, 66, 72] (Fig. 7.4). When V_T reaches approximately 75 % of the prevailing IC (or IRV is 5–10 % of the TLC), there is an inflection or plateau in the V_T/V'_E relation [9, 22, 65, 66] (Fig. 7.4). The V'_E during exercise at which the V_T plateau is discernable depends on the magnitude of the resting IC: in those with a smaller IC, the V_T plateau occurs earlier in exercise at a relatively lower V'_E [9, 22]. This critical volume restriction represents a mechanical limit, and further sustainable increases in V'_E are impossible [9, 22, 65, 66]. Associated tachypnoea further compromises inspiratory muscle function by

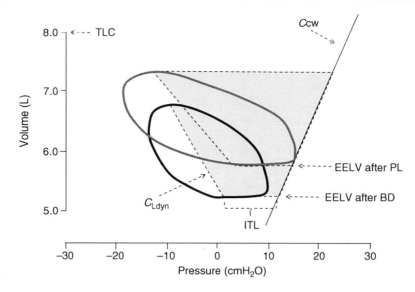

Fig. 7.5 Campbell diagrams are shown at a standardized time during constant work rate cycle exercise testing for a patient with severe COPD. Abbreviations: *CLdyn* dynamic lung compliance, *Ccw* chest wall compliance, *EELV* end-expiratory lung volume, *ITL* the inspiratory threshold load, *TLC* total lung capacity. The *shaded areas* represent the elastic work of breathing, while the resistive work of breathing are the areas within the volume–pressure loops. Please note that after inhaled bronchodilator (*BD, solid black line*) compared with placebo (*PL, solid grey line*), the ITL, elastic and resistive work of breathing are all decreased (Personal data)

the increase in the velocity of shortening of the inspiratory muscles and a reduction in dynamic lung compliance [65, 66, 71, 80]. The rapid shallow breathing pattern in the setting of high physiological dead space that fails to decline as normal can further compromise the efficiency of CO_2 elimination [74]. The V_T plateau marks the onset of the rising disparity between increasing central neural drive and the mechanical/muscular response of the respiratory system [65, 66]. Across the continuum of COPD, from mild to severe disease, the conditions for this neuromechanical dissociation become evident at progressively lower work rates [9, 22, 60, 61, 65, 68, 81].

7.5.4 Mechanical and Muscular Consequences of Dynamic Lung Hyperinflation

The previously mentioned effects of resting lung hyperinflation on respiratory mechanics and muscle function are further aggravated by dynamic increases in EELV during exercise in patients with moderate to severe COPD. As tidal breathing encroaches on the upper alinear extreme of the respiratory system's sigmoidal static pressure–volume relation, there is increased elastic/threshold loading [65, 66, 71, 82–84], and the work and O_2 cost of breathing become very high [40 % of peak oxygen consumption ($V'O_2$)] (Fig. 7.5) [73, 85].

The combination of excessive mechanical loading and increased velocity of shortening of the inspiratory muscles means that V'_E can no longer be sustained. The increased O_2 cost of breathing in the setting of compromised O_2 delivery because of compromised cardiac output or increased respiratory–locomotor muscle competition could precipitate respiratory muscle fatigue or overt mechanical failure in severe COPD. However, the evidence that inspiratory muscle fatigue actually occurs in COPD patients is inconclusive [86, 87], even at the limits of tolerance during both cycle and treadmill exercise [58, 88]. In fact, there is increasing evidence to the contrary and a suggestion that structural adaptations in the inspiratory muscles, particularly the diaphragm, render some degree of resistance to fatigue [54, 56, 58].

7.5.5 Lung Hyperinflation and Cardiac Function During Exercise

The effect of acute-on-chronic lung hyperinflation on dynamic cardiac function during exercise remains unknown. Increases in EELV during exercise could potentially worsen pulmonary hypertension, reduce right ventricular preload (reduced venous return) and, in some cases, increase left ventricular afterload [50, 51, 53, 89, 90]. Patients with severe resting lung hyperinflation (IC/TLC ratio <25 %) have been shown to have a decreased peak exercise O_2 pulse (a crude estimate of stroke volume) [52]. However, in the absence of cardiac disease, other investigators have found that cardiac output increased normally as a function of $V'O_2$ during submaximal exercise in COPD suggesting long-term physiological adaptations: stroke volume is generally smaller, and heart rate correspondingly higher than in health but cardiac output is often preserved [89, 91]. Of note, peak cardiac output reaches a lower maximal value during exercise in COPD, which may be due, in part, to the abnormal ventilatory mechanics [89, 91, 92].

Interventions that reduce lung hyperinflation, such as lung volume reduction surgery, have shown a number of physiological improvements of cardiac function such as increased LV dimensions and filling (assessed by MRI) [93] and improved end-expiratory pulmonary artery wedge pressure [94]. However, the clinical significance of these small improvements is unclear [94]. Similarly, lung deflation following bronchodilator therapy and heliox was associated with modest but consistent improvement in heart rate and O_2 kinetics in the rest-to-exercise transition, but the implications for exercise performance remain unknown [75, 76, 95, 96].

7.5.6 Does Expiratory Muscle Activity Alter Dynamic Lung Hyperinflation During Exercise?

The influence of excessive expiratory muscle activity on the behaviour of dynamic operating lung volumes and on the evolution of the intensity and quality of dyspnoea during exercise remains unknown and has recently been debated [97]. Expiratory muscle activity in more advanced COPD has been shown to be variable (but not dichotomous), and in the majority of small mechanical studies, peak tidal expiratory pressure rose smoothly to ~20–25 % of maximal expiratory pressure at end exercise [98–100]. It has been speculated that increased expiratory muscle pressure generation during exercise may attenuate DH early in the course of COPD and that adaptive expiratory muscle "de-recruitment" characterizes the later phase of the disease [69, 97]. Moreover, it has been postulated that the negative cardiovascular consequences (e.g. reduced venous return and cardiac output) of vigorous expiratory muscle activity in milder COPD may directly impair exercise performance [69, 97]. It is also possible, although still conjectural, that increased expiratory muscle pressure generation, which does not increase expired flow rates in flow-limited patients, aggravates dynamic airway compression and that this, in turn, may directly influence the intensity or quality of exertional dyspnoea [101–103]. In a recent preliminary study, we determined the variability of expiratory muscle activity during symptom-limited incremental cycle exercise in COPD, its relationship with changes in dynamic operating lung volumes, and its influence on the time course of change in the intensity and quality of dyspnoea [104]. We found no evidence that smooth and progressive expiratory muscle recruitment affected the dyspnoea or the dynamic lung volume responses to exercise in moderate to severe COPD [104]. The contention that excessive expiratory muscle activity is not a dominant contributor to dyspnoea is also based on the observation that perceived expiratory difficulty and unsatisfied expiratory effort were rarely selected as representative descriptors by COPD patients who vigorously recruited expiratory muscles and that dyspnoea intensity was more closely correlated with indices of inspiratory effort, neuromechanical uncoupling and mechanical events during exercise (such as critical V_T constraints) that mainly burdened the inspiratory muscles [104].

7.6   Respiratory Mechanical Abnormalities and Dyspnoea

7.6.1   Physiological Correlates of Dyspnoea Intensity in COPD

It is a long-held belief that demand/capacity imbalance fundamentally underscores the intensity and quality of dyspnoea in COPD [105]. The demand/capacity imbalance hypothesis of dyspnoea has been supported by several studies which have shown that dyspnoea intensity ratings correlate well with a number of physiological ratios: (1) the ratio of V'_E to maximal ventilatory capacity (V'_E/MVC), the original "dyspnoea index" [106]; (2) the ratio of tidal oesophageal pressure to maximum pressure (Pes/PImax), an indicator of relative respiratory muscular effort [107]; and (3) the ratio of Poes/PImax to the V_T response (V_T/IC or V_T/VC), the effort/displacement ratio [65, 66, 71]. Dyspnoea intensity ratings also correlate well with indices of DH or its restrictive effects (e.g. V_T/IC ratio) [9, 61, 65, 66, 71]. EILV or IRV, which reflects proximity of V_T to TLC and the "stiffer" portion of the respiratory system's pressure–volume relation, correlates more strongly with dyspnoea intensity ratings than EELV or IC per se [9, 22, 65, 66]. The extent to which increases in EELV during exercise contribute to dyspnoea intensity in COPD will depend on the resting IC and thus the extent of mechanical constraints on V_T expansion [22].

7.6.2   Unsatisfied Inspiration and Lung Hyperinflation

Unsatisfied inspiration ("can't get enough air in") is a dominant qualitative descriptor of dyspnoea during physical exertion in COPD and is not reported in health [71]. This qualitative descriptor is perceived as unpleasant, is recognized as a threat to life and evokes powerful emotive responses (fear, anxiety, panic). It alerts the patient that further increases in V'_E cannot be sustained and demands abrupt behavioural action, e.g. stopping the task. We have postulated that unsatisfied inspiration has its neurophysiological origins in neuromechanical dissociation or uncoupling of the respiratory system [65, 66, 71]. The development of unsatisfied inspiration during exercise coincides with the point where V_T expansion becomes mechanically limited in the setting of increasing central respiratory drive (Fig. 7.6) [65]. This V_T inflection/plateau is an important mechanical event during exercise where dyspnoea intensity rises abruptly to intolerable levels (Fig. 7.6) and the dominant qualitative descriptor changes from increased work/effort to unsatisfied inspiration (Fig. 7.7) [65].

The neurobiology of unsatisfied inspiration remains conjectural. Multiple studies in healthy volunteers have shown that when the V_T response is mechanically constrained in the face of increased chemostimulation of the respiratory centres, unpleasant respiratory discomfort, qualitatively akin to unsatisfied inspiration or air hunger, is the result [108–113]. Perceived unpleasantness associated with the act of breathing is thought to involve affective processing [114]. At the point where unsatisfied inspiration and associated unpleasantness arises during exercise, the central neural drive (and central corollary discharge) has reached near maximal levels while the mechanical/muscular response of the respiratory system has approached or reached physiological limits [115].

7.7   Effects of Interventions on Lung Hyperinflation and Dyspnoea

Indirect evidence of the importance of lung hyperinflation in dyspnoea causation and exercise intolerance in COPD comes from multiple studies which have examined therapeutic interventions [bronchodilators, continuous positive airway pressure (CPAP) oxygen supplementation, exercise training, lung volume reduction surgery] that reduce or counterbalance the effect of lung hyperinflation.

Bronchodilators reduce airway smooth muscle tone, improve airway conductance and accelerate the time constants for lung emptying of heterogeneously distributed alveolar units. Bronchodilators of all classes have consistently been shown to increase the resting IC in patients with COPD by an average of ~0.3 L (or 15 %) (for review, see [116]) which is associated with improvements in dyspnoea and exercise endurance time [59, 117–120]. The magnitude of DH either remains the same or may worsen slightly reflecting the higher levels of V'_E that can be achieved during exercise as a result of the bronchodilation [119–121]. In other words, bronchodilator treatment simply causes a parallel downward shift in the EELV over the

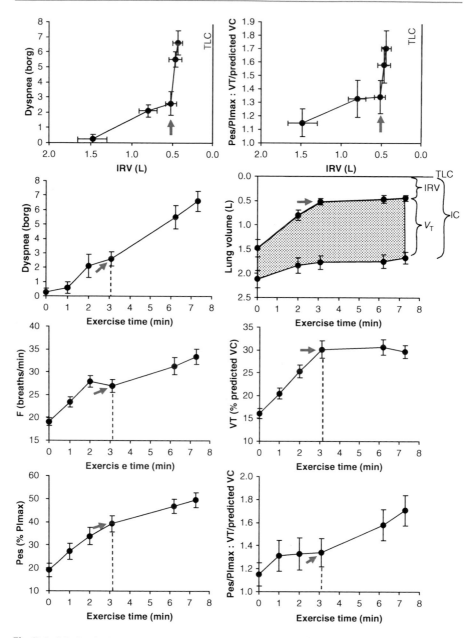

Fig. 7.6 Mechanical threshold of dyspnoea is indicated by the abrupt rise in dyspnoea after a critical "minimal" inspiratory reserve volume (*IRV*) is reached that prevents further expansion of tidal volume (*VT*) during exercise. Beyond this dyspnoea–IRV inflection point during exercise, dyspnoea intensity, breathing frequency (*F*), respiratory effort (Pes/PImax, where *Pes* is oesophageal pressure and *PImax* is maximum values for Pes) and the effort–displacement ratio all continue to rise. *Dashed lines* indicate the threshold where mechanical limitation to VT expansion is reached. *Arrows* indicate the dyspnoea–IRV inflection point. Values are plotted after placebo and expressed as means ± SE. *TLC* total lung capacity, *VC* vital capacity (Data from Ref. [66], with permission (pending))

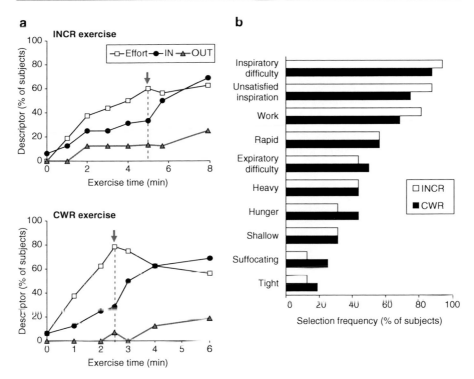

Fig. 7.7 (a) Selection frequency of the three descriptor phrases evaluated during incremental (*INCR*) and constant work rate (*CWR*) exercise: increased work/effort (effort), unsatisfied inspiration (*IN*) and unsatisfied expiration (*OUT*). *Arrows* indicate the point corresponding to the inflection point of the tidal volume–ventilation (*VT/VE*) relation during exercise. (**b**) Selection frequency of the dyspnoea descriptors collected by questionnaire at end exercise. Descriptor choices were similar in both tests with dyspnoea described predominantly as a sense of "inspiratory difficulty", "unsatisfied inspiration" and increased "work" of breathing (Data from Ref. [65], with permission (pending))

course of the exercise test reflecting the reduction in resting IC. This increase in resting IC is beneficial because it delays the onset of critical ventilatory constraints to V'_E. Improvements in dyspnoea and exercise tolerance are closely related with release of V_T restriction [59, 66, 117–120], reduced respiratory effort [66, 122] and enhanced neuromechanical coupling of the respiratory system [66, 122]. In selected individuals non-invasive ventilation using CPAP, carefully titrated to a level below the patients PEEPi, has been shown to improve dyspnoea and exercise endurance presumably by counterbalancing the negative effects of the inspiratory threshold load on the inspiratory muscles [103, 123, 124].

Bullectomy and lung volume reduction surgery by removing redundant bullae or portions of destroyed emphysematous lungs appear to improve lung elastic recoil pressure of the remaining lung tissue [125–129]. The net effect is to reduce the static V_r of the respiratory system. This contributes to reductions in the work and O_2 cost of breathing and enhanced neuromechanical coupling and dyspnoea improvement [128, 130, 131]. As with pharmacological lung volume reduction, the resultant improvement of resting IC delays critical mechanic limits and improves exercise tolerance as already described.

Both hyperoxia and exercise training can reduce V'_E by reducing breathing frequency and potentially the rate of DH in COPD [121, 132–136]. While both these interventions have been associated with reduced DH and dyspnoea relief, via delay in reaching mechanical limits, the dominant effect on dyspnoea amelioration seems to be reduced central neural drive. In other words, reduced DH is not necessarily a prerequisite for subjective relief of dyspnoea with supplemental O_2 or exercise training in COPD but may contribute in some instances.

7.8 Summary

Progressive EFL in COPD and alteration in the elastic properties of the lung are associated with the development of progressive lung hyperinflation and decline in the resting IC. A number of physiological adaptations partially preserve diaphragmatic function in the face of chronic hyperinflation, but the restrictive mechanical effects of a low IC limit the ability to increase V'_E when metabolic demand increases during activity. The situation is further compounded by the deleterious effects of acute dynamic increases in EELV above resting values which forces the respiratory system to approach or reach its physiological limits. During exercise, further reduction of the already diminished IC due to DH critically restricts V_T expansion, mechanically loads and weakens the inspiratory muscles and forces early respiratory mechanical limitation. Additionally, the growing disparity between increased central neural drive and the blunted respiratory muscular/mechanical response (neuromechanical uncoupling) after the V_T inflection likely contributes to perceptions of respiratory discomfort across its intensity, quality and affective distress domains. The corollary is that pharmacological and surgical lung volume reduction increase the resting IC, release V_T restriction, unload the inspiratory muscles and improve neuromechanical coupling of the respiratory system, dyspnoea and exercise intolerance in COPD.

7.9 Financial Disclosure/Acknowledgements

PL and KW have no conflicts of interest to report. DO has received research funding via Queen's University from AstraZeneca, Boehringer Ingelheim, GlaxoSmithKline, Merck, Novartis, Nycomed and Pfizer and has served on speakers bureaus, consultation panels and advisory boards for AstraZeneca, Boehringer Ingelheim, GlaxoSmithKline, Nycomed and Pfizer.

References

1. Barbera JA, Riverola A, Roca J, Ramirez J, Wagner PD, Ros D, Wiggs BR, Rodriguez-Roisin R (1994) Pulmonary vascular abnormalities and ventilation-perfusion relationships in mild chronic obstructive pulmonary disease. Am J Respir Crit Care Med 149(2 Pt 1):423–429

2. Hogg JC, Chu F, Utokaparch S, Woods R, Elliott WM, Buzatu L, Cherniack RM, Rogers RM, Sciurba FC, Coxson HO, Pare PD (2004) The nature of small-airway obstruction in chronic obstructive pulmonary disease. N Engl J Med 350(26):2645–2653
3. McDonough JE, Yuan R, Suzuki M, Seyednejad N, Elliott WM, Sanchez PG, Wright AC, Gefter WB, Litzky L, Coxson HO, Pare PD, Sin DD, Pierce RA, Woods JC, McWilliams AM, Mayo JR, Lam SC, Cooper JD, Hogg JC (2011) Small-airway obstruction and emphysema in chronic obstructive pulmonary disease. N Engl J Med 365(17):1567–1575
4. Rodriguez-Roisin R, Drakulovic M, Rodriguez DA, Roca J, Barbera JA, Wagner PD (2009) Ventilation-perfusion imbalance and chronic obstructive pulmonary disease staging severity. J Appl Physiol 106(6):1902–1908
5. Casanova C, Cote C, de Torres JP, Aguirre-Jaime A, Marin JM, Pinto-Plata V, Celli BR (2005) Inspiratory-to-total lung capacity ratio predicts mortality in patients with chronic obstructive pulmonary disease. Am J Respir Crit Care Med 171(6):591–597
6. Tantucci C, Donati P, Nicosia F, Bertella E, Redolfi S, De Vecchi M, Corda L, Grassi V, Zulli R (2008) Inspiratory capacity predicts mortality in patients with chronic obstructive pulmonary disease. Respir Med 102(4):613–619
7. Celli BR, Decramer M, Lystig T, Kesten S, Tashkin DP (2012) Longitudinal inspiratory capacity changes in chronic obstructive pulmonary disease. Respir Res 13:66
8. Zaman M, Mahmood S, Altaych A (2010) Low inspiratory capacity to total lung capacity ratio is a risk factor for chronic obstructive pulmonary disease exacerbation. Am J Med Sci 339(5):411–414
9. O'Donnell DE, Guenette JA, Maltais F, Webb KA (2012) Decline of resting inspiratory capacity in COPD: the impact on breathing pattern, dyspnea, and ventilatory capacity during exercise. Chest 141(3):753–762
10. Pellegrino R, Viegi G, Brusasco V, Crapo RO, Burgos F, Casaburi R, Coates A, van der Grinten CP, Gustafsson P, Hankinson J, Jensen R, Johnson DC, MacIntyre N, McKay R, Miller MR, Navajas D, Pedersen OF, Wanger J (2005) Interpretative strategies for lung function tests. Eur Respir J 26(5):948–968
11. Pride NB, Macklem PT (1986) Lung mechanics in disease. In: Fishman AP (ed) Handbook of physiology, Part 2: the respiratory system. American Physiological Society, Bethesda, pp 659–692
12. Agostoni E, Hyatt RE (1986) Static behaviour of the respiratory system. In: Macklem PT, Mead J (eds) Handbook of physiology. The respiratory system. American Physiological Society, Bethesda, pp 113–130
13. Henke KG, Sharratt M, Pegelow D, Dempsey JA (1988) Regulation of end-expiratory lung volume during exercise. J Appl Physiol 64(1):135–146
14. Brochard L (2002) Intrinsic (or auto-) positive end-expiratory pressure during spontaneous or assisted ventilation. Intensive Care Med 28(11):1552–1554
15. Vinegar A, Sinnett EE, Leith DE (1979) Dynamic mechanisms determine functional residual capacity in mice. Mus musculus. J Appl Physiol 46(5):867–871
16. Baydur A, Wilkinson L, Mehdian R, Bains B, Milic-Emili J (2004) Extrathoracic expiratory flow limitation in obesity and obstructive and restrictive disorders: effects of increasing negative expiratory pressure. Chest 125(1):98–105
17. Jones RL, Nzekwu MM (2006) The effects of body mass index on lung volumes. Chest 130(3):827–833
18. Pride NB (2005) Ageing and changes in lung mechanics. Eur Respir J 26(4):563–565
19. Albuquerque AL, Nery LE, Villaca DS, Machado TY, Oliveira CC, Paes AT, Neder JA (2006) Inspiratory fraction and exercise impairment in COPD patients GOLD stages II-III. Eur Respir J 28(5):939–944
20. Deesomchok A, Webb KA, Forkert L, Lam YM, Ofir D, Jensen D, O'Donnell DE (2010) Lung hyperinflation and its reversibility in patients with airway obstruction of varying severity. COPD 7(6):428–437
21. Yan S, Kaminski D, Sliwinski P (1997) Reliability of inspiratory capacity for estimating end-expiratory lung volume changes during exercise in patients with chronic obstructive pulmonary disease. Am J Respir Crit Care Med 156(1):55–59

22. Guenette JA, Webb KA, O'Donnell DE (2012) Does dynamic hyperinflation contribute to dyspnoea during exercise in patients with COPD? Eur Respir J 40(2):322–329
23. Fletcher C, Peto R (1977) The natural history of chronic airflow obstruction. Br Med J 1(6077):1645–1648
24. O'Donnell DE, Deesomchok A, Lam YM, Guenette JA, Amornputtisathaporn N, Forkert L, Webb KA (2011) Effects of BMI on static lung volumes in patients with airway obstruction. Chest 140(2):461–468
25. Hogg JC, Macklem PT, Thurlbeck WM (1968) Site and nature of airway obstruction in chronic obstructive lung disease. N Engl J Med 278(25):1355–1360
26. Bates DV, Gordon CA, Paul GI, Place RE, Snidal DP, Woolf CR (1966) Chronic bronchitis. Report on the third and fourth stages of the co-ordinated study of chronic bronchitis in the Department of Veterans Affairs, Canada. Med Serv J Can 22(1):1–59
27. Kikawada M, Ichinose Y, Miyamoto D, Minemura K, Takasaki M, Toyama K (2000) Peripheral airway findings in chronic obstructive pulmonary disease using an ultrathin bronchoscope. Eur Respir J 15(1):105–108
28. Mitzner W (2011) Emphysema–a disease of small airways or lung parenchyma? N Engl J Med 365(17):1637–1639
29. Corbin RP, Loveland M, Martin RR, Macklem PT (1979) A four-year follow-up study of lung mechanics in smokers. Am Rev Respir Dis 120(2):293–304
30. Yuan R, Hogg JC, Pare PD, Sin DD, Wong JC, Nakano Y, McWilliams AM, Lam S, Coxson HO (2009) Prediction of the rate of decline in FEV(1) in smokers using quantitative Computed Tomography. Thorax 64(11):944–949
31. Rambod M, Porszasz J, Make BJ, Crapo JD, Casaburi R (2012) Six-minute walk distance predictors, including CT scan measures, in the COPDGene cohort. Chest 141(4):867–875
32. Washko GR, Dransfield MT, Estepar RS, Diaz A, Matsuoka S, Yamashiro T, Hatabu H, Silverman EK, Bailey WC, Reilly JJ (2009) Airway wall attenuation: a biomarker of airway disease in subjects with COPD. J Appl Physiol 107(1):185–191
33. O'Donnell DE, Parker CM (2006) COPD exacerbations. 3: pathophysiology. Thorax 61(4):354–361
34. Parker CM, Voduc N, Aaron SD, Webb KA, O'Donnell DE (2005) Physiological changes during symptom recovery from moderate exacerbations of COPD. Eur Respir J 26(3):420–428
35. Stevenson NJ, Walker PP, Costello RW, Calverley PM (2005) Lung mechanics and dyspnea during exacerbations of chronic obstructive pulmonary disease. Am J Respir Crit Care Med 172(12):1510–1516
36. Smith J, Bellemare F (1987) Effect of lung volume on in vivo contraction characteristics of human diaphragm. J Appl Physiol 62(5):1893–1900
37. Similowski T, Yan S, Gauthier AP, Macklem PT, Bellemare F (1991) Contractile properties of the human diaphragm during chronic hyperinflation. N Engl J Med 325(13):917–923
38. Polkey MI, Kyroussis D, Hamnegard CH, Mills GH, Green M, Moxham J (1996) Diaphragm strength in chronic obstructive pulmonary disease. Am J Respir Crit Care Med 154(5):1310–1317
39. Decramer M (1997) Hyperinflation and respiratory muscle interaction. Eur Respir J 10(4):934–941
40. Cassart M, Pettiaux N, Gevenois PA, Paiva M, Estenne M (1997) Effect of chronic hyperinflation on diaphragm length and surface area. Am J Respir Crit Care Med 156(2 Pt 1):504–508
41. Laghi F, Harrison MJ, Tobin MJ (1996) Comparison of magnetic and electrical phrenic nerve stimulation in assessment of diaphragmatic contractility. J Appl Physiol 80(5):1731–1742
42. Walsh JM, Webber CL Jr, Fahey PJ, Sharp JT (1992) Structural change of the thorax in chronic obstructive pulmonary disease. J Appl Physiol 72(4):1270–1278
43. Cassart M, Gevenois PA, Estenne M (1996) Rib cage dimensions in hyperinflated patients with severe chronic obstructive pulmonary disease. Am J Respir Crit Care Med 154(3 Pt 1):800–805

44. McKenzie DK, Gorman RB, Tolman J, Pride NB, Gandevia SC (2000) Estimation of dia-phragm length in patients with severe chronic obstructive pulmonary disease. Respir Physiol 123(3):225–234
45. Gauthier AP, Verbanck S, Estenne M, Segebarth C, Macklem PT, Paiva M (1994) Three-dimensional reconstruction of the in vivo human diaphragm shape at different lung volumes. J Appl Physiol 76(2):495–506
46. Zocchi L, Garzaniti N, Newman S, Macklem PT (1987) Effect of hyperinflation and equaliza-tion of abdominal pressure on diaphragmatic action. J Appl Physiol 62(4):1655–1664
47. Rochester DF, Braun NM (1985) Determinants of maximal inspiratory pressure in chronic obstructive pulmonary disease. Am Rev Respir Dis 132(1):42–47
48. Loring SH, Garcia-Jacques M, Malhotra A (2009) Pulmonary characteristics in COPD and mechanisms of increased work of breathing. J Appl Physiol 107(1):309–314
49. Barr RG, Bluemke DA, Ahmed FS, Carr JJ, Enright PL, Hoffman EA, Jiang R, Kawut SM, Kronmal RA, Lima JA, Shahar E, Smith LJ, Watson KE (2010) Percent emphysema, airflow obstruction, and impaired left ventricular filling. N Engl J Med 362(3):217–227
50. Watz H, Waschki B, Magnussen H (2010) Emphysema, airflow obstruction, and left ventricu-lar filling. N Engl J Med 362(17):1638–1639; author reply 1640–1631
51. Watz H, Waschki B, Meyer T, Kretschmar G, Kirsten A, Claussen M, Magnussen H (2010) Decreasing cardiac chamber sizes and associated heart dysfunction in COPD: role of hyper-inflation. Chest 138(1):32–38
52. Vassaux C, Torre-Bouscoulet L, Zeineldine S, Cortopassi F, Paz-Diaz H, Celli BR, Pinto-Plata VM (2008) Effects of hyperinflation on the oxygen pulse as a marker of cardiac perfor-mance in COPD. Eur Respir J 32(5):1275–1282
53. Jorgensen K, Muller MF, Nel J, Upton RN, Houltz E, Ricksten SE (2007) Reduced intratho-racic blood volume and left and right ventricular dimensions in patients with severe emphy-sema: an MRI study. Chest 131(4):1050–1057
54. Orozco-Levi M, Gea J, Llorcta JL, Felez M, Minguella J, Serrano S, Broquetas JM (1999) Subcellular adaptation of the human diaphragm in chronic obstructive pulmonary disease. Eur Respir J 13(2):371–378
55. Supinski GS, Kelsen SG (1982) Effect of elastase-induced emphysema on the force-generating ability of the diaphragm. J Clin Invest 70(5):978–988
56. Levine S, Kaiser L, Leferovich J, Tikunov B (1997) Cellular adaptations in the diaphragm in chronic obstructive pulmonary disease. N Engl J Med 337(25):1799–1806
57. Mercadier JJ, Schwartz K, Schiaffino S, Wisnewsky C, Ausoni S, Heimburger M, Marrash R, Pariente R, Aubier M (1998) Myosin heavy chain gene expression changes in the diaphragm of patients with chronic lung hyperinflation. Am J Physiol 274(4 Pt 1):L527–L534
58. Mador MJ, Kufel TJ, Pineda LA, Sharma GK (2000) Diaphragmatic fatigue and high-intensity exercise in patients with chronic obstructive pulmonary disease. Am J Respir Crit Care Med 161(1):118–123
59. O'Donnell DE, Lam M, Webb KA (1998) Measurement of symptoms, lung hyperinflation, and endurance during exercise in chronic obstructive pulmonary disease. Am J Respir Crit Care Med 158(5 Pt 1):1557–1565
60. O'Donnell DE, Travers J, Webb KA, He Z, Lam YM, Hamilton A, Kesten S, Maltais F, Magnussen H (2009) Reliability of ventilatory parameters during cycle ergometry in multi-centre trials in COPD. Eur Respir J 34(4):866–874
61. O'Donnell DE, Revill SM, Webb KA (2001) Dynamic hyperinflation and exercise intol-erance in chronic obstructive pulmonary disease. Am J Respir Crit Care Med 164(5):770–777
62. Stubbing DG, Pengelly LD, Morse JL, Jones NL (1980) Pulmonary mechanics during exer-cise in subjects with chronic airflow obstruction. J Appl Physiol 49(3):511–515
63. Stubbing DG, Pengelly LD, Morse JL, Jones NL (1980) Pulmonary mechanics during exer-cise in normal males. J Appl Physiol 49(3):506–510
64. Vogiatzis I, Georgiadou O, Golemati S, Aliverti A, Kosmas E, Kastanakis E, Geladas N, Koutsoukou A, Nanas S, Zakynthinos S, Roussos C (2005) Patterns of dynamic hyperinflation

during exercise and recovery in patients with severe chronic obstructive pulmonary disease. Thorax 60(9):723–729

65. Laveneziana P, Webb KA, Ora J, Wadell K, O'Donnell DE (2011) Evolution of dyspnea during exercise in chronic obstructive pulmonary disease: impact of critical volume constraints. Am J Respir Crit Care Med 184(12):1367–1373

66. O'Donnell DE, Hamilton AL, Webb KA (2006) Sensory-mechanical relationships during high-intensity, constant-work-rate exercise in COPD. J Appl Physiol 101(4):1025–1035

67. Guenette JA, Jensen D, Webb KA, Ofir D, Raghavan N, O'Donnell DE (2011) Sex differences in exertional dyspnea in patients with mild COPD: physiological mechanisms. Respir Physiol Neurobiol 177(3):218–227

68. Ofir D, Laveneziana P, Webb KA, Lam YM, O'Donnell DE (2008) Mechanisms of dyspnea during cycle exercise in symptomatic patients with GOLD stage I chronic obstructive pulmonary disease. Am J Respir Crit Care Med 177(6):622–629

69. Aliverti A, Stevenson N, Dellaca RL, Lo Mauro A, Pedotti A, Calverley PM (2004) Regional chest wall volumes during exercise in chronic obstructive pulmonary disease. Thorax 59(3):210–216

70. Iandelli I, Aliverti A, Kayser B, DellacÃ R, Cala SJ, Duranti R, Kelly S, Scano G, Sliwinski P, Yan S, Macklem PT, Pedotti A (2002) Determinants of exercise performance in normal men with externally imposed expiratory flow limitation. J Appl Physiol 92(5): 1943–1952

71. O'Donnell DE, Bertley JC, Chau LK, Webb KA (1997) Qualitative aspects of exertional breathlessness in chronic airflow limitation: pathophysiologic mechanisms. Am J Respir Crit Care Med 155(1):109–115

72. Paoletti P, De Filippis F, Fraioli F, Cinquanta A, Valli G, Laveneziana P, Vaccaro F, Martolini D, Palange P (2011) Cardiopulmonary exercise testing (CPET) in pulmonary emphysema. Respir Physiol Neurobiol 179(2–3):167–173

73. Eves ND, Petersen SR, Haykowsky MJ, Wong EY, Jones RL (2006) Helium-hyperoxia, exercise, and respiratory mechanics in chronic obstructive pulmonary disease. Am J Respir Crit Care Med 174(7):763–771

74. O'Donnell DE, D'Arsigny C, Fitzpatrick M, Webb KA (2002) Exercise hypercapnia in advanced chronic obstructive pulmonary disease: the role of lung hyperinflation. Am J Respir Crit Care Med 166(5):663–668

75. Laveneziana P, Palange P, Ora J, Martolini D, O'Donnell DE (2009) Bronchodilator effect on ventilatory, pulmonary gas exchange, and heart rate kinetics during high-intensity exercise in COPD. Eur J Appl Physiol 107(6):633–643

76. Laveneziana P, Valli G, Onorati P, Paoletti P, Ferrazza AM, Palange P (2011) Effect of heliox on heart rate kinetics and dynamic hyperinflation during high-intensity exercise in COPD. Eur J Appl Physiol 111(2):225–234

77. Chiappa GR, Borghi-Silva A, Ferreira LF, Carrascosa C, Oliveira CC, Maia J, Gimenes AC, Queiroga F Jr, Berton D, Ferreira EM, Nery LE, Neder JA (2008) Kinetics of muscle deoxygenation are accelerated at the onset of heavy-intensity exercise in patients with COPD: relationship to central cardiovascular dynamics. J Appl Physiol 104(5):1341–1350

78. Montes de Oca M, Rassulo J, Celli BR (1996) Respiratory muscle and cardiopulmonary function during exercise in very severe COPD. Am J Respir Crit Care Med 154(5):1284–1289

79. Travers J, Laveneziana P, Webb KA, Kesten S, O'Donnell DE (2007) Effect of tiotropium bromide on the cardiovascular response to exercise in COPD. Respir Med 101(9): 2017–2024

80. Sliwinski P, Kaminski D, Zielinski J, Yan S (1998) Partitioning of the elastic work of inspiration in patients with COPD during exercise. Eur Respir J 11(2):416–421

81. Garcia-Rio F, Lores V, Mediano O, Rojo B, Hernanz A, Lopez-Collazo E, Alvarez-Sala R (2009) Daily physical activity in patients with chronic obstructive pulmonary disease is mainly associated with dynamic hyperinflation. Am J Respir Crit Care Med 180(6): 506–512

82. Mead J (1973) Respiration: pulmonary mechanics. Annu Rev Physiol 35:169–192

83. Roussos C, Macklem PT (1982) The respiratory muscles. N Engl J Med 307(13):786–797

84. Smith TC, Marini JJ (1988) Impact of PEEP on lung mechanics and work of breathing in severe airflow obstruction. J Appl Physiol 65(4):1488–1499
85. Levison H, Cherniack RM (1968) Ventilatory cost of exercise in chronic obstructive pulmonary disease. J Appl Physiol 25(1):21–27
86. Bye PT, Esau SA, Levy RD, Shiner RJ, Macklem PT, Martin JG, Pardy RL (1985) Ventilatory muscle function during exercise in air and oxygen in patients with chronic air-flow limitation. Am Rev Respir Dis 132(2):236–240
87. Sinderby C, Spahija J, Beck J, Kaminski D, Yan S, Comtois N, Sliwinski P (2001) Diaphragm activation during exercise in chronic obstructive pulmonary disease. Am J Respir Crit Care Med 163(7):1637–1641
88. Polkey MI, Kyroussis D, Keilty SE, Hamnegard CH, Mills GH, Green M, Moxham J (1995) Exhaustive treadmill exercise does not reduce twitch transdiaphragmatic pressure in patients with COPD. Am J Respir Crit Care Med 152(3):959–964
89. Light RW, Mintz HM, Linden GS, Brown SE (1984) Hemodynamics of patients with severe chronic obstructive pulmonary disease during progressive upright exercise. Am Rev Respir Dis 130(3):391–395
90. Vizza CD, Lynch JP, Ochoa LL, Richardson G, Trulock EP (1998) Right and left ventricular dysfunction in patients with severe pulmonary disease. Chest 113(3):576–583
91. Morrison DA, Adcock K, Collins CM, Goldman S, Caldwell JH, Schwarz MI (1987) Right ventricular dysfunction and the exercise limitation of chronic obstructive pulmonary disease. J Am Coll Cardiol 9(6):1219–1229
92. Vasilopoulou MK, Vogiatzis I, Nasis I, Spetsioti S, Cherouveim E, Koskolou M, Kortianou EA, Louvaris Z, Kaltsakas G, Koutsoukou A, Koulouris NG, Alchanatis M (2012) On- and off-exercise kinetics of cardiac output in response to cycling and walking in COPD patients with GOLD Stages I-IV. Respir Physiol Neurobiol 181(3):351–358
93. Jorgensen K, Houltz E, Westfelt U, Nilsson F, Schersten H, Ricksten SE (2003) Effects of lung volume reduction surgery on left ventricular diastolic filling and dimensions in patients with severe emphysema. Chest 124(5):1863–1870
94. Criner GJ, Scharf SM, Falk JA, Gaughan JP, Sternberg AL, Patel NB, Fessler HE, Minai OA, Fishman AP (2007) Effect of lung volume reduction surgery on resting pulmonary hemodynamics in severe emphysema. Am J Respir Crit Care Med 176(3):253–260
95. Chiappa GR, Queiroga F Jr, Meda E, Ferreira LF, Diefenthaeler F, Nunes M, Vaz MA, Machado MC, Nery LE, Neder JA (2009) Heliox improves oxygen delivery and utilization during dynamic exercise in patients with chronic obstructive pulmonary disease. Am J Respir Crit Care Med 179(11):1004–1010
96. Berton DC, Barbosa PB, Takara LS, Chiappa GR, Siqueira AC, Bravo DM, Ferreira LF, Neder JA (2010) Bronchodilators accelerate the dynamics of muscle O2 delivery and utilisation during exercise in COPD. Thorax 65(7):588–593
97. Aliverti A, Macklem PT, Debigare R, Maltais F, O'Donnell DE, Webb KA (2008) Point: counterpoint – the major limitations to exercise performance in COPD. J Appl Physiol 105(2):749–757
98. Montes de Oca M, Celli BR (2000) Respiratory muscle recruitment and exercise performance in eucapnic and hypercapnic severe chronic obstructive pulmonary disease. Am J Respir Crit Care Med 161(3 Pt 1):880–885
99. Kyroussis D, Polkey MI, Hamnegard CH, Mills GH, Green M, Moxham J (2000) Respiratory muscle activity in patients with COPD walking to exhaustion with and without pressure support. Eur Respir J 15(4):649–655
100. Marin JM, Montes de Oca M, Rassulo J, Celli BR (1999) Ventilatory drive at rest and perception of exertional dyspnea in severe COPD. Chest 115(5):1293–1300
101. O'Donnell DE, Sanii R, Anthonisen NR, Younes M (1987) Effect of dynamic airway compression on breathing pattern and respiratory sensation in severe chronic obstructive pulmonary disease. Am Rev Respir Dis 135(4):912–918
102. O'Donnell DE, Sanii R, Anthonisen NR, Younes M (1987) Expiratory resistive loading in patients with severe chronic air-flow limitation. An evaluation of ventilatory mechanics and compensatory responses. Am Rev Respir Dis 136(1):102–107

103. O'Donnell DE, Sanii R, Giesbrecht G, Younes M (1988) Effect of continuous positive airway pressure on respiratory sensation in patients with chronic obstructive pulmonary disease during submaximal exercise. Am Rev Respir Dis 138(5):1185–1191

104. Laveneziana P, Ora J, Webb KA, Wadell K, O'Donnell DE (2008) Expiratory muscle recruitment did not attenuate dynamic hyperinflation during cycle exercise in patients with advanced COPD. Eur Respir J 32(Suppl 52):517s

105. Parshall MB, Schwartzstein RM, Adams L, Banzett RB, Manning HL, Bourbeau J, Calverley PM, Gift AG, Harver A, Lareau SC, Mahler DA, Meek PM, O'Donnell DE (2012) An official American Thoracic Society statement: update on the mechanisms, assessment, and management of dyspnea. Am J Respir Crit Care Med 185(4):435–452

106. Gandevia B, Hugh-Jones P (1957) Terminology for measurements of ventilatory capacity; a report to the thoracic society. Thorax 12(4):290–293

107. Leblanc P, Bowie DM, Summers E, Jones NL, Killian KJ (1986) Breathlessness and exercise in patients with cardiorespiratory disease. Am Rev Respir Dis 133(1):21–25

108. Schwartzstein RM, Simon PM, Weiss JW, Fencl V, Weinberger SE (1989) Breathlessness induced by dissociation between ventilation and chemical drive. Am Rev Respir Dis 139(5):1231–1237

109. Harty HR, Corfield DR, Schwartzstein RM, Adams L (1999) External thoracic restriction, respiratory sensation, and ventilation during exercise in men. J Appl Physiol 86(4):1142–1150

110. O'Donnell DE, Hong HH, Webb KA (2000) Respiratory sensation during chest wall restriction and dead space loading in exercising men. J Appl Physiol 88(5):1859–1869

111. Banzett RB, Pedersen SH, Schwartzstein RM, Lansing RW (2008) The affective dimension of laboratory dyspnea: air hunger is more unpleasant than work/effort. Am J Respir Crit Care Med 177(12):1384–1390

112. Evans KC, Banzett RB, Adams L, McKay L, Frackowiak RS, Corfield DR (2002) BOLD fMRI identifies limbic, paralimbic, and cerebellar activation during air hunger. J Neurophysiol 88(3):1500–1511

113. Wright GW, Branscomb BV (1954) The origin of the sensations of dyspnea. Trans Am Clin Climatol Assoc 66:116–125

114. Davenport PW, Vovk A (2009) Cortical and subcortical central neural pathways in respiratory sensations. Respir Physiol Neurobiol 167(1):72–86

115. McKenzie DK, Butler JE, Gandevia SC (2009) Respiratory muscle function and activation in chronic obstructive pulmonary disease. J Appl Physiol 107(2):621–629

116. O'Donnell DE, Laveneziana P (2006) The clinical importance of dynamic lung hyperinflation in COPD. COPD 3(4):219–232

117. Maltais F, Hamilton A, Marciniuk D, Hernandez P, Sciurba FC, Richter K, Kesten S, O'Donnell D (2005) Improvements in symptom-limited exercise performance over 8 h with once-daily tiotropium in patients with COPD. Chest 128(3):1168–1178

118. O'Donnell DE, Fluge T, Gerken F, Hamilton A, Webb K, Aguilaniu B, Make B, Magnussen H (2004) Effects of tiotropium on lung hyperinflation, dyspnoea and exercise tolerance in COPD. Eur Respir J 23(6):832–840

119. O'Donnell DE, Lam M, Webb KA (1999) Spirometric correlates of improvement in exercise performance after anticholinergic therapy in chronic obstructive pulmonary disease. Am J Respir Crit Care Med 160(2):542–549

120. O'Donnell DE, Voduc N, Fitzpatrick M, Webb KA (2004) Effect of salmeterol on the ventilatory response to exercise in chronic obstructive pulmonary disease. Eur Respir J 24(1):86–94

121. Peters MM, Webb KA, O'Donnell DE (2006) Combined physiological effects of bronchodilators and hyperoxia on exertional dyspnoea in normoxic COPD. Thorax 61(7):559–567

122. Belman MJ, Botnick WC, Shin JW (1996) Inhaled bronchodilators reduce dynamic hyperinflation during exercise in patients with chronic obstructive pulmonary disease. Am J Respir Crit Care Med 153(3):967–975

123. Petrof BJ, Calderini E, Gottfried SB (1990) Effect of CPAP on respiratory effort and dyspnea during exercise in severe COPD. J Appl Physiol 69(1):179–188

124. O'Donnell DE, Sanii R, Younes M (1988) Improvement in exercise endurance in patients with chronic airflow limitation using continuous positive airway pressure. Am Rev Respir Dis 138(6):1510–1514

125. Gelb AF, Zamel N, McKenna RJ Jr, Brenner M (1996) Mechanism of short-term improvement in lung function after emphysema resection. Am J Respir Crit Care Med 154(4 Pt 1): 945–951

126. Martinez FJ, de Oca MM, Whyte RI, Stetz J, Gay SE, Celli BR (1997) Lung-volume reduction improves dyspnea, dynamic hyperinflation, and respiratory muscle function. Am J Respir Crit Care Med 155(6):1984–1990

127. O'Donnell DE, Webb KA, Bertley JC, Chau LK, Conlan AA (1996) Mechanisms of relief of exertional breathlessness following unilateral bullectomy and lung volume reduction surgery in emphysema. Chest 110(1):18–27

128. Sciurba FC, Rogers RM, Keenan RJ, Slivka WA, Gorcsan J 3rd, Ferson PF, Holbert JM, Brown ML, Landreneau RJ (1996) Improvement in pulmonary function and elastic recoil after lung-reduction surgery for diffuse emphysema. N Engl J Med 334(17):1095–1099

129. Fishman A, Martinez F, Naunheim K, Piantadosi S, Wise R, Ries A, Weinmann G, Wood DE (2003) A randomized trial comparing lung-volume-reduction surgery with medical therapy for severe emphysema. N Engl J Med 348(21):2059–2073

130. Laghi F, Jubran A, Topeli A, Fahey PJ, Garrity ER Jr, Arcidi JM, de Pinto DJ, Edwards LC, Tobin MJ (1998) Effect of lung volume reduction surgery on neuromechanical coupling of the diaphragm. Am J Respir Crit Care Med 157(2):475–483

131. Laghi F, Jubran A, Topeli A, Fahey PJ, Garrity ER Jr, de Pinto DJ, Tobin MJ (2004) Effect of lung volume reduction surgery on diaphragmatic neuromechanical coupling at 2 years. Chest 125(6):2188–2195

132. O'Donnell DE, Bain DJ, Webb KA (1997) Factors contributing to relief of exertional breathlessness during hyperoxia in chronic airflow limitation. Am J Respir Crit Care Med 155(2):530–535

133. O'Donnell DE, D'Arsigny C, Webb KA (2001) Effects of hyperoxia on ventilatory limitation during exercise in advanced chronic obstructive pulmonary disease. Am J Respir Crit Care Med 163(4):892–898

134. O'Donnell DE, McGuire M, Samis L, Webb KA (1998) General exercise training improves ventilatory and peripheral muscle strength and endurance in chronic airflow limitation. Am J Respir Crit Care Med 157(5 Pt 1):1489–1497

135. Casaburi R, ZuWallack R (2009) Pulmonary rehabilitation for management of chronic obstructive pulmonary disease. N Engl J Med 360(13):1329–1335

136. Somfay A, Porszasz J, Lee SM, Casaburi R (2001) Dose-response effect of oxygen on hyperinflation and exercise endurance in nonhypoxaemic COPD patients. Eur Respir J 18(1):77–84

Lung Recruitment and De-recruitment

8

Göran Hedenstierna and João B. Borges

8.1 Introduction

When we are born, the lungs are completely collapsed or atelectatic and not yet opened up or recruited. The fetus is oxygenated by placental gas exchange, but after birth the newborn has to take over the oxygenation of blood and removal of carbon dioxide within a few minutes. The first inspirations will slowly open up the lungs breath by breath, obviously a necessity for the lungs to take over the gas exchange. These breaths are demanding and respiratory work is heavy but a prerequisite to survive the transition from intra- to extrauterine life that sometimes needs ventilatory support [1]. Under normal conditions, a healthy lung is fully aerated, and no part will be airless or collapsed (or de-recruited). This is essential for optimum gas exchange, i.e., oxygenation of blood and removal of carbon dioxide (CO_2) from the blood. Blood flow through an airless lung causes shunt, i.e., flow of blood that is not oxygenated and cannot eliminate CO_2, resulting in hypoxemia and CO_2 retention [2]. De-recruitment or atelectasis can be seen in 9 of 10 patients during anesthesia [3], more or less all patients in the intensive care setting under ventilator treatment [4], and in lung inflammatory diseases such as pneumonia [5]. It can also be seen in chronic obstructive lung disease (COPD) [6]. The lung may also be de-recruited when exposed to strong external forces, e.g., high gravitational forces [7, 8]. This

G. Hedenstierna, MD, PhD (✉)
Department of Medical Sciences, Hedenstierna Laboratory,
Uppsala University, University Hospital, entrance 40:2, Uppsala S-75185, Sweden
e-mail: goran.hedenstierna@medsci.uu.se

J.B. Borges, MD
Department of Surgical Sciences, Hedenstierna Laboratory,
Uppsala University, University Hospital, Uppsala S-75185, Sweden
e-mail: joao.batista_borges@surgsci.uu.se

A. Aliverti, A. Pedotti (eds.), *Mechanics of Breathing*,
DOI 10.1007/978-88-470-5647-3_8, © Springer-Verlag Italia 2014

chapter will describe mechanisms that keep the lung open and aerated under normal conditions, as well as different causes of de-recruitment, techniques to recruit the lung, and techniques to study de-recruitment and recruitment.

8.2   The Open Lung

The lung consists of elastic tissue that, if not prevented by the surrounding chest wall, will contract the lung until complete airlessness (in an elderly subject airways may close before alveoli have become completely empty). The lungs are kept expanded by the connection to the chest wall via a subatmospheric pressure in the pleural space. This is a small liquid-filled space [9]. When the chest is expanded and the diaphragm contracted, the lungs become further inflated. However, the lung is not uniformly expanded. There is a lower pressure ("negative" compared to atmospheric pressure) in the pleural space (P_{pl}) surrounding upper lung regions than in the pleural space surrounding lower lung regions, i.e., in the gravitational direction [10]. This is mainly an effect of the lung weight itself. P_{pl} increases down the pleural space by approximately 0.3 cmH$_2$O/cm in the healthy lung and more in a sick edematous or fibrotic lung. In a 20 cm high lung, the pleural pressure may be −8 cmH$_2$O at the uppermost lung regions and 0 cmH$_2$O in the bottom of a healthy lung. Since static airway pressure (P_{aw}) is the same all over the lung, the transpulmonary pressure that keeps the lung expanded ($P_{aw} - P_{pl}$) is higher in upper than lower lung regions. The alveoli are larger and airways wider in the upper lung than further down. This is illustrated in Fig. 8.1. Thus, apical regions are more expanded in the upright subject, ventral regions in the supine subject, and the upper lung when subject is in the lateral position. This regional difference in volume applies to moderate lung inflation, but since the pressure–volume curve flattens off at high inspiratory pressures, the difference between dependent and nondependent regions will decrease the more the lung is expanded. At maximum inspiration the alveoli are of equal size all over the lung.

During expiration the alveoli and airways decrease in size more in the lower lung regions than higher up. Airways may eventually close during ongoing expiration as will be discussed in a paragraph further down.

8.3   Causes of Lung Collapse/De-recruitment

8.3.1   Disconnection Lung–Chest Wall (e.g., Pneumothorax)

If there is a leak of air into the pleural space, the lung will collapse as understood from the discussion above, but the chest wall will also expand. This is because its resting position is at higher thoracic volume than that established with an intact pleural function and an inward force from the lung. Thus, the chest wall and the lung balance each other creating what is called the resting lung volume or functional residual capacity (Fig. 8.2).

Fig. 8.1 Pressure–volume (*P–V*) curve of the lung with positioning of a lower (dependent) and an upper (nondependent) region on the *P–V* curve. Note the lower (more negative vs. atmosphere) pleural pressure surrounding upper lung regions. This results in a higher transpulmonary pressure (P_{tp}) in this region, with more expanded alveoli than in dependent regions. Since the *P–V* curve flattens off with increasing P_{tp}, ventilation goes preferentially to dependent regions as indicated by the length of the arrows in the *P–V* curve. With a P_{tp} of 0 cmH$_2$O, airways may close and alveoli become non-ventilated with eventual collapse (de-recruitment)

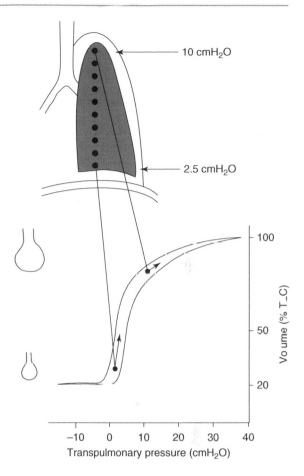

8.3.2   Airway Closure

The walls of the central airways are lined by cartilage and muscle cells that make them resist compression if extramural airway pressure, corresponding to P_{pl}, is increased (although increased muscle tone can also cause bronchoconstriction). The peripheral airway walls have no cartilage and little or no muscle lining and are kept open solely by a higher pressure inside than outside the airway ($P_{aw} - P_{pl}$ must be positive). During expiration P_{pl} increases and may become positive, beginning in the dependent lung. P_{aw} can be approximated to 0 cmH$_2$O during quiet breathing, so when P_{pl} is positive, compression of the airway will occur. This is called airway closure [11].

The resting lung volume, FRC, is decreased in the supine compared to upright position, an effect of the cranial displacement of the diaphragm by the abdominal organs. Airway closure is thus more common or likely in the supine position. The lung volume at which airways close during expiration, called closing capacity, CC, also

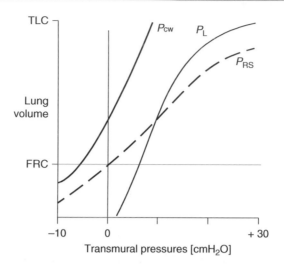

Fig. 8.2 Relationships between the chest and lung. P_{CW} transmural pressure of the chest wall (pleural pressure minus pressure on the body surface), P_L transmural pressure of the lung (intra-alveolar pressure minus pleural pressure), P_{RS} transmural pressure of the respiratory system or "relaxation pressure" (difference between alveolar pressure and pressure on the body surface). Note that at FRC the lung recoils by 6 cmH$_2$O (in this example) and the chest wall is expanding by the same pressure, thus balancing the inward force of the lung. With loss of muscle tone (e.g., by anesthetics, muscle relaxants, and sedatives; c.f. anesthesia and intensive care), lung recoil force is unopposed and the lung volume is reduced and the lung collapses. *TLC* total lung capacity, *FRC* functional residual capacity

increases with age of the subject [11]. This is because of the loss of elastic tissue in the lung (as elsewhere in the body; the skin becomes more twinkled as becomes the lung). FRC is also increasing with age (provided that weight is constant, which is not always true) but less than the CC, and the net effect is more airway closure with age. This is illustrated in Fig. 8.3. It can be seen from the figure that CC is lower than FRC up to an age of approx. 70 years in the upright position and 45 years in the supine posture. Thus, airway closure may occur in middle-aged subjects when supine, e.g., during sleep, but not until higher age in the upright position. If CC is larger than FRC but the breath is larger than CC–FRC, then airways open up during inspiration and close during expiration, causing cyclic airway closure. This may impede oxygenation of blood in the subtended lung unit because of reduced ventilation.

If CC–FRC is larger than the tidal volume, airways will be continuously closed throughout the breath. With continuous airway closure, air will be absorbed from the closed off alveoli, and no replenishment can come from the upper airways. The alveoli decrease in volume and will eventually collapse, causing atelectasis. To go one step further, the alveoli may collapse even with certain inspired ventilation, provided it is minimal compared to the blood flow to the unit. The time it takes to cause atelectasis behind an occluded airway will depend on the gas composition in the closed off unit. Oxygen will be taken up rapidly by the passing capillary blood and nitrogen much slower since there is more or less equilibrium between alveolar nitrogen and nitrogen concentration in different tissues. Dantzker, Wagner, and West [12] calculated the influence of inspired alveolar ventilation/perfusion ratio (V_{AI}/Q) and inspired oxygen

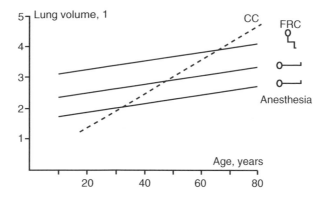

Fig. 8.3 Influence of age on FRC awake in different body positions (sitting and supine) and during anesthesia (supine). Closing capacity (*CC*), the lung volume at which airways begin to close during expiration, is also shown. Note the increase in FRC with increasing age, provided that body height and weight are constant. Note also the decrease in FRC by approximately 0.7–0.8 L when lying down from upright and the further decrease by another 0.4–0.5 L during anesthesia. Closing capacity increases faster with age so that a certain amount of airway closure occurs above FRC in upright position at ages above 65 years and at around 50 years in the supine position. During anesthesia most patients, above 30 years, will suffer from airway closure

concentration on alveolar stability. They found a critical V_{AI}/Q (when alveoli eventually collapse) approaching 0.001 during air breathing, and that was much higher, around 0.07 while breathing 100 % oxygen. They also calculated the minimum time to collapse for units with different V_{AI}/Q ratios at different concentrations of inspired oxygen. As said, the minimum time is much longer during air breathing than during ventilation with oxygen. At a V_{AI}/Q ratio of 0.001, it may take half an hour or more during air breathing but no more than 6 min with an F_IO_2 of 1.0. It was assumed that blood flow through the unit that eventually collapsed was 2 mL/min/mL lung unit. For a homogeneous total lung volume of 2.5 L, this would correspond to a capillary blood flow of 5 L/min, which are reasonable values in the supine subject.

It might be worth mentioning that a breath hold need not cause a de-recruitment, provided that airways are open [13]. Oxygen will be taken up by the capillary blood from the alveoli, and the decrease in alveolar volume reduces alveolar pressure, and fresh gas is sucked down from the airway opening so that the alveolar volume is more or less maintained. The carbon dioxide that is being delivered from capillary blood into the alveolar space adds to the alveolar volume but will be dissolved into the lung tissue and has no lasting effect on the lung volume. Apneic oxygenation, i.e., extended breath hold with oxygen sucked into the lung, can maintain life for many minutes, and death follows not from hypoxemia but from CO_2 retention.

8.3.3   Increased Lung Recoil/Surfactant Deficiency

Surfactant is produced by alveolar type 2 cells and stabilizes the alveolus so that a small alveolus with a higher surface tension will not empty into a larger alveolus with a lower surface tension, which would eventually result in one single alveolus. Surfactant may be affected by anesthesia [14]. Furthermore, a lack of intermittent deep breaths, as is usually the case during mechanical ventilation, may result in a decreased content of active forms of alveolar surfactant [15]. Surfactant production may be decreased or its function impaired in ALI/ARDS and in prematurely born neonates. A decreased production or function of surfactant results in reduced alveolar stability and may contribute to liquid bridging in the airway lumen, promoting airway closure [16]. When the alveolus is reopened by increased airway pressure, e.g., by the application of a positive end-expiratory pressure, PEEP, of 10 cmH$_2$O, the alveolus re-collapses as soon as the PEEP is discontinued [17]. It may then look surprising and even inconsistent when a vital capacity maneuver or the inflation of the lung to +40 cmH$_2$O causes a stable lung so that ventilation can then continue at low or normal airway pressures without the recurrence of atelectasis [18]. However, this can be attributed to the observation that a forceful inflation of the lung releases new surfactant and spreads it out on the alveolar surface and the distal airways, and this makes the lung unit stable again. This may suggest that once PEEP shall be discontinued, it shall be preceded by a forceful inflation of the lung, a vital capacity maneuver. This will again stabilize the lung and will prevent new atelectasis formation, unless high inspired oxygen fraction is used, see below.

8.3.4 External Forces/Lung Compression

Still another possibility for de-recruitment to occur is external forces that reduce the lung volume. Air pilots may develop atelectasis during exposure to high G forces that compress the lung, and this is made worse by oxygen breathing [7, 8]. A similar effect may be exerted by the increased amount of fluid in the lung that increases the weight of the lung and that reduces the gas volume and more so in dependent lung regions, i.e., basal regions in the upright position and the dorsal part when supine [19]. Increased abdominal weight or edema pushes the diaphragm cranially, again promoting lung collapse. Also, laparoscopic surgery with inflation of the abdominal space with gas (CO$_2$) to facilitate visual orientation by the surgeon causes or increases atelectasis [20], surprisingly without increasing shunt or worsening oxygenation of blood, a consequence of increased redistribution of lung blood flow away from the collapsed lung [21].

It may thus be concluded that alveolar collapse may occur when the lung is disconnected from the chest wall (e.g., pneumothorax), by gas absorption from closed off or very poorly ventilated lung units, by reduced surfactant function or production, or by compression of lung tissue (e.g., increased G or lung weight, increased abdominal push on the diaphragm).

8.4 Lung De-recruitment: Location and Amount of Lung Collapse

Lung de-recruitment will occur primarily in the lower lung regions whether the triggering mechanism is airway closure, increased lung recoil, or external lung compression. Thus, de-recruitment or atelectasis can be seen along the dorsal part of the lung in the supine position, in the regions near the diaphragm when upright, and in the lower lung when in the lateral position.

8.4.1 De-recruitment and Recruitment During Anesthesia

Atelectasis occurs in most patients during anesthesia. The size of the atelectasis, measured as area on a CT, in the lung-healthy anesthetized subject may vary from nothing in a few subjects 5 % or so to 25 % or more, the mean being approximately 4 % of the total lung volume [3]. This may not seem impressive or important, but the amount of lung tissue that is collapsed is higher. This is because most of the lung volume is gas and a smaller part is tissue. Around 15 % of the lung tissue is airless or atelectatic during anesthesia, on an average, but this tissue is still perfused and causes shunt, i.e., blood flow through the lung that is not oxygenated, and therefore may cause hypoxemia.

That atelectasis occurs during anesthesia is because the patient is in supine position (lowers FRC), is anesthetized and paralyzed (causes further lowering of FRC to close to residual volume), has presumably received 100 % oxygen during the induction of anesthesia (promotes speed of gas absorption), and is ventilated with rather monotonous ventilation either manually by the anesthetist or with the respirator (no large tidal volume that could have pushed in gas to poorly aerated regions) [22].

Inspired oxygen concentration is of fundamental importance for atelectasis formation [22], a fact that is neglected among anesthetists and intensivists who may feel more comfortable the higher the arterial oxygen tension is [23] (Fig. 8.4). However, atelectasis increases the need of oxygen to compensate for the shunt atelectasis causes, a vicious circle that is created by the anesthetist or intensivist! Subjects, whose anesthesia has been induced during ventilation with lower oxygen concentration, 30 %, do not develop atelectasis although their dependent lung volume is decreased down to residual volume [24]. Indeed, at the time of the rapid eye movement, REM, phase during sleep, the dependent lung regions are decreased in volume to the extent seen during anesthesia, and if we were breathing oxygen during sleep, we would cause de-recruitment of dependent lung regions that have to be reopened when we wake up, breathing air [25].

The use of a sigh maneuver, or a double V_T, has been advocated to reopen any collapsed lung tissue. However, the atelectasis is not decreased by a double V_T or by a sigh up to an airway pressure of 20 cmH$_2$O [26]. Not until an airway pressure of 30 cmH$_2$O is reached does the atelectasis decrease to approximately half the initial size. For complete reopening of all collapsed lung tissue, an inflation pressure of 40 cmH$_2$O is required. Such a large inflation corresponds to a maximum spontaneous inspiration, and it can thus be called a VC maneuver. In adults with healthy lungs, inflation of the lungs to 40 cmH$_2$O maintained for no more than 7–8 s may re-expand all previously collapsed lung tissue. Ventilation of the lungs with pure oxygen after a VC maneuver that had reopened previously collapsed lung tissue will however result in rapid reappearance of the atelectasis. If, on the other hand, a lower oxygen concentration is used, e.g., 40 % O$_2$, atelectasis reappears slowly, and the lung is kept open for about half an hour before any substantial de-recruitment has occurred [25].

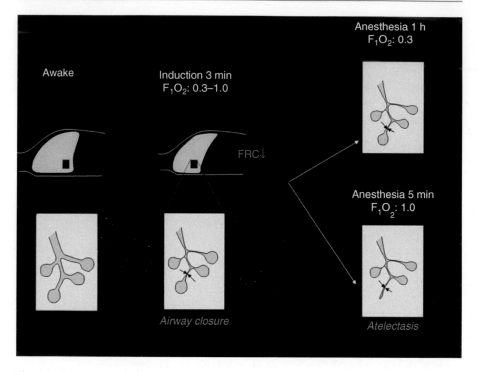

Fig. 8.4 Schematic drawing of the lung (subject in supine position) awake (*left*), after anesthesia induction with ventilation with an inspired oxygen fraction (F_IO_2) of either 0.3 or 1.0 (*middle*) and after a period of anesthesia with an F_IO_2 of 0.3–0.4 but with the previous induction on low or high F_IO_2 (*right*). Note the cranial shift of the diaphragm on induction of anesthesia, causing fall in FRC and airway closure, and de-recruitment (atelectasis) because of gas adsorption behind the closed airway if oxygen concentration is high but not if its concentration is low (and nonabsorbable nitrogen concentration is high)

8.4.2   De-recruitment and Recruitment in Intensive Care

In acute respiratory failure (ARF) and its most severe form, adult respiratory distress syndrome (ARDS), the lung collapse can range from 10 % or less of the lung tissue to 70–80 %. In the latter cases, hypoxemia will be severe and life threatening. It should be clear that some of the airlessness in the ARDS patient might not be collapsed but fluid-filled alveoli. Thus, there are different causes of the airlessness.

Lung collapse is of concern during critical care of patients with acute respiratory distress syndrome (ARDS). Experimental evidence identifies the presence of airspace collapse and cyclic recruitment as important elements in the development of ventilator-induced lung injury (VILI) [27–33]. When compared with injury caused by overdistension, cyclic alveolar recruitment and collapse due to insufficient recruitment and positive end-expiratory pressure (PEEP) seem to have similar or even higher impact on lung injury [29, 33]. Moreover, Otto and colleagues [34] have shown substantial spatial and temporal heterogeneity of indexes of inflammation in

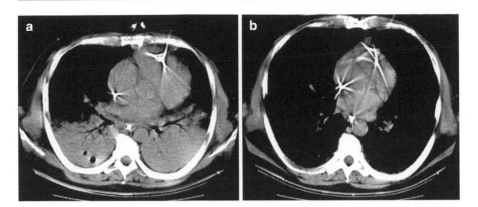

Fig. 8.5 CT scans from a patient with acute respiratory distress syndrome are shown, before (**a**) and after (**b**) the maximal recruitment strategy

a surfactant depletion model of lung injury. In this model, cyclical recruitment was more damaging than stretch. However, other studies suggest that injury [35] occurs predominantly in nondependent regions.

The lung units are mutually interdependent, linked through a meshwork of shared alveolar, interstitial, and connective tissues. Each alveolus is tethered to others so that heightened distending forces are brought to bear on any individual lung unit tending to collapse. This elastic interdependence helps to stabilize the lung and indicates that more atelectrauma may potentiate stretch and more stretch may potentiate atelectrauma. To avoid this deadlock, we must find a strategy able to minimize both mechanisms, instead of selecting one. We must overcome the quest for one key VILI determinant. An alternative strategy is conceivable: perform a safe, individualized, and careful maximum recruitment strategy followed by an appropriate PEEP titration. The subsequent reversal of collapse might promote a more homogeneous distribution of tidal ventilation, making use of the previously collapsed parenchyma to "share" the tidal volume, and possibly relieving nondependent lung hyperinflation.

Reinforcing the importance of minimizing tidal hyperinflation, Tschumperlin and colleagues showed that tidal stretch can be attenuated if the net deformation of the alveolar epithelial cell is minimal [33]. A recent study [28] showed that a key factor in alveolar epithelial type 2 cells death is amplitude exceeding 37 % of the membrane surface area rather than peak deformation. Although their results show that the alveolar epithelial cell injury is modest when the deformation amplitudes are less than a level associated with total lung capacity (37 % of the membrane surface area), the severe deformation exceeding this level is likely to occur in certain areas of the lung during mechanical ventilation. In particular, it could easily occur for ARDS patients. As observed by CT imaging, closed and overinflated alveoli can occur simultaneously in different parts of the lung parenchyma during mechanical ventilation [36] (Figs. 8.5a and 8.7a). The overinflation may induce large alveolar epithelial deformations, resulting in alveolar epithelial cell death, and trigger the inflammatory process related to VILI primarily in the baby lung.

Perlman and colleagues utilized real-time confocal microscopy to determine the micromechanics of alveolar perimeter distension in perfused rat lungs [37]. They were able to image a 2 µm thick optical section under the pleura. Five to eight segments were identified within each alveolus. The average length of these segments was compared for normal and hyperinflated conditions. They found the segment distension to be heterogeneous within the single alveolus. Rausch et al. [27] recently showed, employing synchrotron-based x-ray tomographic microscopy on isolated rat lungs, that local strains developing in alveolar walls are much higher than the global extension. Their method allowed them, for the first time, to determine local three-dimensional strain states in real highly resolved alveolar geometries. It turned out the local strains are up to four times higher than the global strains. Additionally, they found strain hot spots to occur within the thinnest parts. This seems feasible since there is less tissue to resist the deformation. This leads to an uneven strain distribution throughout the parenchymal tissue. Thin regions become overstretched, whereas regions with tissue accumulation remain unchallenged. These elegant data suggest that an overextension of the "healthy" parts (baby lung) of the heterogeneous aerated ARDS lungs can play a primary role on the activation of the inflammatory signaling cascade (biotrauma). Thus, in the ARDS lung the collapsed dependent and the statically hyperinflated nondependent regions may act as stress raisers toward open "healthy" regions that become exposed to tidal stretch. In other words, the local consequences of static stretch in nondependent regions and the local consequences of the mechanisms related to collapse in dependent ones are less important than the consequent stresses driven to the remaining aerated and ventilated but small "baby" lung in terms of regional inflammation. An important message of these findings is that we cannot choose which mechanism of VILI is more critical to oppose, but rather they emphasize the importance of strategies capable of minimizing both end-inspiratory and end-expiratory stresses, unloading the baby lung. Three major studies investigated the lung-protective strategy as a whole [38–40], including both low tidal volumes–pressures and optimum PEEP after recruitment maneuvers. They all reported significant clinical benefits.

A difficulty in testing the open lung hypothesis is related to the efficacy of recruitment maneuvers as conventionally proposed. Various studies have suggested that the success rate of such maneuvers is just modest and dependent on initial disease. In addition, the oxygenation/mechanical benefits have hardly been sustained over time [41–49]. Without a significant reduction of alveolar collapse, and without sustained effects, it is always possible to allege that the negative results were related to suboptimal strategy.

Among the main reasons probably causing and promoting lung tissue de-recruitment in intensive care are (1) inadequate evaluation of potential of recruitment; (2) application of partial and inefficacious recruitment maneuvers; (3) absence of any specific, independent, and coupled strategy to keep the lung open during and after the recruitment maneuver; (4) mechanical ventilation strategies based on incremental PEEP as a recruitment maneuver and/or a PEEP titration procedure, instead of titrate, and apply PEEP to keep the lung open after and adequate and specific recruitment strategy; (5) and or suboptimal PEEP titration. It is of questionable benefit to perform insufficient lung recruitments, and it is useless to perform maximum lung recruitment without adding an appropriate open lung PEEP strategy.

Studies proposing a maximum recruitment strategy [36, 50, 51] have found that it was possible to reverse lung collapse and to stabilize lung recruitment in the majority of patients with early ARDS, regardless of etiology (primary or secondary) (Fig. 8.5). The success rate and magnitude of lung recruitment reported in these studies were unusual when compared with previous investigations, especially considering the high proportion of patients with primary ARDS, including patients with *Pneumocystis* pneumonia [19, 52]. Among the reasons explaining this efficacy, one must consider the anti-de-recruitment strategy [36] with PEEP levels kept at 25 cmH$_2$O during the whole recruiting phase. Such high PEEP levels were intended to work as a recruitment keeper, while the patient-specific closing pressures were undetermined. After recruitment, a careful decremental PEEP titration detected and individualized the optimum PEEP level. This optimum level was still above the average lower inflection point found in previous studies [38] and also far exceeded PEEP levels used in previous studies of lung recruitment [43–48]. Of note, despite the prolonged use of hypercapnia and low tidal volumes, it was possible to maintain a stable open lung confirmed by CT analysis (i.e., collapsed lung mass <5 %) at 30 min after recruitment and confirmed by maintenance of oxygenation during the first few days of mechanical ventilation. Importantly, it was not needed to perform repetitive recruitment maneuvers [36, 51].

The distribution of threshold-opening pressures provides insight into the reasons for previous negative recruitment studies [53]. The bimodal shape of the curve of the distribution of threshold-opening pressures suggests that there are two main populations of alveoli in terms of opening pressures. As observed visually during CT scanning, zones of sticky and completely degassed atelectasis, at the most dependent lung [54], frequently require airway opening pressures above 35–40 cmH$_2$O to recruit [55, 56] (Fig. 8.6). If one does not challenge the lung to airway pressures $\cong$ of 60 cmH$_2$O, you might conclude that less than 50 % of early ARDS can be recruited [57]. The combination of insufficient opening pressures and time of application, associated with suboptimal PEEP levels, results in significant collapse on CT and moderate PaO$_2$.

Major side effects anticipated for an intense recruitment strategy are barotrauma, hemodynamic impairment, and hyperinflation. In fact, only a transient decrease in cardiac index during such recruitment maneuver has been found, not accompanied by deterioration in mixed-venous saturation, or by decrease in systemic arterial blood pressure. No direct clinical consequence of such perturbation was seen [36, 51]. Three major precautions minimized potential side effects: (1) all patients were previously optimized in terms of vascular volume [58–62] and vasopressor infusion; (2) pressure-controlled cyclic ventilation was used instead of vital capacity maneuvers (sustained pressures) during the high stress phases, theoretically minimizing hemodynamic impairment [63–66]; and (3) a stepwise protocol was applied that was capable of individualizing the opening pressures applied, using the minimum necessary for each individual. Despite recruitment with high pressures, or

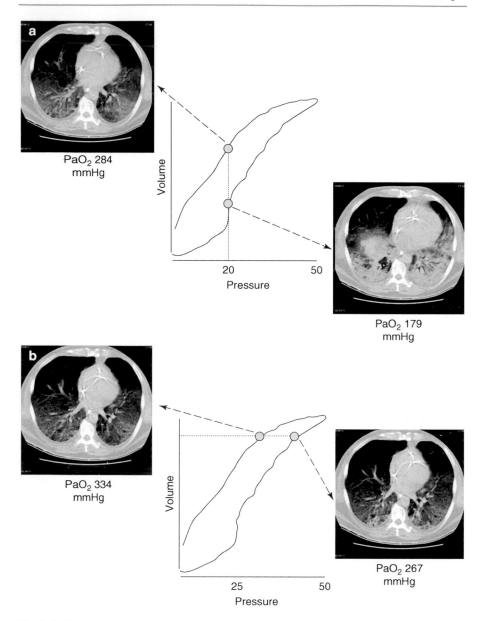

Fig. 8.6 Forceful, aggressive versus partial recruitment of the lung. Inspiratory and expiratory pressure–volume curves during a slow-flow inflation and deflation maneuver in a supine patient with acute respiratory distress syndrome are shown. Inflation was stopped at an airway pressure enough to obtain a maximal recruitment. Partial pressures of oxygen (PaO_2) at corresponding situations, in the same patient, are shown. (**a**) CT scans are shown at the same airway pressure, before (inflation limb) and after (deflation limb) the maximal recruitment. PaO_2 and total lung volume are higher, and the amount of atelectasis is less after the maximal recruitment. (**b**) CT scans are shown at the same total lung volume, also before and after the maximal recruitment. PaO_2 is 25 % higher after the maximal recruitment. This could possibly be explained by lower lung inflation pressure and less squeeze of blood flow downward in the lung, which still has collapsed lung tissue

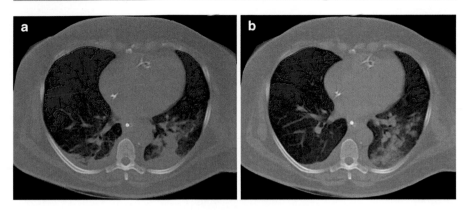

Fig. 8.7 CT analyses are shown of pulmonary voxels presenting hyperinflation (in *red*) before (**a**) and after (**b**) the maximal recruitment in a patient with acute respiratory distress syndrome. Both measurements were done during inspiratory pause at the same airway pressure. Note the decrease of hyperinflation in intermediate and nondependent lung zones after massive recruitment

thanks to it, no hyperinflation may be seen on CT. In fact, the opposite may be seen: decrease of hyperinflation in nondependent lung zones [36] (Fig. 8.7). Massive recruitment with an overall increase in pleural pressure, and thus decrease in trans-pulmonary pressure in nondependent regions [67], may explain such findings.

In conclusion, the challenge is not to answer a simplistic question about whether to do or not to do recruitment, or simply to apply higher versus lower PEEP [68], but rather how to perform a physiology-based protective open lung strategy.

8.5 Techniques to Study Recruitment and De-recruitment

8.5.1 Conventional Chest X-ray

At the bedside, accurate evaluation of lung pathologic entities and pulmonary aeration in critically ill patients ventilated for acute respiratory distress syndrome (ARDS) remain problematic. Technical limitations reduce the quality of bedside chest radiography, which, nevertheless, remains the daily reference for lung imaging. These limitations include movements of the chest wall, patient rotation, supine position with the x-ray film cassette placed posterior to the thorax, and an x-ray beam originating anteriorly at a shorter distance than recommended and not tangentially to the apex of the hemidiaphragm. All of these various factors contribute to poor-quality x-ray films and mistaken assessment of pleural effusion, alveolar consolidation, interstitial markings, mediastinum, and cardiac dimensions. Even with careful control of exposure factors, radiographic images remain suboptimal in more than one third of cases and are poorly correlated to lung computed tomographic images [69]. Lichtenstein and colleagues have shown that lung ultrasonography is better than bedside chest radiography for diagnosing pleural effusion, alveolar consolidation, and alveolar–interstitial syndrome and for assessing the extent of lung injury [70]. It has been suggested that the routine use of lung ultrasonography for critically ill patients with ARDS could reduce the indications of bedside chest radiography.

8.5.2 Computed Tomography, CT

Computed x-ray tomography, CT, has been frequently used for clinical and research purposes. Modern equipment has high temporal resolution enabling, for example, intra-tidal breath analysis and high spatial resolution and can cover the full lung from apex to base using spiral technique. Because of three-dimensional reconstruction, volumetric analysis of the lung can be done which is not possible or less reliable with conventional chest x-ray. The atelectasis that has been shown in the anesthetized subject with CT has not been possible to visualize on conventional chest x-ray – it has needed the 3D reconstruction made available with CT [17].

The CT image shows the density of each volume element (voxel) of the image. In the lung, aeration, or rather the gas/tissue ratio, in each voxel is usually described as the Hounsfield number (HU), the number ranging from +1,000 (bone) to blood (+30/40 HU) water (±0 HU) to air (−1,000 HU). For practical purposes, the HU divided by −10 gives the percentage of air in a particular voxel. Thus, as an example, −700 HU corresponds to 70 % air (−700 HU ÷ −10=70 %). This is in general good enough. However, to be more exact, lung tissue has a specific density of 1,065 on an average, and the calculation of the gas/tissue ratio in a voxel will be HU × 1,065 ÷ −10 [71].

The standard definition of atelectasis by CT is a lung region with a density of −100>HU>+100 [72]. This implies that there will be voxels that contain small amount of air, up to 10 % of the total volume. Atelectasis will thus be slightly overestimated. On the other hand, the voxels with small amount of air up to 10 % indicate poor aeration and presumably poor ventilation. The upper limit, +100 HU, is not critical and, if it is changed to +50 or +200 HU, will not affect the calculation of atelectasis to any extent [73]. It is also common practice to calculate poorly aerated regions from HU −100 to HU −500, normally aerated lung regions from HU −500 to HU −900, and over-aerated regions from HU −900 to HU −1,000. These values are rather arbitrarily chosen and can be discussed. Thus, a normally aerated lung may rather be some −400 to −800 HU. For research purposes, it can also be of interest to partition the voxels into ten percentiles of 100 HU each from −1,000 to 0 (or +100).

When calculating the amount of atelectasis, one should subtract larger vessels that can be seen in the lower half of the lungs and that may sometimes be difficult to separate from pure atelectasis. Manual delineation of vessels will be necessary since there is no software that can do that automatically. Also, the separation of de-recruited collapsed lung in the bottom of the lung from the chest wall can be difficult and requires manual delineation. The remaining lung borders against atmosphere and mediastinal organs are mostly obvious and can be done with computer software.

Most presentations of de-recruitment are done by describing the area of the atelectasis in the CT cut as percent of the lung area or, by covering the whole lung by continuous exposure while the subject is moving through the gantry of the CT scanner ("spiral CT"), by volume of atelectasis in percent of total lung volume. This is again a simplification, although frequently used, because the volume of the collapsed lung will reflect more or less pure tissue, whereas the aerated lung will contain both gas and tissue. The best estimation of de-recruited lung may thus be to relate its tissue amount to the total amount of lung tissue [36]. The result of such a calculation will be a larger share of the lung that is atelectatic, and the difference between an area measurement of atelectasis and its share of the total lung tissue can be large. Thus, an average area of atelectasis at a cut near the diaphragm during anesthesia is 4 % of the lung area, but the tissue is about 15 % of the lung tissue in that cut.

There are several computer programs that can be used for analyzing the lung CT. Some are freeware (Maluna), Osiris Medical Imaging Software program®, and others are very advanced and commercially available (e.g., G.G. IOWA program).

8.5.3 Spirometry and Respiratory Mechanics

With de-recruitment the lung volume will be reduced. Thus, a spirometry measuring total gas volume might give information. However, the normal range of volumes even after taking age, body size, and height into account is too large to allow conclusions regarding atelectasis unless one third or more of the lung has collapsed. If, on the other hand, an initial volume has been measured before any de-recruitment, a comparison may be more precise. Thus, the FRC or the expiratory reserve volume (the volume that can be expired from FRC to maximum expiration, ERV) will be reduced approximately in proportion to the amount of atelectasis. A vital capacity maneuver is the most reproducible volume measurement with spirometry; however, the maximum inspiration that is part of the VC recording will recruit lung tissue [26, 36] and thus interfere with what is aimed at to study. In theory, the expiratory flow should be higher at a given lung volume when part of the lung has collapsed since the lung will behave as if it is stiffer (lower compliance), but in practice measurements will be poorly reliable.

A "stress index" method has been developed to detect recruitment and de-recruitment. The rate of change of the airway pressure–time (P_{aw}–t) curve during constant flow inspiration corresponds to the rate of change of compliance of the respiratory system during tidal inflation [74]. A progressive increase in the slope of the P_{aw}–t curve indicates that compliance is progressively increasing, suggestive of recruitment, and a progressive decrease in slope of the P_{aw}–t curve indicates that compliance is decreasing with tidal inflation, suggestive of overdistension. This could also be demonstrated by CT measurements in experimental lung injury [75]. One should however realize that the stress index might be affected by simultaneous recruitment and overdistension, making it less sensitive to regional events, as for all global measurements.

The forced oscillation technique (FOT) is a noninvasive technique that allows the measurement of pulmonary mechanical properties at a given lung volume, independent of tidal volume and spontaneous breathing, with high temporal resolution [76]. Briefly, it consists of evaluating the response of the respiratory system to small amplitude pressure oscillations in terms of impedance (Z_{rs}). Z_{rs} is made up of two terms, resistance (R_{rs}) and reactance (X_{rs}), which is in turn related to the dynamic elastance (reflecting tissue elasticity, size of the lung, amount of alveolar units connected to the airways opening) and inertia (reflecting the energy that has to be spent to accelerate gas and tissues) of the respiratory system. X_{rs} measured at the oscillatory frequency of 5 Hz is strongly related to the fraction of recruited tissue irrespective of its spatial distribution [77] and is effective in guiding PEEP titration through the identification of the optimal trade-off between recruitment and lung tissue distention in experimental acute lung injury [78].

8.5.4   Gas Exchange

The de-recruited lung will still be perfused, but the blood will not be oxygenated. Thus, the PaO_2 will be reduced. If ventilation is provided with high oxygen concentration, above 50 %, any oxygen impairment is primarily by shunt [2]. With decreasing inspired oxygen concentration, ventilation/perfusion mismatch will play an increasing role in causing gas exchange impairment. Thus, increasing the oxygen concentration in the inspired gas enables a recording of PaO_2 that is mainly affected by shunt. However, high oxygen concentration will transfer regions with a low VA/Q ratio, as discussed above [12], to atelectasis and shunt. We may thus measure more shunt and assume a larger atelectasis by our effort to measure lung collapse. Another aspect is that most devices for measuring PaO_2 are less reliable at high oxygen tensions. Careful calibration with high oxygen tension gases will be needed, and they are not routine in the critical care setting.

The pulmonary shunt increases and decreases by cyclic alveolar recruitment and de-recruitment. This induces respiratory-dependent oscillations of the PaO_2 as described by means of ultrafast, invasive measurement of the PaO_2 [79, 80]. The oxygen probe used for these studies is a fiber-optic one, measuring PaO_2 based on oxygen-sensitive fluorescence quenching with a time resolution up to 10 Hz. The occurrence and amplitudes of PaO_2 oscillations could be elegantly used to quantify the extent of cyclic alveolar recruitment and de-recruitment. However, there are other potential causes of respiratory-dependent oscillation in PaO_2, e.g., varying perfusion distribution and respiratory variations in alveolar PO_2. The oscillation may be in or out of phase with the breath, and the amplitude of the PO_2 oscillation can vary. All these observations are of importance when identifying the mechanism behind the oscillation.

A standard tool in anesthesia and intensive care is pulse oximetry. It measures the arterial saturation with certain reliability. It is a simple and easy to use tool. The major problem with saturation is that shunt must be large before it affects saturation unless the patient or the subject is breathing air or a low oxygen concentration. A safety limit is often set at 94 % saturation of the hemoglobin (SaO_2 or $SpO_2 = 94$ %). However, an SpO_2 of 94 % when breathing air, and assuming "normal" values for the other variables in the shunt equation, will correspond to a shunt fraction of approximately 15 %. With higher inspired oxygen concentration, shunt can be much larger before a decrease in saturation will be seen. Thus, saturation measurements are not very helpful in quantifying shunt and atelectasis except for the most severe cases.

8.5.5   Electrical Impedance Tomography, EIT

Electrical impedance tomography (EIT) has emerged as a new functional imaging method potentially meeting many clinical needs [81]. Subjecting the chest to minute electrical currents, this radiation-free, noninvasive technique measures the electric potentials at the chest wall surface to produce two-dimensional images that reflect the impedance distribution within the thorax. Cyclic variations in pulmonary air and blood content are the major determinants for the changes in thoracic impedance, the former usually of much larger magnitude. Because cyclic changes in local impedance mainly correspond to changes in lung aeration, recent studies have shown that EIT can reliably assess imbalances in the distribution of regional ventilation in critically ill patients [82].

Collapsed and overdistended lung compartments commonly coexist, and a method capable of assessing both, simultaneously, would be invaluable as a tool to titrate PEEP. Regarding this, an EIT-based method was recently described for estimating alveolar collapse at the bedside, pointing out its regional distribution [83]. A good correlation was found between EIT and CT estimates of lung collapse during decremental PEEP trials after a maximal lung recruitment maneuver. Combining data obtained from EIT and respiratory mechanics, it was also possible to estimate the amount of overdistension during a PEEP trial

8.5.6   Lung Ultrasound

In critically ill patients with ALI/ARDS, lung ultrasound appears to be an attractive alternative to bedside chest radiography; it is noninvasive, easily repeatable, and provides an accurate assessment of lung morphology, pneumothorax, lung consolidation, alveolar–interstitial syndrome, and pleural effusion [84].

A recent study has shown that transthoracic lung ultrasound can detect nonaerated lung area reduction during PEEP increases from 5 to 15 cmH$_2$O in patients with ARDS [85]. Recent data also pointed out that lung ultrasound is equivalent to the pressure–volume curve method for quantitative assessment of PEEP-induced lung recruitment [86]. In this study, lung ultrasound allowed regional assessment of lung recruitment and close monitoring of treatments and maneuvers aimed at improving lung aeration. However, it did not allow an accurate assessment of PEEP-induced lung hyperinflation, and further studies are needed to evaluate the benefit of ultrasound monitoring in patients with ARDS/ALI in terms of morbidity and mortality.

References

1. Lista G, Castoldi F, Cavigioli F, Bianchi S, Fontana P (2012) Alveolar recruitment in the delivery room. J Matern Fetal Neonatal Med 25:39–40
2. West JB, Wagner PD (1991) Ventilation-perfusion relationships. Raven Press, New York, pp 1289–1305
3. Hedenstierna G, Edmark L (2010) Mechanisms of atelectasis in the perioperative period. Best Pract Res Clin Anaesthesiol 24(2):157–169

4. Gattinoni L, Caironi P, Pelosi P, Goodman LR (2001) What has computed tomography taught us about the acute respiratory distress syndrome? Am J Respir Crit Care Med 164(9):1701–1711
5. Rodriguez-Roisin R, Roca J (1996) Update '96 on pulmonary gas exchange pathophysiology in pneumonia. Semin Respir Infect 11(1):3–12
6. Ley-Zaporozhan J, Puderbach M, Kauczor H-U (2008) MR for the evaluation of obstructive pulmonary disease. Magn Reson Imaging Clin N Am 16(2):291–308, ix
7. Tacker WA, Balldin UI, Burton RR, Glaister DH, Gillingham KK, Mercer JR (1987) Induction and prevention of acceleration atelectasis. Aviat Space Environ Med 58(1):69–75
8. Haswell MS, Tacker WA, Balldin UI, Burton RR (1986) Influence of inspired oxygen concentration on acceleration atelectasis. Aviat Space Environ Med 57(5):432–437
9. Lee KF, Olak J (1994) Anatomy and physiology of the pleural space. Chest Surg Clin N Am 4(3):391–403
10. Lai-Fook SJ, Rodarte JR (1991) Pleural pressure distribution and its relationship to lung volume and interstitial pressure. J Appl Physiol 70(3):967–978
11. Milic-Emili J, Torchio R, D'Angelo E (2007) Closing volume: a reappraisal (1967-2007). Eur J Appl Physiol 99(6):567–583
12. Dantzker DR, Wagner PD, West JB (1974) Proceedings: instability of poorly ventilated lung units during oxygen breathing. J Physiol (Lond) 242(2):72P
13. Frumin MJ, Epstein RM, Cohen G (1959) Apneic oxygenation in man. Anesthesiology 20:789–798
14. Wollmer P, Schairer W, Bos JA, Bakker W, Krenning EP, Lachmann B (1990) Pulmonary clearance of 99mTc-DTPA during halothane anaesthesia. Acta Anaesthesiol Scand 34(7): 572–575
15. Otis DR, Johnson M, Pedley TJ, Kamm RD (1993) Role of pulmonary surfactant in airway closure: a computational study. J Appl Physiol 75(3):1323–1333
16. Oyarzun MJ, Iturriaga R, Donoso P, Dussaubat N, Santos M, Schiappacasse ME, Lathrop ME, Larrain C, Zapata P (1991) Factors affecting distribution of alveolar surfactant during resting ventilation. Am J Physiol 261(2):L210–L217
17. Brismar B, Hedenstierna G, Lundquist H, Strandberg A, Svensson L, Tokics L (1985) Pulmonary densities during anesthesia with muscular relaxation–a proposal of atelectasis. Anesthesiology 62(4):422–428
18. Rothen HU, Sporre B, Engberg G, Wegenius G, Hedenstierna G (1995) Reexpansion of atelectasis during general anaesthesia may have a prolonged effect. Acta Anaesthesiol Scand 39(1):118–125
19. Gattinoni L, Pelosi P, Suter PM, Pedoto A, Vercesi P, Lissoni A (1998) Acute respiratory distress syndrome caused by pulmonary and extrapulmonary disease. Different syndromes? Am J Respir Crit Care Med 158(1):3–11
20. Andersson LE, Bååth M, Thörne A, Aspelin P, Odeberg-Wernerman S (2005) Effect of carbon dioxide pneumoperitoneum on development of atelectasis during anesthesia, examined by spiral computed tomography. Anesthesiology 102(2):293–299
21. Strang CM, Freden F, Maripuu E, Hachenberg T, Hedenstierna G (2010) Ventilation-perfusion distributions and gas exchange during carbon dioxide-pneumoperitoneum in a porcine model. Br J Anaesth 105(5):691–697
22. Joyce CJ, Williams AB (1999) Kinetics of absorption atelectasis during anesthesia: a mathematical model. J Appl Physiol 86(4):1116–1125
23. Edmark L, Kostova-Aherdan K, Enlund M, Hedenstierna G (2003) Optimal oxygen concentration during induction of general anesthesia. Anesthesiology 98(1):28–33
24. Rothen HU, Sporre B, Engberg G, Wegenius G, Reber A, Hedenstierna G (1995) Prevention of atelectasis during general anaesthesia [see comments]. Lancet 345(8962):1387–1391
25. Appelberg J, Pavlenko T, Bergman H, Rothen HU, Hedenstierna G (2007) Lung aeration during sleep. Chest 131(1):122–129
26. Rothen HU, Sporre B, Engberg G, Wegenius G, Hedenstierna G (1993) Re-expansion of atelectasis during general anaesthesia: a computed tomography study. Br J Anaesth 71(6): 788–795

27. Rausch SMK, Haberthur D, Stampanoni M, Schittny JC, Wall WA (2011) Local strain distribution in real three-dimensional alveolar geometries. Ann Biomed Eng 39(11):2835–2843
28. Ye H, Zhan Q, Ren Y, Liu X, Yang C, Wang C (2012) Cyclic deformation-induced injury and differentiation of rat alveolar epithelial type II cells. Respir Physiol Neurobiol 180(2):237–246
29. Muscedere JG, Mullen JB, Gan K, Slutsky AS (1994) Tidal ventilation at low airway pressures can augment lung injury. Am J Respir Crit Care Med 149(5):1327–1334
30. Taskar V, John J, Evander E, Robertson B, Jonson B (1997) Surfactant dysfunction makes lungs vulnerable to repetitive collapse and reexpansion. Am J Respir Crit Care Med 155(1): 313–320
31. Webb HH, Tierney DF (1974) Experimental pulmonary edema due to intermittent positive pressure ventilation with high inflation pressures. Protection by positive end-expiratory pressure. Am Rev Respir Dis 110(5):556–565
32. Tremblay L, Valenza F, Ribeiro SP, Li J, Slutsky AS (1997) Injurious ventilatory strategies increase cytokines and c-fos m-RNA expression in an isolated rat lung model. J Clin Invest 99(5):944–952
33. Tschumperlin DJ, Oswari J, Margulies AS (2000) Deformation-induced injury of alveolar epithelial cells. Effect of frequency, duration, and amplitude. Am J Respir Crit Care Med 162(2):357–362
34. Otto CM, Markstaller K, Kajikawa O, Karmrodt J, Syring RS, Pfeiffer B, Good VP, Frevert CW, Baumgardner JE (2008) Spatial and temporal heterogeneity of ventilator associated lung injury after surfactant depletion. J Appl Physiol 104(5):1485–1494
35. Tsuchida S, Engelberts D, Peltekova V, Hopkins N, Frndova H, Babyn P, McKerlie C, Post M, McLoughlin P, Kavanagh BP (2006) Atelectasis causes alveolar injury in nonatelectatic lung regions. Am J Respir Crit Care Med 174(3):279–289
36. Borges JB, Okamoto VN, Matos GFJ, Caramez MPR, Arantes PR, Barros F, Souza CE, Victorino JA, Kacmarek RM, Barbas CSV, Carvalho CRR, Amato MBP (2006) Reversibility of lung collapse and hypoxemia in early acute respiratory distress syndrome. Am J Respir Crit Care Med 174(3):268–278
37. Perlman CE, Bhattacharya J (2007) Alveolar expansion imaged by optical sectioning microscopy. J Appl Physiol 103(3):1037–1044
38. Amato MB, Barbas CS, Medeiros DM, Magaldi RB, Schettino GP, Lorenzi Filho G, Kairalla RA, Deheinzelin D, Munoz C, Oliveira R, Takagaki TY, Carvalho CR (1998) Effect of a protective-ventilation strategy on mortality in the acute respiratory distress syndrome. N Engl J Med 338(6):347–354
39. Ranieri VM, Suter PM, Tortorella C, De Tullio R, Dayer JM, Brienza A, Bruno F, Slutsky AS (1999) Effect of mechanical ventilation on inflammatory mediators in patients with acute respiratory distress syndrome: a randomized controlled trial. JAMA 282(1):54–61
40. Villar J, Kacmarek RM, Pérez-Méndez L, Aguirre-Jaime A (2006) A high positive end-expiratory pressure, low tidal volume ventilatory strategy improves outcome in persistent acute respiratory distress syndrome: a randomized, controlled trial. Crit Care Med 34(5): 1311–1318
41. Moran I, Zavala E, Fernandez R, Blanch L, Mancebo J (2003) Recruitment manoeuvres in acute lung injury/acute respiratory distress syndrome. Eur Respir J Suppl 42:37s–42s
42. Blanch L, Villagrá A (2004) Recruitment maneuvers might not always be appropriate in ARDS. Crit Care Med 32(12):2540–2541
43. Povoa P, Almeida E, Fernandes A, Mealha R, Moreira P, Sabino H (2004) Evaluation of a recruitment maneuver with positive inspiratory pressure and high PEEP in patients with severe ARDS. Acta Anaesthesiol Scand 48(3):287–293
44. Villagrá A, Ochagavía A, Vatua S, Murias G, Del Mar Fernández M, Lopez Aguilar J, Fernández R, Blanch L (2002) Recruitment maneuvers during lung protective ventilation in acute respiratory distress syndrome. Am J Respir Crit Care Med 165(2):165–170
45. Oczenski W, Hörmann C, Keller C, Lorenzl N, Kepka A, Schwarz S, Fitzgerald RD (2004) Recruitment maneuvers after a positive end-expiratory pressure trial do not induce sustained effects in early adult respiratory distress syndrome. Anesthesiology 101(3):620–625

46. Pelosi P, Cadringher P, Bottino N, Panigada M, Carrieri F, Riva E, Lissoni A, Gattinoni L (1999) Sigh in acute respiratory distress syndrome. Am J Respir Crit Care Med 159(3):872–880

47. Foti G, Cereda M, Sparacino ME, De Marchi L, Villa F, Pesenti A (2000) Effects of periodic lung recruitment maneuvers on gas exchange and respiratory mechanics in mechanically ventilated acute respiratory distress syndrome (ARDS) patients. Intensive Care Med 26(5):501–507

48. Lapinsky SE, Aubin M, Mehta S, Boiteau P, Slutsky AS (1999) Safety and efficacy of a sustained inflation for alveolar recruitment in adults with respiratory failure. Intensive Care Med 25(11):1297–1301

49. Grasso S, Mascia L, Del Turco M, Malacarne P, Giunta F, Brochard L, Slutsky AS, Marco Ranieri V (2002) Effects of recruiting maneuvers in patients with acute respiratory distress syndrome ventilated with protective ventilatory strategy. Anesthesiology 96(4):795–802

50. Medoff BD, Harris RS, Kesselman H, Venegas J, Amato MB, Hess D (2000) Use of recruitment maneuvers and high-positive end-expiratory pressure in a patient with acute respiratory distress syndrome. Crit Care Med 28(4):1210–1216

51. de Matos GFJ, Stanzani F, Passos RH, Fontana MF, Albaladejo R, Caserta RE, Santos DCB, Borges JB, Amato MBP, Barbas CSV (2012) How large is the lung recruitability in early acute respiratory distress syndrome: a prospective case series of patients monitored by computed tomography. Crit Care 16(1):R4

52. D'Angelo E, Calderini E, Robatto FM, Puccio P, Milic-Emili J (1997) Lung and chest wall mechanics in patients with acquired immunodeficiency syndrome and severe Pneumocystis carinii pneumonia. Eur Respir J 10(10):2343–2350

53. Crotti S, Mascheroni D, Caironi P, Pelosi P, Ronzoni G, Mondino M, Marini JJ, Gattinoni L (2001) Recruitment and derecruitment during acute respiratory failure: a clinical study. Am J Respir Crit Care Med 164(1):131–140

54. Yap DY, Liebkemann WD, Solway J, Gaver DP (1994) Influences of parenchymal tethering on the reopening of closed pulmonary airways. J Appl Physiol 76(5):2095–2105

55. Takeuchi M, Goddon S, Dohlnikoff M, Shimaoka M, Hess D, Amato MBP, Kacmarek RM (2000) Determination of optimal PEEP level following recruitment maneuvers (RMs) in an ARDS sheep model (abstract). Am J Respir Crit Care Med 161(3):A48

56. Fujino Y, Goddon S, Dolhnikoff M, Hess D, Amato MB, Kacmarek RM (2001) Repetitive high-pressure recruitment maneuvers required to maximally recruit lung in a sheep model of acute respiratory distress syndrome. Crit Care Med 29(8):1579–1586

57. Borges JB, Carvalho CRR, Amato MBP (2006) Lung recruitment in patients with ARDS. N Engl J Med 355(3):319–320; author reply 321–322

58. Perel A, Minkovich L, Preisman S, Abiad M, Segal E, Coriat P (2005) Assessing fluid-responsiveness by a standardized ventilatory maneuver: the respiratory systolic variation test. Anesth Analg 100(4):942–945

59. De Backer D, Heenen S, Piagnerelli M, Koch M, Vincent J-L (2005) Pulse pressure variations to predict fluid responsiveness: influence of tidal volume. Intensive Care Med 31(4):517–523

60. Michard F, Boussat S, Chemla D, Anguel N, Mercat A, Lecarpentier Y, Richard C, Pinsky MR, Teboul JL (2000) Relation between respiratory changes in arterial pulse pressure and fluid responsiveness in septic patients with acute circulatory failure. Am J Respir Crit Care Med 162(1):134–138

61. Michard F, Chemla D, Richard C, Wysocki M, Pinsky MR, Lecarpentier Y, Teboul JL (1999) Clinical use of respiratory changes in arterial pulse pressure to monitor the hemodynamic effects of PEEP. Am J Respir Crit Care Med 159(3):935–939

62. Magder S (2004) Clinical usefulness of respiratory variations in arterial pressure. Am J Respir Crit Care Med 169(2):151–155

63. Odenstedt H, Aneman A, Kárason S, Stenqvist O, Lundin S (2005) Acute hemodynamic changes during lung recruitment in lavage and endotoxin-induced ALI. Intensive Care Med 31(1):112–120

64. Lim S–C, Adams AB, Simonson DA, Dries DJ, Broccard AF, Hotchkiss JR, Marini JJ (2004) Intercomparison of recruitment maneuver efficacy in three models of acute lung injury. Crit Care Med 32(12):2371–2377

65. Lim S–C, Adams AB, Simonson DA, Dries DJ, Broccard AF, Hotchkiss JR, Marini JJ (2004) Transient hemodynamic effects of recruitment maneuvers in three experimental models of acute lung injury. Crit Care Med 32(12):2378–2384

66. Frank JA, McAuley DF, Gutierrez JA, Daniel BM, Dobbs L, Matthay MA (2005) Differential effects of sustained inflation recruitment maneuvers on alveolar epithelial and lung endothelial injury. Crit Care Med 33(1):181–188; discussion 254–255

67. Amato MBP, Marini JJ (1998) Barotrauma, volutrauma, and the ventilation of acute lung injury. In: Marini JJ, Slutsky AS, Lenfant C (eds) Physiological basis of ventilatory support, vol 118, 1st edn. Marcel Dekker, Inc, New York/Basel/Hong Kong, pp 1187–1245

68. Brower RG, Lanken PN, MacIntyre N, Matthay MA, Morris A, Ancukiewicz M, Schoenfeld D, Thompson BT, National Heart Lung, and Blood Institute ARDS Clinical Trials Network (2004) Higher versus lower positive end-expiratory pressures in patients with the acute respiratory distress syndrome. N Engl J Med 351(4):327–336

69. Rouby JJ, Puybasset L, Cluzel P, Richecoeur J, Lu Q, Grenier P (2000) Regional distribution of gas and tissue in acute respiratory distress syndrome. II. Physiological correlations and definition of an ARDS Severity Score. CT Scan ARDS Study Group. Intensive Care Med 26(8):1046–1056

70. Lichtenstein D, Goldstein I, Mourgeon E, Cluzel P, Grenier P, Rouby J-J (2004) Comparative diagnostic performances of auscultation, chest radiography, and lung ultrasonography in acute respiratory distress syndrome. Anesthesiology 100(1):9–15

71. Rosenblum LJ, Mauceri RA, Wellenstein DE, Thomas FD, Bassano DA, Raasch RN, Chamberlain CC, Heitzman ER (1980) Density patterns in the normal lung as determined by computed tomography. Radiology 137(2):409–416

72. Gattinoni L, Pesenti A, Bombino M, Baglioni S, Rivolta M, Rossi F, Rossi G, Fumagalli R, Marcolin R, Mascheroni D, Torresin A (1988) Relationship between lung computed tomographic density, gas exchange, and PEEP in acute respiratory failure. Anesthesiology 69(6):824–832

73. Lundquist H, Hedenstierna G, Strandberg A, Tokics L, Brismar B (1995) CT-assessment of dependent lung densities in man during general anaesthesia. Acta Radiol 36(6):626–632

74. Ranieri VM, Giuliani R, Fiore T, Dambrosio M, Milic-Emili J (1994) Volume-pressure curve of the respiratory system predicts effects of PEEP in ARDS: "occlusion" versus 'constant flow' technique. Am J Respir Crit Care Med 149(1):19–27

75. Grasso S, Terragni P, Mascia L, Fanelli V, Quintel M, Herrmann P, Hedenstierna G, Slutsky AS, Ranieri VM (2004) Airway pressure–time curve profile (stress index) detects tidal recruitment/hyperinflation in experimental acute lung injury. Crit Care Med 32(4):1018–1027

76. Kaczka DW, Dellacá RL (2011) Oscillation mechanics of the respiratory system: applications to lung disease. Crit Rev Biomed Eng 39(4):337–359

77. Dellacá RL, Andersson Olerud M, Zannin E, Kostic P, Pompilio PP, Hedenstierna G, Pedotti A, Frykholm P (2009) Lung recruitment assessed by total respiratory system input reactance. Intensive Care Med 35(12):2164–2172

78. Dellacá RL, Zannin E, Kostic P, Olerud MA, Pompilio PP, Hedenstierna G, Pedotti A, Frykholm P (2011) Optimisation of positive end-expiratory pressure by forced oscillation technique in a lavage model of acute lung injury. Intensive Care Med 37(6):1021–1030

79. Baumgardner JE, Markstaller K, Pfeiffer B, Doebrich M, Otto CM (2002) Effects of respiratory rate, plateau pressure, and positive end-expiratory pressure on PaO2 oscillations after saline lavage. Am J Respir Crit Care Med 166(12):1556–1562

80. Hartmann EK, Boehme S, Bentley A, Duenges B, Klein KU, Elsaesser A, Baumgardner JE, David M, Markstaller K (2012) Influence of respiratory rate and end-expiratory pressure variation on cyclic alveolar recruitment in an experimental lung injury model. Crit Care 16(1):R8

81. Costa EL, Lima RG, Amato MB (2009) Electrical impedance tomography. Curr Opin Crit Care 15(1):18–24

82. Victorino JA, Borges JB, Okamoto VN, Matos GF, Tucci MR, Caramez MP, Tanaka H, Sipmann FS, Santos DC, Barbas CS, Carvalho CR, Amato MB (2004) Imbalances in regional lung ventilation: a validation study on electrical impedance tomography. Am J Respir Crit Care Med 169(7):791–800

83. Costa ELV, Borges JB, Melo A, Suarez-Sipmann F, Toufen C, Bohm SH, Amato MBP (2009) Bedside estimation of recruitable alveolar collapse and hyperdistension by electrical impedance tomography. Intensive Care Med 35(6):1132–1137
84. Arbelot C, Ferrari F, Bouhemad B, Rouby J-J (2008) Lung ultrasound in acute respiratory distress syndrome and acute lung injury. Curr Opin Crit Care 14(1):70–74
85. Stefanidis K, Dimopoulos S, Tripodaki E-S, Vitzilaios K, Politis P, Piperopoulos P, Nanas S (2011) Lung sonography and recruitment in patients with early acute respiratory distress syndrome: a pilot study. Crit Care 15(4):R185
86. Bouhemad B, Brisson H, Le-Guen M, Arbelot C, Lu Q, Rouby J-J (2011) Bedside ultrasound assessment of positive end-expiratory pressure-induced lung recruitment. Am J Respir Crit Care Med 183(3):341–347

Part II

Assessment of Mechanics of Breathing

Lung Function Testing, Spirometry, Diffusion Capacity and Interpretation

9

Flemming Madsen, Jann Mortensen, Birgitte Hanel, and Ole F. Pedersen

9.1 Background

Lung function covers several physiological measures of respiratory function and structure. Ventilation, distribution of ventilation, gas diffusion, and lung perfusion are the most common terms.

Measurement of lung function is used for diagnostics, monitoring, and research, but irrespective of the purpose, the methods, i.e., equipment and measurement technique, must be standardized [1] and must be subjected to continuous quality control.

9.2 Spirometry

FEV_1, FVC, FEV_6, VC, and PEF

F. Madsen, DMSc
Pulmonary Function Laboratory, Allergy & Lung Clinic Helsingør,
Sct. Olai Gade 39, Helsingør, Capital Region 3000, Denmark
e-mail: flem-mad@dadlnet.dk

J. Mortensen
Department of Clinical Physiology, Nuclear Medicine & PET,
Rigshospitalet, University of Copenhagen, Copenhagen, Denmark
e-mail: jann.mortensen@regionh.dk

B. Hanel
Pediatric Pulmonary Service and CF-Center Copenhagen, 5003,
Copenhagen University Hospital, Rigshospitalet, Copenhagen, Denmark
e-mail: birgitte.hanel@regionh.dk

O.F. Pedersen (✉)
Institute of Public Health, University of Aarhus, Aarhus, Denmark
e-mail: ofp@mil.au.dk

A. Aliverti, A. Pedotti (eds.), *Mechanics of Breathing*,
DOI 10.1007/978-88-470-5647-3_9, © Springer-Verlag Italia 2014

9.2.1 Equipment

The ATS/ERS standard from 2005 [2] describes the requirements regarding equipment and measurement technique. New initiatives indicate that there is a demand for a more systematic quality control of both equipment and measurement techniques [3] in primary care as well as in secondary care including research laboratories.

Spirometry is a physiological test with measurement of inspiration and expiration of air, either as dynamic spirometry, with volume or flow measured as a function of time, or statically with only gas volume measured. Spirometry requires a good collaboration between the person tested and the person testing. The results, therefore, depend both on technical and biological factors, among other things the equipment, which must be standardized and calibrated.

9.2.2 Procedure

There are three steps in an FVC test:
1. A complete inspiration
2. A forceful expiration
3. A continued and complete expiration with complete emptying of the lungs
   These three steps must be demonstrated before the test.

The test person inhales fast and completely from the functional residual capacity (FRC), and the mouthpiece is taken into the mouth if not already done. Tube-formed mouthpieces must pass between the teeth into the mouth. It is assured that the lips closed tightly around the mouthpiece, and the FVC maneuver begins shortly after. A certain reduction in PEF is found if there is a short pause (>2 s) at TLC and in FEV_1 if the pause is 4–6 s, before the expiration is initiated [4]. It is therefore important that the start of the test is with no hesitation, so that the pause before the expiration is minimal, i.e., less than 1 s.

9.2.3 Correct Spirometry

In order for a spirometry maneuver to be accepted, it is required that both start and end of test criteria are acceptable.

9.2.3.1 Start Criteria
Even though the maximally forced expiration is performed correct, there is an interval from the beginning of the expiration where the flow is 0 and until the flow becomes maximal. It has been decided to adjust the registration of 0-time for the forced expiration by back extrapolation of time. This is in practice performed by applying an extrapolation line to the steepest part of the forced expiratory curve, and where the line intersects with the time axis, the new 0-time is located and from this new 0-time, the expiratory volumes should be calculated, e.g., FEV_1. If the interval

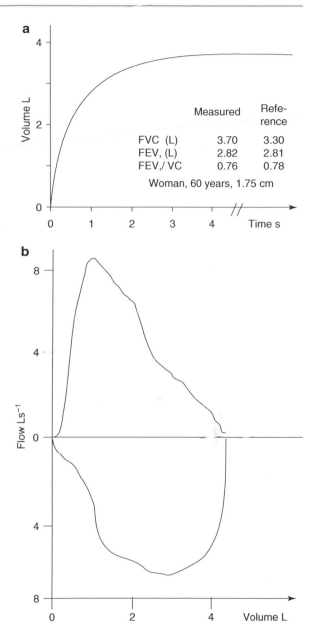

Fig. 9.1 Spirometry. (**a**) Normal volume-time curve. (**b**) Formalized flow-volume curve. Not from the same person

between the start of expiration and the new 0-time becomes too long, the volume expired during the interval becomes too large to be acceptable, and, therefore, it has been decided that maneuvers where the expired volume in this interval exceeds 150 ml or 5 % of FVC, resulting from too slow a start of the maneuver (Fig. 9.1), are not acceptable. The software of the equipment should report this "back extrapolated volume."

9.2.3.2 End of Test Criteria

The end of test is not instantaneous just as the start in the forced expiratory maneuver is not. Therefore, explicit criteria have been decided to determine the time for the end of test. When the flow for at least 1 s has been below 25 mL $\cdot$ s^{-1} and the expiration has lasted at least 6 s, the end of test criteria has been fulfilled, and, thus, the volume corresponding to this end time can be calculated, e.g., the FVC.

In practice most patients learn after a few training maneuvers to fulfill the start criteria, whereas many patients keep on having trouble fulfilling the end of test criteria. One problem is that some patients with normal ventilatory capacity empty their lungs before 6 s has passed. Another and bigger problem is that some patients cannot expire long time enough to get the flow below 25 mL $\cdot$ s^{-1} since they become uncomfortable during the maneuver of maximal expiration. Therefore, the test has to be repeated until at least eight maneuvers have been performed and not until then the testing can be stopped [2]. This is only a minor problem in studies where spirometry is performed once or twice, i.e., aiming at a diagnosis, but in patient with, e.g., COPD and asthma, where the test is performed many times as part of the monitoring of a chronic condition, the demand for at least eight maneuvers might be too strenuous for some patients and impractical for the laboratory.

Therefore, the FEV$_6$ might constitute a good alternative to the FVC when spirometry is used for the monitoring of patients since the patients experiencing difficulties keeping on expiring until the flow is below 25 mL $\cdot$ s^{-1} can stop the expiration after only 6 s. The FEV$_6$ has been validated and is accepted in the international standards as an alternative to the FVC [5–7]. Except for end of test criteria, selection criteria's for the FEV$_6$ and FVC maneuvers are identical [7].

For the evaluation of a spirometry, it is necessary with a minimum of three correctly made measurements. The uniformity of the curves is acceptable if the difference between the largest FVC or FEV$_6$ and the second largest FVC or FEV$_6$ is smaller than 0.150 L and the difference between the largest FEV$_1$ and the next largest FEV$_1$ <0.150 L. If FVC or FEV$_6$ <1.00 L, the differences for both FEV$_1$ and FVC or FEV$_6$ must be <0.100 L.

9.2.4 Equipment

It is a prerequisite for a correctly performed spirometry that the volume is correctly measured, irrespective of measurement with a volume recording or a flow recording spirometer. Correct volume measurement are ensured by comparing the recording of the volume of the calibration syringe with the measured volume. The volume of the syringe is stable for several years with careful handling of the syringe [8]. But at least once a year, the volume of the syringes must be controlled in order to fulfill the ATS/ERS standard, and it must be assured that the syringes are calibrated by a method acceptable for volume determination [8, 9]. Security for optimal volume and time registration can be obtained by using flow calibration as a supplement to the volume calibration. There are commercially available flow calibrators which can generate ATS test flow-volume curves [10–12], but there are more simple calibrators using decompression [13].

The software must immediately after the forced expiration be able to show the values necessary for evaluation of whether the maneuver fulfills the ATS/ERS criteria for start, end of test, and reproducibility so that is it possible to judge whether additional maneuvers are necessary.

9.2.4.1 The Most Common Errors, Problems, and Questions

- Insufficient maximal deep inspiration
- Lacking calibration of spirometer
- Inadequate reference material
- Use of bacterial filters? For political reasons, the answer is yes. Does it protect against infection? The answer is that the evidence is weak [1].
- Is it necessary to make corrections for temperature and barometric pressure? This depends on the spirometer.

9.2.4.2 Peak Expiratory Flow (PEF)

- The patient takes a complete breath in.
- The patient inserts the mouthpiece between the teeth and closes the lips around it.
- The neck must be extended (not hyperextended). A bent neck may change the mechanical conditions in the upper airways and consequently decrease PEF. The measuring device must be held correctly so that the reading is not compromised.
- The expiration should start without hesitation, and the force must be maximal from the beginning and last for 1–2 s.

At least three correctly performed maneuvers are needed. When the patient performs measurements on his/her own, it is important that he/she is correctly instructed. Regular control of the PEF technique and the PEF meter is an important part of the examination.

Ninety five percent of untrained subjects can reproduce the two highest PEF with a difference of 40 L $\cdot$ min^{-1} or below [2].

9.3   Diffusion Capacity

9.3.1   The Pulmonary Diffusion Capacity for CO:D$_L$CO

D$_L$CO is measured by a gas dilution technique where the principle is that an inert gas, e.g., He or CH_4, is used to determine the dilution volume and CO is used to measure the diffusion from air to blood. With the test, the CO uptake in the lungs is measured as the decrease of CO (from start to end) of a 10 s breath hold at TLC. The decrease is measured per L alveolar gas, per time unit, and per unit pressure difference across alveolar membrane (K_{CO}). When K_{CO} is multiplied by the alveolar volume V_A, which is single-breath TLC minus dead space, we get D$_L$CO, which is determined as mmol $\cdot$ min$^{-1} \cdot$ kPa^{-1} performed at TLC.

Table 9.1 Frequent causes of typical changes in D_LCO, K_{CO}, and V_A

Condition or disease	D_LCO	K_{CO}	V_A
Diffuse alveolar destruction			
Emphysema	Low	Very low	High
Pulmonary fibrosis, sarcoidosis	Low	Low	Low
Lung volume decrease			
Poor cooperation (submaximal inspiration)	Low	High	Low
Extrapulmonary restriction/neuromuscular disease	Low	High/normal	Low
Lung resection	Low	High	Low
Severe obesity	Normal/high	High	Low
Change in perfusion			
Primary pulmonary hypertension, pulmonary embolism	Low	Low	Normal
During exercise, left-right shunt	High	High	Normal

Different conditions and diseases can influence D_LCO (Table 9.1). They may influence both V_A and K_{CO} as well as either V_A or K_{CO}. V_A and K_{CO} are inversely correlated. In a less than optimally performed test with, e.g., insufficient inspiration to TLC, this may lead to a fall in V_A and an increase of K_{CO}, but only a modest fall in D_LCO.

The method has been subjected to considerable standardization and automation and can be executed in a short time. Despite the fact that several variations of the method have been introduced such as intrabreath, rebreathing, and steady-state techniques, the single-breath technique is still the most common method for clinical purposes [14].

1. After steady-state tidal breathing, the subject expires to RV.
2. Inhalation as fast as possible and 85 % of VI should be inspired in maximally 4 s of a calibrated gas mixture (e.g., 0.3 % CO, 10–14 % He, 18–21 % O_2 in N_2).
3. Hold the breath for 10($\pm$2) s at TLC.
4. Expiration as fast as possible and for max. 4 s. The first part contaminated with anatomical dead space and gas from the dead space of the equipment is discarded (V_D), typically 0.75–1 L. Then a sample of the alveolar gas is collected (sample volume (V_S) typically 0.5–1.0 L). If V_C is below 2 L, V_D and V_S may be reduced.
5. After at least 4 min, the procedure is repeated. The D_LCO values must differ less than 10 %, and 1 mmol min^{-1} kPa^{-1} or additional tests are performed. Finally, the mean value of the highest two values is reported.

The present brief description does not include children, where a number of special conditions, like equipment dead space and sampling volume, must be taken into account.

Sources of error which the clinician should pay attention to (when the laboratory is behind the quality control) should be contained in the report indicating the technical quality of the test.

Other points that should be recorded:
- Hb correction (because anemia reduces and polycythemia increases D_LCO).
- Smoking increases CO hemoglobin and back pressure and thereby reduces D_LCO.
- Oxygen supply increases F_IO_2 and causes reduction of D_LCO.

9.3.2   Determination of Diffusion Capacity from NO ($D_L NO$)

$D_L NO$ expresses like $D_L CO$ the ability of the lungs to transport oxygen from the alveoli to the lung capillaries. D_L is the total contribution from two components and can be expressed as $D_L = D_M + \Theta Vc$, where D_M is the membrane component (the alveolar-capillary component) and ΘV_c is the blood component with the reaction velocity Θ with hemoglobin in the capillary volume (V_c). In the classical method from 1957, Roughton and Foster [15] separated D_M and V_c by using a low and a high oxygen concentration, a method that requires arterial puncture preceded by oxygen breathing. In 1987 Guernard introduced a single-breath method which simultaneously measured $D_L CO$ and $D_L NO$ [16]. This method makes it possible to measure D_M and V_C and is based on the physiological assumption that the much higher reaction velocity of NO than of CO with hemoglobin causes the blood component to be neglected so that $D_L NO$ becomes a measure of D_M. This method is easy, fast, and relatively cheap. The inhaled gas consists of an inert gas and CO, O_2, and N_2, which is mixed with NO just before the measurement. The breath-hold time is between 4 and 8 s. But as breath-hold time is more critical for determination of $D_L NO$ than for $D_L CO$, it is important to standardize the procedure and to record this time both for healthy and diseased subjects. Furthermore, it is important to define the diffusion constants (alpha) based on molecular weight and solubility of CO and NO to 1.97 [16] or 2.42 [17]. $D_L NO$ is independent of the partial pressure of oxygen [18]. Regarding quality control, the same rules as for $D_L CO$ are required.

Application of D_M and V_C as markers of the severity of changes in the alveolar epithelium and/or the lung capillaries and ventilation/perfusion relationship has been more common after the introduction of $D_L NO$.

9.3.2.1 Selected Findings
- *Idiopathic interstitial pneumonia* ($n = 32$). D_M And V_c contribute equally to the decrease of D_L [19].
- *Cystic fibrosis* (CF) ($n = 17$) and *healthy controls* ($n = 17$). $D_L NO$ is significantly lower in CF than in resting controls. This difference is increased during exercise. Peak SaO_2, during exercise, is related to $D_L NO$ [20].
- *Cystic fibrosis* (CF) ($n = 21$). $D_L NO$ is significantly lower than $D_L CO$. Computed tomography Brody score correlates better with $D_L NO$ than with FEV_1, $_sRaw$, and RV/TLC [21].
- *Fontan patients* ($n = 87$) and *healthy controls* ($n = 9$). The study assessed possible determinants in the etiology of the reduction in diffusing capacity and found a reduced V_c (53 %) and a normal Dm (97 %) [22].

9.3.3   Calibration of Equipment for Measurement of $D_L CO$

Traditionally, the quality of measurement of diffusion capacity has only been secured by repeatability of the measurements and by the use of biological controls. It is, however, evident that in this way, you cannot secure no systematic errors in the accuracy of the measurements. Only by the use of a method that can be traced to international standards it is possible to evaluate the accuracy of the method. Hans Rudolph Inc. has developed equipment for calibration of diffusion capacity, based on traceable standards.

The method is based on the use of gas mixtures that simulate expired gas from a patient who has inspired a test gas similar to that applied in the measuring equipment, typically a mixture of CO and CH_4 (or He), O_2 and CO_2 in N_2. A calibrated 5.5 L syringe is used to simulate the D_LCO maneuvers: tidal breathing, maximal expiration, maximal inspiration, and breath hold. After breath-hold expiration from a 2.5 L syringe simulates low, middle, or high D_LCO depending on the calibration gas. V_I is known from the 5.5 L syringe; the expired gas concentration is known from the content of the 2.5 L syringe. The measured gas concentrations are known from the analyzers and breath-hold time from the software. It is now possible to calculate V_A and D_LCO and directly check the accuracy of the gas analyzers.

The calibration test gas is at ATPD, but results should be converted to BTPS, and breath-holding time must be well defined. There are different definitions of breath-holding time, and it is most common to define the breath-hold time according to Meade and Jones [23]. The breath-hold time starts after 1/3 of the inspired volume has been completed. As in spirometry [2], the back-extrapolation technique should be used to establish time zero.

The time when 90 % of the VI has been inspired is a reasonable end point for defining inspiratory time according to the ATS/ERS standard [14]. Breath-hold time ends when half of the expired sample has been exhaled.

9.4   Lung Volumes

9.4.1   Lung Volumes: Total Lung Capacity (TLC), Residual Volume (RV), Functional Residual Capacity (FRC), and Vital Capacity (VC)

Lung volumes are most often determined by the use of a body plethysmograph, but can also be measured by gas dilution techniques and by X-ray. Measurements take less than 10 min, and only claustrophobia and lacking ability of the patient to perform the test are relative contraindications. Determination of lung volumes is often necessary for the interpretation of lung function. Determination of lung volumes is extensively described in the ATS/ERS document: "Standardization of the measurement of lung volumes" [24] which should be consulted for further information.

9.5   Indication and Interpretation

The interpretation of lung function test is often complex. The desire to make a simple definition of COPD (FEV_1/FVC <0.7) is not based on scientific grounds, because FEV_1/FVC is age dependent, and too many false positives will be included.

COPD should be defined if both FEV_1 and FEV_1/FVC are less than the lower limit of normal (LLN), of the age and gender corrected reference material [25]. It is, however, our impression that sharp borders between normal and pathological conditions do not exist from a biological point of view, but might be useful to work with in guidelines. In practice this means that a subject suffers from COPD if FEV_1/FVC <0.4 (irreversibly decreased) and the subject does not suffer from COPD if FEV_1/FVC >0.8 [26]. In the interval between 0.4 and 0.8 one has to be careful. Values near LLN should cause suspicion and supplementary examination, or a visit to a specialist may be necessary.

The interpretation is further complicated, because spirometry alone in many cases is a sufficient examination, but not in other situations. Attempts to simplify the interpretation of a complex problem will lead to problems (as in the case of COPD above). It is only the clinician and the patient who together can decide how large a risk can be allowed in the individual case. Fortunately the complex of problems is straightforward in most cases, but in case of doubt or with spirometric values near LLN, the patient should be referred to D_LCO and lung volume measurements and/or repeat examination and consultation with a specialist in lung physiology (pulmonology or clinical physiology).

9.5.1 Indications for Pulmonary Function Testing

9.5.1.1 Symptoms
- Dyspnea at rest and during exercise
- Wheezing
- Cough
- Expectoration of phlegm and blood
- Thoracic pain that cannot be explained by other diseases

9.5.1.2 Pulmonary Disease, Disease in the Airways, Diagnostics, Monitoring, Classification of Severity, and Prognosis
- Asthma
- COPD
- Neoplasms
- Neuromuscular diseases
- Obliterating bronchiolitis
- Interstitial lung disease (for instance, sarcoidosis and pulmonary fibrosis)
- Occupational disease (for instance, asthma, asbestosis, allergic alveolitis)
- Medically induced lung diseases (for instance, by the use of nitrofurantoin or bleomycin)
- Bronchiectasis
- Ciliary dyskinesia
- Intrapulmonary hemorrhage
- Intra- and/or extrathoracic fixed or variable airway stenosis

9.5.1.3 Diseases with Lung Manifestations
- Tobacco dependence
- Infectious diseases (HIV and aspergillosis)
- Autoimmune diseases (for instance, arthritis and Sjôgren's disease)
- Immunodeficiency (for instance, serum-IgA deficiency)
- Cystic fibrosis
- Serum $alpha_1$-antitrypsin deficiency
- Graft versus host reaction

9.5.1.4 Legal Indications
- Insurance
- Occupational disease
- Doping and antidoping

9.5.1.5 Prevention and Treatment
- Preoperative risk assessment
- Prevention and treatment in diving
- Prevention and treatment in flying
- Advice in choice of inhalation equipment
- Advice in choice of ventilation strategy in ventilator insufficiency
- Advice regarding rehabilitation
- Advice regarding lung transplantation and lung volume reduction

9.5.2   Interpretation

All physicians treating patients with respiratory diseases must be familiar with the classification of ventilatory impairments as described in Fig. 9.2 (primary level). COPD and asthma are the most common obstructive diseases. They are seen with varying degrees of decreased diffusion capacity and/or increased TLC. Restrictively decreased ventilatory capacity is defined by decreased TLC. Take care always to evaluate all the curves and check them for errors. The repeatability criteria must be fulfilled.

9.6   Reference Material

We recommend the use of the ECCS reference material [27] for adult Caucasians until updated local reference values have been obtained. The stature must always be measured, and not told by the subject. Be aware of racial difference.

9.6.1   The Bronchodilatator Test (the Reversibility Test)

9.6.1.1 Indications
- Diagnostic: decreased FEV_1/VC and FEV_1/FVC ratio. Decreased FEV_1, VC, and PEF and/or increased RV
- Unclear response to previously done reversibility tests

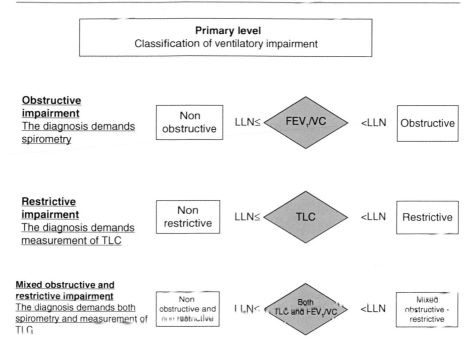

Fig. 9.2 Simplified algorithm representing typical patterns for changes in lung function and lung disease. This algorithm can be used in the clinic provided all values near the LLN are carefully interpreted. Some patients present typical patterns and others present atypical patterns and deviations from normal. The decision about how far the algorithm can be followed is clinical and depends on the questions you want to have answered and on the clinical information that is already available. The algorithm is not suited for clarifications of extrathoracic obstructions. When the results of the lung function tests are close to the border between normal and abnormal, more information is needed, and the evaluation may be in accordance with the specialist level (Fig. 9.3)

- Diagnosis of asthma
- Diagnosis, classification, and reclassification of COPD
- Determination of the maximal FEV_1 and FVC

9.6.1.2 Relative Contraindications
- Cardiac arrhythmia
- Pregnancy
- Cerebrovascular disease
- Known paradox reaction to bronchodilator

9.6.1.3 Be Aware of the Following
- A bronchodilator test cannot be used to evaluate whether a COPD patient has a benefit from bronchodilator treatment.
- Remember pause in medicine administration before the test.
- The test has a relatively low reproducibility and must therefore be repeated.
- An increase in FEV_1 and/or FVC >12 % and 200 ml is statistically significant.

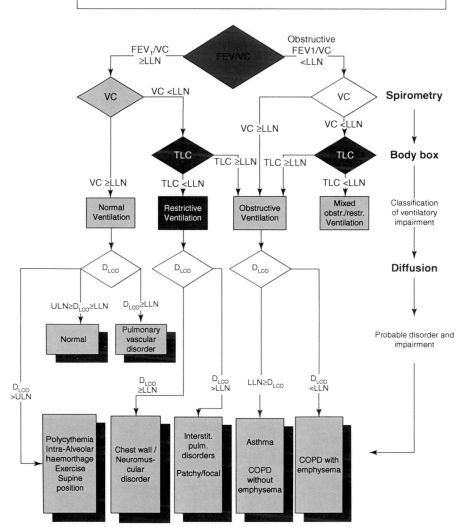

Fig. 9.3 Advanced algorithm including $D_L CO$

• The dose of bronchodilator must be sufficient to ensure maximal bronchodilation (for instance, inhalation of salbutamol pressurized metered dose inhaler given as four individual doses 0.1 mg each given via spacer and measurement of response after 15–30 min).

For simplification, FVC is used in the primary-level algorithm, whereas the more correct V_C is used in the more advanced algorithms in Fig. 9.3.

Conclusion

Lung function testing gives an idea about the functional status for the lungs but may not provide an etiological diagnosis of lung disease. Functional abnormalities may be present if the lung function values are outside the confidence limits of the reference values. This chapter only deals with spirometry and determination of D_LCO and K_{CO}, whereas determination of lung volumes is only superficially considered. The advantage of using D_LNO instead of D_LCO is mentioned. By this method the blood component can be neglected, and D_LNO will become a measure of the membrane component of the diffusing capacity and can be determined without arterial puncture. It is emphasized that rigorous calibration is necessary to obtain optimal results. Even the calibration syringes should be regularly checked and the volumes should be traceable to well-known standards.

References

1. Miller MR, Crapo R, Hankinson J, Brusasco V, Burgos F, Casaburi R, Coates A, Enright P, Grinten CPM, Gustafsson P, Jensen R, Johnson DC, Macintyre N, McKay R, Navajas D, Pedersen OF, Pellegrino R, Viegi G, Wanger J (2005) General considerations for lung function testing. Eur Respir J 26:153–161
2. Miller MR, Hankinson J, Brusasco V, Burgos F, Casaburi R, Coates A, Crapo R, Enright P, van der Grinten CP, Gustafsson P, Jensen R, Johnson DC, Macintyre N, McKay R, Navajas D, Pedersen OF, Pellegrino R, Viegi G, Wanger J (2005) Standardisation of spirometry. Eur Respir J 26:319–338
3. Cooper B, Steenbruggen I, Mitchell S, Severin T, Oostveen E, Burgos F, Mathys H, Normand H, Kivastik J, Leuppi J, Flezar M, Agnew M, Pedersen OF, Sorichter S, Brusasco V, Tonalk W, Palange P (2011) Hermes spirometry: the European spirometry driving licence. Breathe 7: 259–275
4. D'Angelo E, Prandi E, Milic-Emili J (1993) Dependence of maximal flow-volume curves on time course of preceding inspiration. J Appl Physiol 75:1155–1159
5. Akpinar-Elci M, Fedan KB, Enright PL (2006) FEV6 as a surrogate for FVC in detecting airways obstruction and restriction in the workplace. Eur Respir J 27:374–377
6. Pedersen OF (2006) FEV6: a shortcut in spirometry? Eur Respir J 27:245–247
7. Bellia V, Sorino C, Catalano F, Augugliaro G, Scichilone N, Pistelli R, Pedone C, Antonelli-Incalzi R (2008) Validation of FEV6 in the elderly: correlates of performance and repeatability. Thorax 63:60–66
8. Madsen F. Validation of spirometer calibration syringes. http://informahealthcare.com/doi/pdf/10.3109/00365513.2012.723739. Accessed 10 Oct 2012
9. NCCLS (1993) Determining performance of volumetric equipment, 1st edn. NCCLS, Villanova. Proposed guideline series NCCLS vol 4 nr 6, Villanova Pa: National Committee for Clinical laboratory standards. Date of first publication 1984. http://find.lib.uts.edu.au/search.do;jsessionid=0A4C9450890FA52CA19C75BD828BAB77?R=OPAC_b1179813
10. Hankinson JL, Gardner RM (1982) Standard waveforms for spirometric testing. Am Rev Respir Dis 126:362–364
11. Hankinson JL, Crapo RO (1995) Standard flow-time waveforms for testing of PEF meters. Am J Respir Crit Care Med 152:696–701
12. Hankinson JL, Reynolds JS, Das MK, Viola JO (1997) Method to produce American Thoracic Society flow-time waveforms using a mechanical pump. Eur Respir J 10:690–694

13. Pedersen OF, Naeraa N, Lyager S, Hilberg C, Larsen L (1983) A device for evaluation of flow recording equipment. Bull Eur Physiopathol Respir 19:515–520
14. Macintyre N, Crapo RO, Viegi G, Johnson DC, van der Grinten CP, Brusasco V, Burgos F, Casaburi R, Coates A, Enright P, Gustafsson P, Hankinson J, Jensen R, McKay R, Miller MR, Navajas D, Pedersen OF, Pellegrino R, Wanger J (2005) Standardisation of the single-breath determination of carbon monoxide uptake in the lung. Eur Respir J 26:720–735
15. Roughton FJ, Forster RE (1957) Relative importance of diffusion and chemical reaction rates in determining rate of exchange of gases in the human lung, with special reference to true diffusing capacity of pulmonary membrane and volume of blood in the lung capillaries. J Appl Physiol 11:290–302
16. Guenard H, Varene N, Vaida P (1987) Determination of lung capillary blood volume and membrane diffusing capacity in man by the measurements of NO and CO transfer. Respir Physiol 70:113–120
17. Tamhane RM, Johnson RL Jr, Hsia CC (2001) Pulmonary membrane diffusing capacity and capillary blood volume measured during exercise from nitric oxide uptake. Chest 120:1850–1856
18. Borland CD, Higenbottam TW (1989) A simultaneous single breath measurement of pulmonary diffusing capacity with nitric oxide and carbon monoxide. Eur Respir J 2:56–63
19. Wemeau-Stervinou L, Perez T, Murphy C, Polge AS, Wallaert B (2012) Lung capillary blood volume and membrane diffusion in idiopathic interstitial pneumonia. Respir Med 106:564–570
20. Wheatley CM, Foxx-Lupo WT, Cassuto NA, Wong EC, Daines CL, Morgan WJ, Snyder EM (2011) Impaired lung diffusing capacity for nitric oxide and alveolar-capillary membrane conductance results in oxygen desaturation during exercise in patients with cystic fibrosis. J Cyst Fibros 10:45–53
21. Dressel H, Filser L, Fischer R, Marten K, Muller-Lisse U, de la Motte D, Nowak D, Huber RM, Jorres RA (2009) Lung diffusing capacity for nitric oxide and carbon monoxide in relation to morphological changes as assessed by computed tomography in patients with cystic fibrosis. BMC Pulm Med 9:30
22. Idorn L, Hanel B, Jensen AS, Juul K, Reimers JI, Nielsen KG, Søndergaard L (2012) New insights into aspects of pulmonary diffusing capacity in Fontan patients. Cardiol Young 24:311–320
23. Jones RN, Meade F (1961) A theoretical and experimental analysis of anomalies in the estimation of pulmonary diffusing capacity by the single breath method. Q J Exp Physiol Cogn Med Sci 46:131–143
24. Wanger J, Clausen JL, Coates A, Pedersen OF, Brusasco V, Burgos F, Casaburi R, Crapo R, Enright P, van der Grinten CP, Gustafsson P, Hankinson J, Jensen R, Johnson D, Macintyre N, McKay R, Miller MR, Navajas D, Pellegrino R, Viegi G (2005) Standardisation of the measurement of lung volumes. Eur Respir J 26:511–522
25. Swanney MP, Ruppel G, Enright PL, Pedersen OF, Crapo RO, Miller MR, Jensen RL, Falaschetti E, Schouten JP, Hankinson JL, Stocks J, Quanjer PH (2008) Using the lower limit of normal for the FEV1/FVC ratio reduces the misclassification of airway obstruction. Thorax 63:1046–1051
26. Enright P, Studnica M, Zielinski J (2005) Spirometry to detect and manage chronic obstructive pulmonary disease and asthma in the primary care setting. Eur Respir Mon 10:1–14
27. Quanjer PH, Tammeling GJ, Cotes JE, Pedersen OF, Peslin R, Yernault J-C (1993) Lung volumes and forced ventilatory flows 1993 update. Eur Respir J 6(Suppl 16):5–40

Forced Oscillation Technique

10

Daniel Navajas, Raffaele L. Dellacà, and Ramon Farré

10.1 Introduction

Normal tidal breathing is produced by cyclic muscular pressure applied to the chest wall. The breathing flow generated by the driving pressure is determined by the mechanical properties of the respiratory system. Therefore, information on the mechanical properties of the airways and lung and chest wall tissues can be derived from the relationship between the driving pressure and the resulting flow. Airflow and volume changes are easily recorded with a pneumotachograph placed at the airway opening. Muscular pressure, however, cannot be directly measured. An alternative procedure is to place an esophageal balloon and to regard this recording as an estimate of pleural pressure. A noninvasive approach is to apply low-amplitude pressure oscillation with a loudspeaker connected to the mouth during spontaneous breathing. By using external excitation, it is possible to measure both the driving

D. Navajas (✉)
Unitat de Biofísica i Bioenginyeria, Universitat de Barcelona,
Casanova 143, E-08036 Barcelona, Spain

CIBER de Enfermedades Respiratorias, Bunyola, Spain

Institut de Bioenginyeria de Catalunya, Barcelona, Spain
e-mail: dnavajas@ub.edu

R.L. Dellacà
Bioengineering Department, Politencino di Milano, Milano, Italy
e-mail: raffaele.dellaca@polimi.it

R. Farré
Unitat de Biofísica i Bioenginyeria, Universitat de Barcelona,
Casanova 143, E-08036, Barcelona, Spain

CIBER de Enfermedades Respiratorias, Bunyola, Spain

Institut d'Investigacions Biomèdiques August Pi Sunyer, Barcelona, Spain
e-mail: rfarre@ub.edu

A. Aliverti, A. Pedotti (eds.), *Mechanics of Breathing*,
DOI 10.1007/978-88-470-5647-3_10, © Springer-Verlag Italia 2014

Fig. 10.1 Setup for measuring respiratory impedance (Z_{rs}) in spontaneous breathing patients. *LS* loudspeaker, *PN* pneumotachograph, *PT* pressure transducer, *BR* bias resistor, *MC* microcomputer

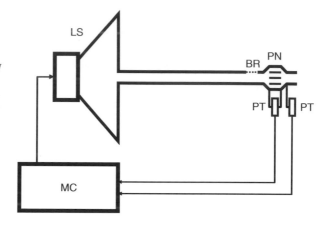

oscillatory pressure and the resulting oscillatory flow. This approach is known as the forced oscillation technique (FOT) [1, 2].

10.2   Forced Oscillation Technique Setup

A common FOT setup [3] used in clinical studies is shown in Fig. 10.1. The low-amplitude pressure oscillation (~2 cmH$_2$O, peak-to-peak) is generated by a loud-speaker attached to a chamber. The forced oscillation is applied to the mouth by means of a flexible hose (diameter of ~2 cm). The flow at the mouth (V'_{mo}) is measured with a pneumotachograph connected to a differential pressure transducer. A similar pressure transducer is used to measure mouth pressure (P_{mo}). A bias resistor (~1 cmH$_2$O $\cdot$ s/l) connected between the hose and the pneumotachograph allows the spontaneous breathing of the patient and avoids CO$_2$ rebreathing. A microcomputer generates the excitation signal to the loudspeaker. The same microcomputer is used for recording P_{mo} and V'_{mo} and for data processing. The oscillatory frequency (f_{os}) must be high enough to be separable from respiration. The equipment must be designed in accordance with published recommendations [4].

10.3   Data Processing

Figure 10.2 shows simultaneous pressure and flow recordings of 20 s obtained in a healthy subject with 2 Hz sinusoidal excitation superimposed onto the spontaneous breathing. The sinusoidal flow generated by the sinusoidal pressure excitation is clearly observed by zooming a 1 s fragment of the recording. In this example, a sinusoidal pressure amplitude (P_{os}) of 0.61 cmH$_2$O produced an oscillatory flow with amplitude (V'_{os}) of 0.19 l/s. Since the maximums and minimums of flow appear before those of pressure, it is said that flow leads pressure ($\Delta t = -0.070$ s). The corresponding phase lag of the oscillatory flow is $\varphi = 2\pi f_{os} \Delta t$ (−50.7°). The modulus of

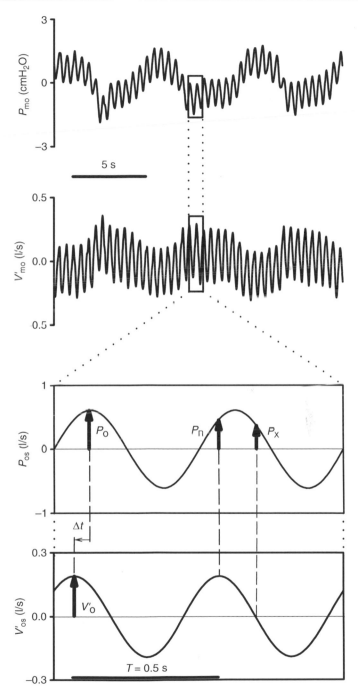

Fig. 10.2 Pressure (P_{mo}) and flow (V'_{mo}) recorded (20 s) at the mouth of a healthy subject during 2 Hz forced oscillation superimposed onto the spontaneous breathing. *Bottom*: zoom of a 1 s fragment of the oscillatory pressure (P_{os}) and flow (V'_{os}) obtained by digital filtering of P_{mo} and V'_{mo}. T period of oscillation, P'_o amplitude of pressure oscillation, V'_o amplitude of flow oscillation, Δt time lag between flow and pressure, P_R pressure at maximum oscillatory flow, P_X pressure at maximum oscillatory volume

impedance ($|Z|$) is defined as the amplitude ratio of applied oscillatory pressure and resulting oscillatory flow $|Z|=P_o/V'_o$ (3.1 cmH$_2$O·s/l). The amplitude and the phase lag of the induced flow oscillation depend on the mechanical load of the respiratory system. The greater the mechanical load, the lower the induced flow. The modulus and the phase lag define respiratory impedance (Z_{rs}), which fully characterizes the oscillatory mechanics of the respiratory system at this frequency. Nevertheless, Z_{rs} is more usually characterized by means of the oscillatory resistance (R_{rs}) and reactance (X_{rs}) which are more directly related to mechanical parameters of the respiratory system. R_{rs} accounts for the pressure component in phase with flow and can be computed as $R_{rs}=P_R/V'_o$, where P_R is the pressure at maximum flow and zero oscillatory volume (Fig. 10.2, bottom). X_{rs} is defined as $-P_X/V'_o$, where P_X is pressure at zero flow and maximum oscillatory volume. Therefore, X_{rs} accounts for the component of pressure out-of-phase with flow (in-phase with volume). In the example of Fig. 10.2, $R_{rs}=2.45$ cmH$_2$O·s/l and $X_{rs}=-2.00$ cmH$_2$O·s/l.

10.4   Modeling

Figure 10.3 shows the oscillatory impedance measured in the same subject at frequencies ranging from 2 to 16 Hz. R_{rs} varies little with frequency. By contrast, X_{rs} exhibits negative values at low frequencies and a marked frequency dependence, reaching positive values at frequencies higher than ~10 Hz. In healthy subjects, oscillation mechanics can be roughly represented by a simple model of the respiratory system composed of a series combination of resistance, elastance, and inertance (*R-I-E* model) (Fig. 10.3). Accordingly, R_{rs} is interpreted as the resistance of the total respiratory system (airways and tissues). In this simple model, $X_{rs}=I\cdot 2\pi f - E/2\pi f$, and, therefore, X_{rs} accounts for the elastic and inertial properties of the respiratory system. At low frequencies, X_{rs} is dominated by lung and chest wall elastance ($I\cdot 2\pi f \approx 0$) and at high frequencies by airway inertance ($E/2\pi f \approx 0$). The frequency where the elastic and inertial loads are counterbalanced ($X_{rs}=0$) is called frequency of resonance (f_R).

Fig. 10.3 Frequency dependence of respiratory impedance measured in a healthy subject. *Solid symbols*: respiratory resistance (R_{rs}); *hollow symbols*: respiratory reactance (X_{rs}). *Solid lines*: fit of the resistance-elastance-inertance (*REI*) model of the respiratory system (*right*)

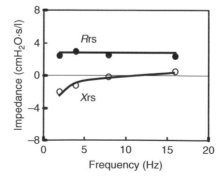

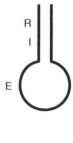

Fig. 10.4 Change in Z_{rs} due to upper airway obstruction

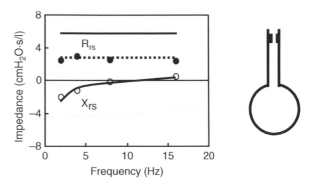

Fig. 10.5 Change in Z_{rs} due to peripheral airways obstruction or nonhomogeneous time constant distribution of lung units

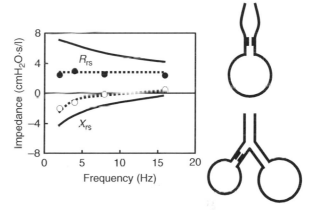

Changes in Z_{rs} observed in patients are interpreted by more complex mechanical models. An obstruction in upper or central airway resistance results in a parallel upward shift in R_{rs} with no change in X_{rs} (Fig. 10.4). By contrast, peripheral airway obstruction causes pendelluft between central airways and peripheral lung units. This leads to an increase in R_{rs}, which is more marked at low frequencies, and a decrease in X_{rs} with higher f_R (Fig. 10.5). A similar pattern of change can be observed in parallel pendelluft caused by nonhomogeneous time constant distribution of lung units.

10.5 Clinical Applications

FOT allows the assessment of respiratory mechanics, requiring no active patient cooperation during the physiological conditions of spontaneous breathing. Therefore, the technique is suitable for clinical applications [5, 6], particularly in infants/children [2] and in patients with severe cognitive or breathing impairment [7]. A number of studies have obtained reference values of R_{rs} and X_{rs} from adult and children populations with different anthropometric characteristics [8–11]. It should be pointed out, however, that the reference values published were collected by FOT methodologies which were not fully standardized. Accordingly, the reference values available at present should be considered only as indicative, particularly, in view of diagnostic applications.

The frequency dependence of R_{rs} and X_{rs} in different respiratory diseases, such as asthma, COPD, chronic bronchitis, early emphysema, interstitial disease, kyphoscoliosis, ankylosing spondylitis, neuromuscular diseases, obesity, and tracheostenosis, has been investigated and compared with normal controls [12–25]. FOT has also been used to characterize respiratory mechanics in occupational epidemiology [26–30]. The variations in R_{rs} and X_{rs} induced by postural changes, by modifying the mouth/nose route of breathing and by the phase of the breathing cycle, have also been evaluated in healthy subjects and in patients [31–37]. Although most clinical studies have been carried out in the frequency range ~4–30 Hz, a number of works have pointed out that extending FOT to frequencies lower and/or higher than usual may be of clinical interest [17, 38–46].

10.5.1 Assessment of Airway Obstruction in Responsiveness Tests

In contrast to forced spirometry, which is the most conventional technique for assessing lung mechanics, FOT does not require the performance of deep inspiration and expiration maneuvers. As the FOT measurement is carried out during spontaneous breathing, the bronchial tone is not modified. This makes FOT particularly useful in assessing the changes in respiratory mechanics induced by the inhalation of bronchodilator and bronchoconstrictor drugs. In this application, post- and pre-challenge R_{rs} and X_{rs} values are compared. As the patient is his/her own control, the need for accurate reference values is not critical to evaluate the effect of the inhaled agent. FOT has been used to assess the increase in airway obstruction induced by bronchial challenges with histamine, methacholine, cold air hyperventilation, carbachol, and glutathione [15, 47–61]. The technique has also been employed to measure the changes in respiratory impedance induced by bronchodilatation drugs [62–67]. As FOT provides a high-time resolution in the assessment of respiratory mechanics, it is useful in dose-response tests [68–70]. In these applications, FOT has a sensitivity and specificity similar to that of conventional spirometric and plethysmographic indices [71]. A number of studies report that, given the theoretical considerations, the capability of FOT in detecting changes after bronchial challenge may be improved by modifying the conventional setup and data analysis [72–76].

10.5.2 Assessment of Respiratory Mechanics in Patients Subjected to Ventilatory Support

Although the most conventional applications of FOT are carried out in spontaneously breathing patients, the technique can also be applied to patients subjected to ventilatory support though a nasal/facial mask or an endotracheal tube [77]. To this end, the typical FOT setup shown in Fig. 10.1 is modified so that it can be connected in parallel to an external positive pressure ventilator [78–80]. Alternatively, it has been suggested that the conventional ventilator is modified to generate the oscillation pressure simultaneously with the artificial ventilation waveform [81]. FOT has been applied in patients with the sleep apnea-hypopnea syndrome (SAHS) subjected to continuous positive airway pressure (CPAP) [82]. The technique has also been applied during invasive and noninvasive mechanical ventilation of patients with acute or chronic respiratory failure [78, 83].

An FOT feature that makes it particularly useful for quantifying the degree of airway obstruction during sleep is the time resolution of the technique. Indeed, when applying a single-frequency oscillation, the signal-to-noise ratio achieved is high enough to allow a time resolution capable of accurately tracking the changes in R_{rs} and X_{rs} along the breathing cycle [84, 85]. This possibility and the fact that FOT does not interfere with sleep [86] make it useful in the diagnosis of SAHS [84] and in the titration of the treatment CPAP value [87]. Moreover, it has been shown that FOT can be easily implemented to control automatic CPAP treatment adapted to the degree of patient impedance [3, 88]. Applications of FOT during mechanical ventilation, which are described in detail in another chapter of this book, may allow us to automatically monitor the mechanical status of ventilated patients and to adapt the ventilator settings to the evolution of the patient's respiratory mechanics.

10.5.3 Routine Monitoring of Respiratory Mechanics

Research data obtained in recent years suggest that FOT may be a useful tool for the routine management of chronic respiratory diseases such as asthma and COPD. Indeed, it has been shown that the short- and midterm variability of respiratory impedance measured by FOT can provide interesting information about the pathophysiology and progress of respiratory diseases, particularly asthma [89, 90]. Moreover, within-breath variability of FOT data, specifically respiratory reactance, provides an index to assess expiratory flow limitation, which is of special interest in COPD since these patients are prone to this respiratory alteration mainly in supine body posture [91, 92]. The fact that periodic monitoring of respiratory mechanics using FOT, both in the very short- and midterm, is informative of the potential response to treatments (such as bronchodilators or CPAP) suggests that this noninvasive technique could play an important role in monitoring the respiratory status of patients at home. This is indeed possible since it was shown that portable FOT devices [93] allow the patients to self-perform reliable measurements of R_{rs} and X_{rs} at home without intervention of healthcare staff [94]. Moreover, the application of information and communication technology tools into portable FOT devices has opened the door to telemetrically assessing respiratory mechanics at the patient's home [95].

Conclusions

FOT is a noninvasive method to assess respiratory mechanics without patient cooperation during spontaneous breathing and during mechanical ventilation. This technique is a tool for characterizing in detail the mechanics of the respiratory system to investigate the mechanisms of respiratory diseases [96]. In fact, there are considerable data available demonstrating that FOT is easily implemented and useful in a number of routine clinical applications. Published technical recommendations for FOT devices and measurement procedures [97], together with new developments in telemedicine applications, may increase the widespread use of this technique in clinical routine.

Acknowledgments This work was supported in part by the Spanish Ministry of Economy and Competitiveness (SAF2011-22576, FIS-PI11/00089).

References

1. Navajas D, Farré R (1999) Oscillation mechanics. Eur Respir Mon 12:112–140
2. Marchal F, Loos N (1997) Respiratory oscillation mechanics in infants and preschool children. Eur Respir Mon 5:58–87
3. Farré R, Rigau J, Montserrat JM, Ballester E, Navajas D (2001) Evaluation of a simplified oscillation technique for assessing airway obstruction in sleep apnea. Eur Respir J 17: 456–461
4. Van de Woestijne KP, Desager KN, Duiverman EJ, Marchal F (1994) Recommendations for measurement of respiratory input impedance by means of the forced oscillation method. Eur Respir Rev 4:235–237
5. Johnson BD, Beck KC, Zeballos RJ, Weisman IM (1999) Advances in pulmonary laboratory testing. Chest 116:1377–1387
6. Kaminsy DA, Irvin CG (2001) New insights from lung function. Curr Opin Allergy Clin Immunol 1:205–209
7. Carvalhaes-Neto N, Lorino H, Gallinari C, Escolano S, Mallet A, Zerah F, Harf A, Macquin-Mavier I (1995) Cognitive function and assessment of lung function in the elderly. Am J Respir Crit Care Med 152:1611–1615
8. Gimeno F, van-der Weele LT, Koeter GH, van Altena R (1992) Forced oscillation technique. Reference values for total respiratory resistance obtained with the Siemens Siregnost FD5. Ann Allergy 68:155–158
9. Pasker HG, Mertens I, Clement J, Van de Woestijne KP (1994) Normal values of total respiratory input resistance and reactance for adult men and women. Eur Respir Rev 4(19):134–137
10. Peslin R, Teculescu D, Locuty J, Gallina C, Duvivier C (1994) Normal values of total respiratory input impedance with the head generator technique. Eur Respir Rev 4(19):138–142
11. Ducharme FM, Davis GM, Ducharme GR (1998) Pediatric reference values for respiratory resistance measured by forced oscillation. Chest 113:1322–1328
12. Shindoh C, Sekizawa K, Hida W, Sasaki H, Takishima T (1985) Upper airway response during bronchoprovocation and asthma attack. Am Rev Respir Dis 132:671–678
13. Van Noord NJ, Clement J, Van-de Woestijne KP, Demedts M (1991) Total respiratory resistance and reactance in patients with asthma, chronic bronchitis, and emphysema. Am Rev Respir Dis 143:922–927
14. Cuijpers CE, Wesseling GJ, Swaen GM, Sturmans F, Wouters EF (1994) Asthma-related symptoms and lung function in primary school children. J Asthma 31:301–312
15. Klug B, Bisgaard H (1996) Measurement of lung function in awake 2–4 year old asthmatic children during methacholine challenge and acute asthma: a comparison of the impulse oscillation technique, the interrupter technique, and transcutaneous measurement of oxygen versus whole-body plethysmography. Pediatr Pulmonol 21:290–300
16. Lebecque P, Stanescu D (1997) Respiratory resistance by the forced oscillation technique in asthmatic children and cystic fibrosis patients. Eur Respir J 10:891–895

17. Chalker RB, Celli BR, Habib RH, Jackson AC (1992) Respiratory input impedance from 4 to 256 Hz in normals and chronic airflow obstruction: comparisons and correlations with spirometry. Am Rev Respir Dis 146:570–576

18. Wesseling GJ, Wouters EF (1992) Analysis of respiratory impedance characteristics in chronic bronchitis. Respiration 59:81–88

19. Govaerts E, Demedts M, Van-de WK (1993) Total respiratory impedance and early emphysema. Eur Respir J 6:1181–1185

20. Van Noord JA, Cauberghs M, Van de Woestijne KP, Demedts M (1989) Total respiratory resistance and reactance in patient with diffuse interstitial lung disease. Eur Respir J 2:846–852

21. Van Noord NJ, Cauberghs M, Van de Woestujne K, Demedts M (1991) Total respiratory resistance and reactance in ankylosing spondylitis and kyphoscoliosis. Eur Respir J 4:945–951

22. Wesseling G, Quaedvlieg FC, Wouters EF (1992) Oscillatory mechanics of the respiratory system in neuromuscular disease. Chest 102:1752–1757

23. Zerah LF, Lofaso F, Coste A, Ricolfi F, Goldenberg F, Harf A (1997) Pulmonary function in obese snorers with or without sleep apnea syndrome. Am J Respir Crit Care Med 156: 522–527

24. Horan T, Mateus S, Beraldo P, Araujo L, Urschel J, Urmenyi E, Santiago F (2001) Forced oscillation technique to evaluate tracheostenosis in patients with neurologic injury. Chest 120:69–73

25. Pankor HG, Schepers R, Clement J, Van-de Woestijne WK (1996) Total respiratory impedance measured by means of the forced oscillation technique in subjects with and without respiratory complaints. Eur Respir J 9:131–139

26. Wouters EF (1990) Total respiratory impedance measurement by forced oscillations: a noninvasive method to assess bronchial response in occupational medicine. Exp Lung Res 16: 25–40

27. Pairon JC, Iwatsubo Y, Hubert C, Lorino H, Nouaigui H, Gharbi R, Brochard P (1994) Measurement of bronchial responsiveness by forced oscillation technique in occupational epidemiology. Eur Respir J 7:484–489

28. Pham QT, Bourgkard E, Chau N, Willim G, Megherbi SE, Teculescu D, Bohadana A, Bertrand JP (1995) Forced oscillation technique (FOT): a new tool for epidemiology of occupational lung diseases? Eur Respir J 8:1307–1313

29. Cuijpers CE, Swaen GM, Wesseling G, Hoek G, Sturmans F, Wouters EF (1995) Acute respiratory effects of low level summer smog in primary school children. Eur Respir J 8:967–975

30. Pasker HG, Peeters M, Genet P, Clement J, Nemery B, Van-de- Woestijne KP (1997) Short-term ventilatory effects in workers exposed to fumes containing zinc oxide: comparison of forced oscillation technique with spirometry. Eur Respir J 10:1523–1529

31. Lorino AM, Lofaso F, Abi NF, Drogou I, Dahan E, Zerah F, Harf LH (1998) Nasal airflow resistance measurement: forced oscillation technique versus posterior rhinomanometry. Eur Respir J 11:720–725

32. Cauberghs M, Van-de-Woestijne K (1992) Changes of respiratory input impedance during breathing in humans. J Appl Physiol 73:2355–2362

33. Peslin R, Ying Y, Gallina C, Duvivier C (1992) Within-breath variations of forced oscillation resistance in healthy subjects. Eur Respir J 5:86–92

34. Davidson RN, Greig CA, Hussain A, Saunders KB (1986) Within-breath changes of airway calibre in patients with airflow obstruction by continuous measurement of respiratory impedance. Br J Dis Chest 80:335–352

35. Farré R, Peslin R, Rotger M, Barbera JA, Navajas D (1999) Forced oscillation total respiratory resistance and spontaneous breathing lung resistance in COPD patients. Eur Respir J 14: 172–178

36. Navajas D, Farré R, Rotger M, Milic-Emili J, Sanchis J (1988) Effect of body posture on respiratory impedance. J Appl Physiol 61:194–199

37. Michels A, Decoster K, Derde L, Vleurinck C, Van de Woestijne K (1991) Influence of posture on lung volumes and impedance of respiratory system in healthy smokers and nonsmokers. J Appl Physiol 71:294–299

38. Hall GL, Hantos Z, Wildhaber JH, Sly PD (2002) Contribution of nasal pathways to low-frequency respiratory impedance in infants. Thorax 57(5):396–399
39. Lutchen KR, Yang K, Kaczka DW, Suki B (1993) Optimal ventilation waveforms for estimating low-frequency respiratory impedance. J Appl Physiol 75:478–488
40. Kaczka DW, Ingenito EP, Suki B, Lutchen KR (1997) Partitioning airway and lung tissue resistances in humans: effects of bronchoconstriction. J Appl Physiol 82:1531–1541
41. Kaczka DW, Ingenito EP, Israel E, Lutchen KR (1999) Airway and lung tissue mechanics in asthma. Effects of albuterol. Am J Respir Crit Care Med 159:169–178
42. Kaczka IEP, Lutchen KR (1999) Technique to determine inspiratory impedance during mechanical ventilation: implications for flow limited patients. Ann Biomed Eng 27:340–355
43. Frey U, Suki B, Kraemer R, Jackson AC (1997) Human respiratory input impedance between 32 and 800 Hz, measured by interrupter technique and forced oscillations. J Appl Physiol 82:1018–1023
44. Frey U, Silverman M, Kraemer R, Jackson AC (1998) High frequency respiratory impedance in infants by forced oscillations. Am J Respir Crit Care Med 158:363–370
45. Frey U, Silverman M, Kraemer R, Jackson AC (1998) High frequency input impedance in infants assessed with the high speed interrupter technique. Eur Respir J 12:148–158
46. Frey U, Jackson AC, Silverman M (1998) Differences in airway wall compliance as a possible mechanism for wheezing disorders in infants. Eur Respir J 12:136–142
47. Holmgren D, Engstrom I, Bjure J, Sixt R, Aberg N (1993) Respiratory resistance and transcutaneous PO2 during histamine provocation in children with bronchial asthma. Pediatr Pulmonol 15:168–174
48. Van Noord JA, Clement J, Van de Woestijne KP, Demedts M (1989) Total respiratory resistance and reactance as a measurement of response to bronchial challenge with histamine. Am Rev Respir Dis 139:921–926
49. Snashall PD, Parker S, Phil M, Ten Haave P, Simmons D, Noble MIM (1991) Use of an impedance meter for measuring airways responsiveness to histamine. Chest 99:1183–1185
50. Echazarreta AL, Gomez FP, Ribas J, Sala E, Barbera JA, Roca J, Rodriguez-Roisin R (2001) Pulmonary gas exchange responses to histamine and methacholine challenges in mild asthma. Eur Respir J 17:609–614
51. Rodriguez-Roisin R, Ferrer A, Navajas D, Agusti AGN, Wagner PD, Roca J (1991) Ventilation-perfusion mismatch after methacholine challenge in patients with mild bronchial asthma. Am Rev Respir Dis 144:88–94
52. Weersink EJ, Elshout FJ, Van Herwaarden C, Folgering H (1995) Bronchial responsiveness to histamine and methacholine measured with forced expirations and with the forced oscillation technique. Respir Med 89:351–356
53. Wilson NM, Bridge P, Phagoo SB, Silverman M (1995) The measurement of methacholine responsiveness in 5 year old children: three methods compared. Eur Respir J 8:364–370
54. Ducharme FM, Davis GM (1998) Respiratory resistance in the emergency department: a reproducible and responsive measure of asthma severity. Chest 113:1566–1572
55. Decramer M, Demedts M, Van de Woestijne KP (1984) Isocapnic hyperventilation with cold air in healthy non-smokers, smokers and asthmatic subjects. Bull Eur Physiopathol Respir 20: 237–243
56. Wesseling GJ, Wouters EFM (1992) Respiratory impedance measurements in a dose-response study of isocapnic hyperventilation with cold air. Respiration 59:259–264
57. Wesseling GJ, Vanderhoven AI, Wouters EF (1993) Forced oscillation technique and spirometry in cold air provocation tests. Thorax 48:254–259
58. Schmekel B, Smith HJ (1997) The diagnostic capacity of forced oscillation and forced expiration techniques in identifying asthma by isocapnic hyperpnoea of cold air. Eur Respir J 10:2243–2249
59. Pennings HJ, Wouters EF (1997) Effect of inhaled beclomethasone dipropionate on isocapnic hyperventilation with cold air in asthmatics, measured with forced oscillation technique. Eur Respir J 10:665–671
60. Lorino AM, Lofaso F, Lorino H, Harf A (1994) Changes in respiratory resistance to low dose carbachol inhalation and to pneumatic trouser inflation are correlated. Eur Respir J 7: 2000–2004

61. Marrades RM, Roca J, Barbera JA, de Jover L, MacNee W, Rodriguez-Roisin R (1997) Nebulized glutathione induces bronchoconstriction in patients with mild asthma. Am J Respir Crit Care Med 156:425–430

62. Wouters EF, Landser FJ, Polko AH, Visser BF (1992) Impedance measurement during air and helium-oxygen breathing before and after salbutamol in COPD patients. Clin Exp Pharmacol Physiol 19:95–101

63. Van Noord JA, Smeets J, Clement J, Van de Woestijne KP, Demedts M (1994) Assessment of reversibility of airflow obstruction. Am J Respir Crit Care Med 150:551–554

64. Zerah F, Lorino AM, Lorino H, Harf A, Macquin MI (1995) Forced oscillation technique vs spirometry to assess bronchodilatation in patients with asthma and COPD. Chest 108:41–47

65. Pauwels JH, Desager KN, Creten WL, Van-der VJ, Van BH (1997) Study of the bronchodilating effect of three doses of nebulized oxitropium bromide in asthmatic preschool children using the forced oscillation technique. Eur J Pediatr 156:329–332

66. Hellinckx J, De BK, Demedts M (1998) No paradoxical bronchodilator response with forced oscillation technique in children with cystic fibrosis. Chest 113:55–59

67. Delacourt C, Lorino H, Herve-Guillot M, Reinert P, Harf A, Housset B (2000) Use of the forced oscillation technique to assess airway obstruction and reversibility in children. Am J Respir Crit Care Med 161:730–736

68. Sekizawa K, Sasaki H, Shimizu Y, Takishima T (1986) Dose-response effects of methacholine in normal and in asthmatic subjects. Relationship between the site of airway response and overall airway hyperresponsiveness. Am Rev Respir Dis 133:593–599

69. Duiverman EI, Neijens HJ, Van der Snee-van Smaalen M, Kerrebijn KF (1986) Comparison of forced oscillometry and forced expirations for measuring dose-related responses to inhaled methacholine in asthmatic children. Bull Eur Physiopathol Respir 22:433–436

70. Chinet T, Pelle G, Macquin-Mavier I, Lorino H, Harf A (1988) Comparison of the dose-response curves obtained by forced oscillation and plethysmography during carbachol inhalation. Eur Respir J 1:600–605

71. Mazurek HK, Marchal F, Derelle J, Hatahet R, Moneret VD, Monin P (1995) Specificity and sensitivity of respiratory impedance in assessing reversibility of airway obstruction in children. Chest 107:996–1002

72. Peslin R, Duvivier C, Didelon J, Gallina C (1985) Respiratory impedance measured with head generator to minimize upper airway shunt. J Appl Physiol 59:1790–1795

73. Cauberghs M, Van de Woestijne K (1989) Effect of upper airway shunt and series properties on respiratory impedance measurements. J Appl Physiol 66:2274–2279

74. Iwatsubo Y, Lorino H, Hubert C, Duvivier C, Peslin R, Pham QT, Moreau T, Hosselet JJ, Brochard P (1994) Measurement of respiratory impedance by forced oscillation: comparison of the standard and head generator methods. Eur Respir J 7:901–906

75. Marchal F, Mazurek H, Habib M, Duvivier C, Derelle J, Peslin R (1994) Input respiratory impedance to estimate airway hyperreactivity in children: standard method versus head generator. Eur Respir J 7:601–607

76. Farré R, Rotger M, Marchal F, Peslin R, Navajas D (1999) Assessment of bronchial reactivity by forced oscillation admittance avoids the upper airway artifact. Eur Respir J 13:761–766

77. Van de Woestijne K (1993) The forced oscillation technique in intubated, mechanically-ventilated patients [editorial]. Eur Respir J 6:767–769

78. Peslin R, Felicio-da SJ, Duvivier C, Chabot F (1993) Respiratory mechanics studied by forced oscillations during artificial ventilation. Eur Respir J 6:772–784

79. Farré R, Ferrer M, Rotger M, Navajas D (1995) Servocontrolled generator to measure respiratory impedance from 0.25 to 26 Hz in ventilated patients at different PEEP levels. Eur Respir J 8:1222–1227

80. Farré R, Rotger M, Montserrat JM, Navajas D (1997) A system to generate simultaneous forced oscillation and continuous positive airway pressure. Eur Respir J 10:1349–1353

81. Farré R, Manzini M, Rorger M, Ferrer M, Roca J, Navajas D (2001) Oscillatory resistanse measured during noninvasive proportional assist ventilation. Am J Respir Crit Care Med 164:790–794

82. Navajas D, Farré R, Rotger M, Puig-de-Morales M, Montserrat JM (1998) Assessment of air-flow obstruction during CPAP by means of forced oscillation in patients with sleep apnea. Am J Respir Crit Care Med 157:1526–1530

83. Farré R, Gavela E, Rotger M, Ferrer M, Roca J, Navajas D (2000) Non-invasive assessment of respiratory resistance in severe chronic respiratory patients with nasal CPAP. Eur Respir J 15:314–319

84. Badia JR, Farré R, Montserrat JM, Ballester E, Hernandez L, Rotger R, Rodriguez RR, Navajas D (1998) Forced oscillation technique for the evaluation of severe sleep apnoea/hypopnoea syndrome: a pilot study. Eur Respir J 11:1128–1134

85. Lorino AM, Lofaso F, Duizabo D, Zerah F, Goldenberg F, Pia d'Ortho M, Harf A, Lorino H (1998) Respiratory resistive impedance as an index of airway obstruction during nasal continuous positive airway pressure titration. Am J Respir Crit Care Med 158:1465–1470

86. Badia R, Farré R, Rigau J, Uribe L, Navajas D, Montserrat JM (2001) Forced oscillation measurements do not affect upper airway muscle tone or sleep in clinical studies. Eur Respir J 18:335–339

87. Montserrat JM, Badia JR, Farré R, Ballester E, Hernandez L, Navajas D (1999) Routine application of the forced oscillation technique (FOT) for CPAP titration in the sleep apnea/hypopnea syndrome. Am J Respir Crit Care Med 160:1550–1554

88. Randerath WJ, Parys K, Feldmeyer F, Sanner B et al (1999) Self adjusting nasal continuous positive airway pressure therapy base on measurement of impedance: a comparison of two different maximum pressure levels. Chest 116:991–999

89. Reddel HK, Taylor DR, Bateman ED, Boulet LP, Boushey HA, Busse WW, Casale TB, Chanez P, Enright PL, Gibson PG, de Jongste JC, Kerstjens HA, Lazarus SC, Levy ML, O'Byrne PM, Partridge MR, Pavord ID, Sears MR, Sterk PJ, Stoloff SW, Sullivan SD, Szefler SJ, Thomas MD, Wenzel SE, American Thoracic Society/European Respiratory Society Task Force on Asthma Control and Exacerbations (2009) An official American Thoracic Society/European Respiratory Society statement: asthma control and exacerbations: standardizing endpoints for clinical asthma trials and clinical practice. Am J Respir Crit Care Med 180:59–99

90. Frey U, Maksym G, Suki B (2011) Temporal complexity in clinical manifestations of lung disease. J Appl Physiol 110:1723–1731

91. Dellacà RL, Rotger M, Aliverti A, Navajas D, Pedotti A, Farré R (2006) Noninvasive detection of expiratory flow limitation in COPD patients during nasal CPAP. Eur Respir J 27:983–991

92. Dellacà RL, Pompilio PP, Walker PP, Duffy N, Pedotti A, Calverley PM (2009) Effect of bronchodilation on expiratory flow limitation and resting lung mechanics in COPD. Eur Respir J 33:1329–1337

93. Rigau J, Farré R, Roca J, Marco S, Herms A, Navajas D (2002) A portable forced oscillation device for respiratory home monitoring. Eur Respir J 19:146–150

94. Rigau J, Burgos F, Hernández C, Roca J, Navajas D, Farré R (2003) Unsupervised self-testing of airway obstruction by forced oscillation at the patient's home. Eur Respir J 22:668–671

95. Gulotta C, Suki B, Brusasco V, Pellegrino R, Gobbi A, Pedotti A, Dellacà RL (2012) Monitoring the temporal changes of respiratory resistance: a novel test for the management of asthma. Am J Respir Crit Care Med 185:1330–1331

96. Bates JHT, Irvin CG, Farre R, Hantos Z (2011) Oscillation mechanics of the respiratory system. Compr Physiol 1:1233–1272

97. Oostveen E, McLeod D, Lorino H, Farré R, Hantos Z, Desager K, Marchal F, ERS Task Force (2003) The forced oscillation technique in clinical practice: methodology, recommendations and future developments. Eur Respir J 22:1026–1041

Optoelectronic Plethysmography: Principles of Measurements and Recent Use in Respiratory Medicine

11

Andrea Aliverti and Antonio Pedotti

11.1 Introduction

Although the measurement of pulmonary ventilation by a spirometer or a pneumo-tachograph may appear to be a simple procedure, it is much more complicated than most realize. Temperature, humidity, pressure, viscosity, and density of gas influence the recording of its volume. Mouthpieces, face masks, and noseclips may introduce leaks and therefore cause losses, are impractical for prolonged measurement, limit the subject's mobility, introduce additional dead space, and thereby increase tidal volume. They also make the subject aware that his breathing is being measured and therefore interfere with the natural pattern of breathing and its neural control [1, 2]. Breathing through a mouthpiece and flowmeter or from a spirometer is extremely difficult in children or uncooperative adults; it cannot be used during sleep, to analyze phonation, and during weaning from mechanical ventilation may require excessive patient cooperation. During exercise, rebreathing from a spirometer or a bag-in-box system can only be done for short time periods, while integration of flow at the mouth suffers from integration drift, so that changes in absolute lung volume are not accurately recorded. A possible approach to solve this problem is to collect the expired gas, breath by breath, in a large spirometer (e.g., a Tissot spirometer) or in a large, gas-tight bag (e.g., a Douglas bag), which are then emptied through a precision gasometer. But even emptying the spirometer or the bag causes problems due to the gasometer, which may require intermittent calibration over time.

A. Aliverti, PhD (✉) • A. Pedotti
Dipartimento di Elettronica, Informazione e Bioingegneria,
Politecnico di Milano, Piazza Leonardo da Vinci, 32,
I-20133 Milano, Italy
e-mail: andrea.aliverti@polimi.it

A. Aliverti, A. Pedotti (eds.), *Mechanics of Breathing*,
DOI 10.1007/978-88-470-5647-3_11, © Springer-Verlag Italia 2014

11.1.1 Measurements of Chest Wall Motion

All these problems have induced investigators to attempt to measure ventilation indirectly by external measurement of chest wall surface motion [3]. The chest wall is defined by all the anatomical structures surrounding the lung and moving with it: the rib cage, diaphragm, abdominal content, and abdominal wall. Displacements of the lung are transmitted to the chest wall and vice versa, and, therefore, measurements of thoracoabdominal surface movement can be used to estimate lung volume variations. In the last decades, a number of devices and methods have been developed in order to allow measurements of the rib cage and abdominal motion, and, in parallel, several attempts have been made to define calibration methods able to estimate volume changes of the single compartments of the entire chest wall and of the lung from measurements of diameters, circumferences, or cross-sectional areas, such as the isovolume method [4], changing posture [5], natural breathing [6]. The validity of the calibration coefficients obtained experimentally to convert one or two dimensions to volume is generally limited to the estimation of tidal volume under conditions matched to those during which the calibration was performed. Numerous devices based on sensing belts positioned on the rib cage and abdomen or wearable garments embedding different kinds of sensors have been proposed. The sensor technology used in sensing belts can be quite different and includes mechanical transducers, such as capacitive elastic strain gauges [7] and piezoelectric films [8], ultrasound waves in rubber tubes [9], and optical fibers [10]. Respiratory inductive plethysmography (RIP) allows to measure changes of rib cage and abdominal cross-sectional areas, by two coils of insulated wire sewn inside elastic bands which are usually placed below the axillary line and above the umbilicus [11]. Variations in the self-inductance of the coil are proportional to the cross-sectional area enclosed by the coil, and, therefore, it varies as the rib cage and the abdomen expand and contract during respiration.

A variety of optical techniques using multiple video cameras combined with either light projected on the chest surface or reflective markers positioned on it have been proposed to track the changing shape of the thoracoabdominal surface during breathing and from this to calculate the enclosed volume. Optical methods based on structured light to analyze chest wall movement during breathing have been pioneered by Peacock et al. [12] and Saumarez [13], who proposed a technique for mapping the size and shape of the thoracoabdominal wall by projecting a grid on sheets of light creating contour lines on the visible surface of the torso, recording them by still or video cameras and reconstructing the shape from digital information. These systems, however, remained confined in few research applications. More recent advances, including color structured light systems [14], are nowadays opening new perspectives for the development of more automatic procedures to process the data and to obtain chest wall surface movement and volume variations during breathing. These systems are still in their development phase, however.

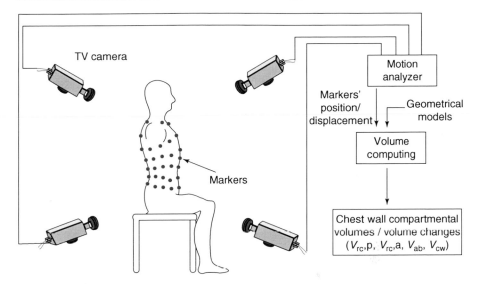

Fig. 11.1 Optoelectronic plethysmography (OEP): principle of measurement

11.1.2 Optoelectronic Plethysmography

Optoelectronic plethysmography (Fig. 11.1) is a now-established technique, based on typical methods for optical motion analysis, that allows to measure the variations of the volume of the chest wall and its compartments during breathing [15, 16]. A number of reflective markers are positioned by a hypoallergenic tape on the trunk of the subject in selected anatomical reference sites of the rib cage and the abdomen.

A set of cameras is placed nearby the subject under analysis. Each camera is equipped with an illuminator (infrared light-emitting diodes) that determines a high contrast between the reflective marker and the rest of the scene on the recorded image, thus allowing the fully automatic recognition of the markers. When a single marker is seen by two or more cameras, its position (defined by the three-dimensional coordinates in the reference system of the laboratory) can be calculated by stereophotogrammetry, being known the position, orientation, and the internal parameters of each camera. Once the 3D coordinates (X, Y, Z) of the points belonging to the chest wall surface are acquired with reference to an arbitrary coordinate system (Fig. 11.2), a closed surface is defined by connecting the points to form triangles (mesh of triangles) (Fig. 11.3). For each triangle, the area (A_i) and the direction of the normal of the plane defined by that triangle are determined. Successively, the internal volume of the shape is computed using Gauss' theorem (or divergence theorem, or Green's theorem in space).

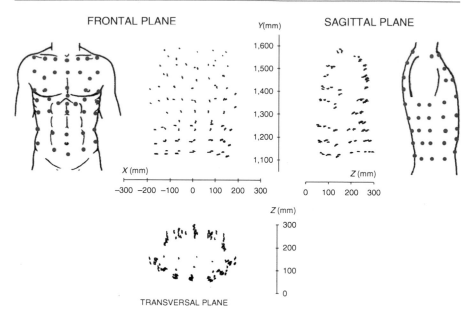

Fig. 11.2 Trajectories in the frontal (*X-Y* axes), sagittal (*Y-Z* axes), and transversal (*X-Z* axes) planes of the markers placed on the chest wall surface (during quiet spontaneous breathing). From markers' displacement, the variations of the enclosed volume is computed (see Fig. 11.3)

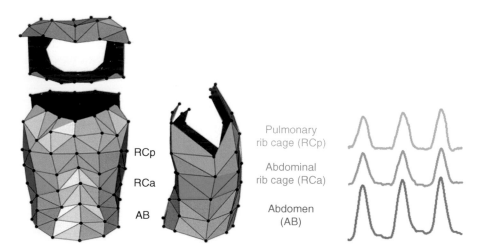

Fig. 11.3 Geometrical models of the three chest wall compartments: pulmonary rib cage (*RCp*), abdominal rib cage (*RCa*), and abdomen (*AB*) (*left*, three views) and their volume changes during quiet spontaneous breathing, respectively, $V_{rc,p}$; $V_{rc,a}$; and V_{ab}. Chest wall volume (V_{cw}) is equal to $V_{rc,p} + V_{rc,a} + V_{ab}$

Let S_{cw} be the closed chest wall surface S_{cw} enclosing the volume V_{cw}, and let $\vec{F}$ be a vector field defined at every point of V_{cw} then

$$\int_{S_{cw}} \vec{F} \cdot \vec{n} \, dS_{cw} = \int_{V_{cw}} \nabla \vec{F} \, dV_{cw} \tag{11.1}$$

where:

S_{cw} is the chest wall surface

V_{cw} is the volume enclosed by S_{cw}

$\vec{F}$ is an arbitrary vector

$\vec{n}$ is the outward-pointing unit normal vector at the different points of S_{cw}

∇ is the divergence operator

If we choose an arbitrary vector with a unit divergence, Eq. 11.1 becomes

$$\int_{S_{cw}} \vec{F} \cdot \vec{n} \, dS_{cw} = \int_{V_{cw}} dV_{cw} = V_{cw} \tag{11.2}$$

and the volume integral is computed by means of an easier surface integral.

Passing from continuous to discrete form, Eq. 11.2 becomes

$$\sum_{i=1}^{K} \vec{F} \cdot \vec{n}_i A_i = V_{cw} \tag{11.3}$$

where:

K is the total number of the triangles

A_i is the area of the ith triangle

$\vec{n}$ is the normal unit vector of the ith triangle

This procedure allows the direct computation of the volume enclosed by the thoracoabdominal surface approximated by a closed mesh of triangles.

11.2 Measurement of Chest Wall Compartmental Volumes

The markers are positioned on approximately horizontal rows at the levels of the clavicular line, the manubriosternal joint, the nipples, the xiphoid process, the lower costal margin, the umbilicus, and the anterior superior iliac crest [15]. Surface landmarks for the vertical lines are the midlines, both anterior and posterior axillary lines, the midpoint of the interval between the midline and the anterior axillary line, the midpoint of the interval between the midline and the posterior axillary line, and the midaxillary lines. Extra markers are added bilaterally at the midpoint between the xiphoid and the most lateral portion of the 10th rib and in corresponding posterior positions.

Markers' positioning is designed to allow an adequate sampling of the complex shape of the thoracoabdominal surface and an adequate subdivision of total chest

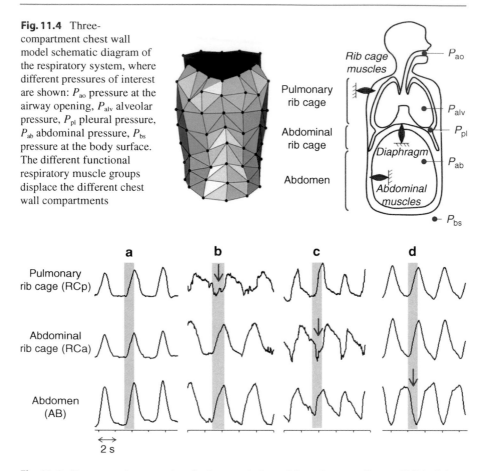

Fig. 11.4 Three-compartment chest wall model schematic diagram of the respiratory system, where different pressures of interest are shown: P_{ao} pressure at the airway opening, P_{alv} alveolar pressure, P_{pl} pleural pressure, P_{ab} abdominal pressure, P_{bs} pressure at the body surface. The different functional respiratory muscle groups displace the different chest wall compartments

Fig. 11.5 Representative examples of volume variations of the pulmonary rib cage (*RCp*), abdominal rib cage (*RCa*), and abdomen (*AB*) during quiet breathing. (**a**) Normal healthy subject. (**b**) Patient with type III osteogenesis imperfecta, presenting inspiratory paradoxical inward motion of the RCp. (**c**) Patient with chronic obstructive pulmonary disease (COPD), presenting inspiratory paradoxical inward motion of the RCa. (**d**) Patient with late-onset type II glycogenosis, presenting inspiratory paradoxical inward motion of the AB due to diaphragmatic severe weakness. *Gray area*: inspiration. Paradoxical motion is shown by the *red arrows*

wall volume into different compartments. The geometrical models of the compartments that have been developed for OEP volume measurements follow the three-compartment model, composed by the pulmonary rib cage (RCp), the abdominal rib cage (RCa), and the abdomen (AB) [15–18]. The rib cage is separated from the abdomen by the line of markers placed on the lower costal margin. The subdivision of the rib cage into RCp ad RCa is defined by the transverse section at the level of the xiphoid [19]. Precisely, the surface that encloses RCp extends from the clavicles to the line of markers extending transversely at the level of the xiphisternum, while RCa extends from this line to the lower costal margin. AB extends caudally from the lower costal margin to the level of the anterior superior iliac crest.

The three-compartment model of the chest wall takes into consideration that the lung- and diaphragm-apposed parts of the rib cage (RCp and RCa, respectively) are exposed to substantially different pressures on their inner surface during inspiration (pleural pressure and abdominal pressure, respectively), that the diaphragm acts directly only on RCa and not on RCp, and that non-diaphragmatic inspiratory muscles (i.e., external intercostal, parasternals, scalene, neck muscles) act largely on RCp and not on RCa. Abdominal volume change is defined as the volume swept by the abdominal wall, as described by Konno and Mead [20], and it is the result of the action of the diaphragm and expiratory abdominal muscles (internal and external obliques, rectus, and transversus) (Fig. 11.4). As these three compartments are exposed to different pressures and to the action of different respiratory muscle groups, their movement is in principle independent. This is shown in Fig. 11.5. While in healthy subjects the three compartments generally move synchronously, in different diseases, different asynchronous movement between the three chest wall compartments can be found, typically as paradoxical inward motion in either the pulmonary rib cage (e.g., in osteogenesis imperfecta, due to rib cage deformities), the abdominal rib cage (e.g., in chronic obstructive pulmonary disease, COPD, due to lung hyperinflation and the consequent flattened diaphragm), or the abdomen (e.g., in late-onset type II glycogenosis, due to diaphragm paralysis). OEP allows also to split each compartment into its right and left parts, where asynchronies can also be found, e.g., in the presence of diaphragm hemiparalysis or hemiplegia.

11.3 Accuracy of Measurement of Lung Volume Variations

In the last years, different protocols of OEP have been developed for different experimental and clinical situations. The validation of these measurement protocols was always performed by comparing the chest wall volume variation, measured by OEP, with lung volume variations measured by a spirometer or integrating a flow measurement at the airway opening. In the first studies, volume changes were compared in healthy subjects while sitting or standing and wearing 89 markers, during quiet breathing, slow vital capacity maneuvers [15], and incremental exercise on a cycle ergometer [18]. In these conditions, the coefficient of variation of the two signals was always lower than 4 %. Successively, OEP was validated in constrained postures, like the supine and prone position. In these situations, the analysis is performed placing the markers only in the visible part of the trunk surface, while the inferior part is considered fixed with the support (e.g., the bed). The volumes measured using OEP were also compared with measurements taken using spirometry and pneumotachography both in healthy subjects during quiet and deep breathing on rigid and soft supports in supine and prone position [16] and in sedated and paralyzed patients with acute lung injury and acute respiratory distress syndrome while receiving continuous positive pressure ventilation or pressure support ventilation [21]. Tidal volume measurements of OEP, spirometry, and pneumotachography were always highly correlated with discrepancies lower than 5 %.

More recently, simultaneous measurements of tidal volume by OEP and pneumotachography demonstrated that OEP is able to provide accurate measurements of tidal volume values in newborns at rest [22] and in healthy men and women during submaximal (-2.0 ± 7.2 %) and maximal (2.4 ± 3.9 %) cycling exercise [23]. OEP has also recently shown to accurately evaluate vital capacity in the supine position in patients with respiratory muscle dysfunction of variable severity, including those with paradoxical abdominal movements [24]. Intra-rater and inter-rater reliability of OEP was evaluated on at rest and during cycle-ergometer submaximal exercise [25], and results showed intraclass correlation coefficient values higher than 0.75 and coefficient of variation of method error values less than 10 % for most variables in both conditions.

11.4 Double Plethysmography

Although the results obtained in all the above-cited validation studies have shown a very good agreement between chest wall and lung volume variations, it is important to remind that the two measurements are not necessarily equal. Gas compression and dilation and possible blood shifts into and out of the thorax might produce relevant differences between variation of gas and chest volumes, particularly during maneuvers in which intrathoracic pressures change significantly. When, for example, the respiratory system is subjected to large positive or negative pressures (e.g., during mechanical ventilation, during active expiration with occluded airways or in the presence of expiratory flow limitation, during inspiratory efforts with occluded airways), changes in V_{cw} equal changes in lung gas volume (ΔV_L), plus the volume of any blood shifts from the thorax to extremities or vice versa (V_B): $\Delta V_{cw} = \Delta V_L + V_B + \Delta V_L$ is the sum of the volume of gas expired (or inspired) at the mouth (V_M) plus the volume of gas compressed (or dilated) in the lung (V_C) and therefore $\Delta V_{cw} = V_M + V_B + V_C$. Recently, OEP was combined to whole-body plethysmography (WBP) which measures changes in body volume which are equal to $V_M + V_C$. WBP is insensitive to blood shifts, whereas OEP measures the same variables as WBP plus any blood shifts between the trunk and the extremities (Fig. 11.6).

In a series of experiments, simultaneous measurements of OEP and WBP allowed to measure VB continuously with the so-called double plethysmography [26, 27]. It was shown that outflow from the splanchnic blood reservoir is controlled by abdominal pressure, and that during quiet breathing with diaphragm descent, the diaphragm serves two functions, i.e., to ventilate the lung and to shift blood from the splanchnic vascular bed to the extremities. With simultaneous contraction of abdominal muscles, such as occurs during exercise [17], the circulatory function of the diaphragm can be considerably enhanced. Under appropriate circumstances, the diaphragm's circulatory function combined with abdominal muscle contraction can act as an abdominal circulatory pump, capable of acting as an auxiliary heart.

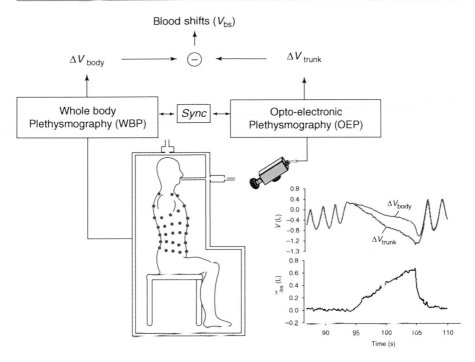

Fig. 11.6 Double plethysmography: principle of measurement (see text). The graphs on the bottom right show simultaneous recordings of total body volume variations (*red line*) and trunk volume variations (*blue line*) (top tracings) during a ramp increase in P_{ab}, while P_{pl} remained unchanged. The volume of blood shifted from the trunk to the extremities (V_{bs}) is shown in the bottom tracing (Modified from Aliverti et al. [26])

11.5 Measurement of End-Expiratory Lung Volume Variations

The measurement of end-expiratory lung volume (EELV) is of scientific and clinical importance in understanding respiratory mechanics. Unfortunately, continuous monitoring of EELV in normals and patients presents technical difficulties. Gas dilution techniques cannot be used for continuous monitoring because of the long wash-in/washout time, while the accuracy of RIP in monitoring EELV has also been questioned. Flowmeters cannot be used for long periods, mainly because integration of flow at the mouth suffers from integrator drift, so that changes in absolute lung volume are not accurately recorded. In fact, when flow is integrated to provide volume, an upward or downward drift in the volume baseline is invariably seen due to both physiological reasons and methodological errors: not unitary respiratory exchange ratio, differences in temperature and gas composition between inspiration and expiration, leaks between the airway opening and pneumotachometer, zero offset in flow calibration, and imperfections in the pneumotachometer response. In principle, it might be possible to avoid drift in volume by preconditioning the inspired gas to BTPS conditions, continuously monitoring gas partial pressures in both the alveoli and the pulmonary arterial and venous blood to correct for respiratory exchange ratios not equal to unity, and eliminating all the factors mentioned above. However, this is extremely difficult, if not impossible, in practice. Consequently, it is never known how much of the baseline drift in volume is due to drift and how much represents a true change in absolute lung volume. Drift correction algorithms first assess the upward or downward trend in functional residual capacity (FRC) over a period containing many breaths in which the subject is assumed to be in the physiological steady state and the assumption generally made is that FRC remains more or less constant; successively, the algorithm removes the trend. Although OEP cannot provide the absolute lung volume unless the subdivisions of lung volumes are known, it appears to be a suitable method for estimating its variations and measuring breath-by-breath EELV changes, as well as its distribution in the different chest wall compartments. End-expiratory volume variations of the chest wall (ΔEEV_{cw}) measured breath by breath by OEP before, during, and after an increase/decrease in positive end-expiratory pressure were compared with the corresponding variations of EEVL measured by the helium (He) dilution technique [28]. The regression line between EEVL changes measured by He and EEV_{cw} changes measured by OEP was very close to identity. OEP measurements of EEV_{cw} accurately reflect the changes of EEVL. Furthermore, OEP allows a continuous compartmental analysis, even during unsteady conditions, and this feature to track end-expiratory and end-inspiratory chest wall volume is extremely useful during incremental exercise as an alternative to serial measurements of inspiratory capacity (IC). This procedure, usually adopted for determining EELV changes during exercise, has inherent problems, namely, (a) the requirement of a high level of patient's collaboration, (b) the assumption that total lung capacity is reached at every maneuver performed by the subject, (c) that the maneuver is started from a volume that is representative of EELV, (d) the assumption that TLC does not change, and (e) the impossibility of track EELV on a breath-by-breath basis. Vogiatzis et al. [29] compared simultaneous measurements of inspiratory capacity (IC) at rest and during incremental cycle exercise in a group of male and female patients with stable COPD. Changes in IC from quiet breathing measured by the spirometer were in good relationship with end-expiratory chest wall volume variations obtained by OEP during exercise and recovery from exercise, with a mean difference between these two measurements throughout all stages equal to 7.0 (5.8)% or 35 (24) ml.

11.5.1 Studies Based on Optoelectronic Plethysmography in Health

In the last decade, a high number of studies employing OEP to study chest wall kinematics in various conditions have been performed, both in health and disease.

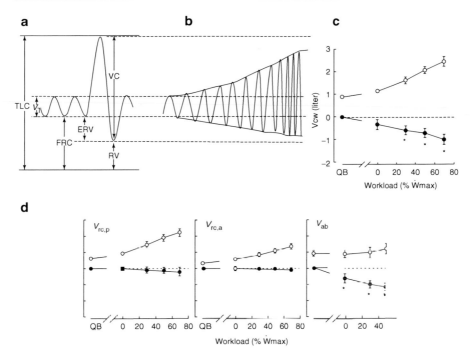

Fig. 11.7 (a) Normal spirogram (*TLC* total lung capacity, *FRC* functional residual capacity, *ERV* expiratory reserve volume, *RV* residual volume, *VC* vital capacity, V_T tidal volume). (b) Schematic diagram of the variations of V_T during incremental exercise in healthy subjects. (c) Chest wall volume (V_{cw}) during exercise. The difference between end-inspiratory (*open circles*) and end-expiratory V_{cw} (*closed circles*) is V_T. *Dashed line*, end-expiratory V_{cw} during quiet breathing (*QB*). (d) End-inspiratory (*open symbols*) and end-expiratory (*closed symbols*) mean volumes of the pulmonary rib cage ($V_{rc,p}$), abdominal rib cage ($V_{rc,a}$), and abdomen (V_{ab}) during exercise (Modified from Aliverti et al. [17])

Here below is not provided a comprehensive literature analysis, but only a summary of the main findings achieved so far.

Healthy subjects were analyzed during exercise, both on a cycle ergometer [17, 18, 30, 31] and during walking on a treadmill [32]. In both modalities, end-expiratory lung volume is reduced because of the recruitment of the expiratory muscles, and this reduction increases with the intensity of exercise. During heavy exercise, about one third of the tidal volume is accomplished below FRC, and about 40 % of the increase in tidal volume is attributable to the recruitment of expiratory reserve volume. The reduction in end-expiratory total chest wall volume is almost entirely due to a decrease in end-expiratory volume of the abdomen (Fig. 11.7).

End-expiratory volumes of both rib cage compartments do not change significantly. As the end-inspiratory displacement of the abdomen is nearly constant during exercise, the increase in end-inspiratory lung volume is almost entirely due to rib cage expansion. In other words, during exercise, the increase in rib cage tidal volume results from recruiting only its inspiratory reserve volume, while the increase in abdominal tidal volume largely resulted from recruiting only its expiratory reserve volume. Despite different recruitment patterns, the relative contributions to tidal volume from the different compartments remain nearly constant, although the tidal volume more than triples during exercise.

In other conditions than exercise, a detailed analysis of total and compartmental chest wall volumes allows to better understand mechanisms underlying different functions provided by the respiratory muscles. In a recent study investigating cough mechanics in health, it was shown how operating total and compartmental chest wall volumes are the most important determinant of the peak flow achieved and volume expelled during coughing [33]. Binazzi et al. [34] studied chest wall kinematics during reading, singing, and whispering. They found that the activity of the control of expiration during phonation is more complex than during exercise and all the three chest wall compartments contribute to the decrease of the total end-expiratory chest wall volume. Similar complex mechanisms of interaction between non-diaphragmatic inspiratory muscles and expiratory muscles are adopted during professional flute playing and allow the control of sound production that results in "breath support" which in turn is associated with high-quality playing [35].

11.5.2 Optoelectronic Plethysmography Studies in Disease

11.5.2.1 Chronic Obstructive Pulmonary Disease (COPD)

OEP has been extensively used to evaluate total and compartmental volume variations during incremental exercise in COPD patients. It was found that the patients with more severe COPD showed dynamic hyperinflation during incremental exercise, but other patients, specifically those with a greater expiratory flow reserve at rest, adopted the more "normal" approach of reducing EEV_{cw} when they exercised [36]. The presence in COPD patients of two distinct groups, those that strongly recruited abdominal muscles and those that did not, was confirmed in a subsequent study [37]. Among the patients who developed DH at maximal exercise, at least two significantly different patterns of change in EEV_{cw} were observed during the test [29, 38]. Some patients had a progressive significant increase in end-expiratory volume of the chest wall ("early hyperinflators") (Fig. 11.8), while in other patients, this remained unchanged up to about 66 % of maximum workload and increased significantly only in the last third period of exercise ("late hyperinflators").

The essential difference between euvolumics and hyperinflators is the degree of expiratory muscle recruitment. The kinematic difference, in fact, is in the behavior of the abdomen. During exercise, in some patients with COPD, excessive expiratory muscle recruitment occurs and the high expiratory pressures have adverse circulatory effects, namely, decreased cardiac output and blood shifts from the trunk to extremities. In addition, the oxygen cost of breathing is so high in COPD that it can become a very large percentage of total body oxygen uptake. This can establish competition between respiratory and locomotor muscles for the available oxygen supply at low exercise workloads and this can be a potent factor limiting exercise

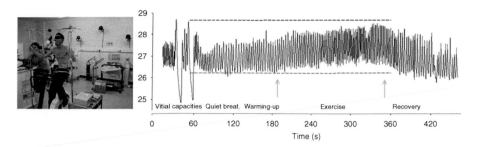

Fig. 11.8 *Left*: a COPD patient analyzed by OEP during exercise on a cycle ergometer at Aintree University Hospital, Liverpool, UK. *Right*: representative tracing showing chest wall volume variations during two vital capacity maneuvers, spontaneous quiet breathing at rest, warming up, incremental exercise, and recovery from exercise. Note dynamic hyperinflation of the chest wall during the period of exercise. *Red dashed* tracings indicate chest wall volume at FRC and TLC

performance in COPD [39]. In a series of complex experiments employing OEP, cardiac output, and peripheral muscle oxygen measurements, it has been recently shown that the heliox breathing during exercise improves peripheral muscle oxygen availability with different mechanisms in hyperinflator and non-hyperinflator COPD patients. In hyperinflators, heliox increases arterial oxygen content and quadriceps blood flow at similar cardiac output, whereas in non-hyperinflators, heliox improves central hemodynamics and increases systemic vascular conductance and quadriceps blood flow at similar arterial oxygen content [40, 41].

It is not yet clear why COPD patients adopt different patterns of end-expiratory rib cage and abdominal volume variations during exercise. Nevertheless, this seems at least partially dependent of the presence of lower ribcage inspiratory inward paradoxical motion that is present at rest in several COPD patients [42, 43]. In a recent study, it was shown that total end-expiratory chest wall volume increased immediately when exercise began ("early hyperinflation") in patients presenting lower rib cage paradox at rest, but later ("late hyperinflation") in patients with synchronous rib cage motion [42].

11.5.2.2 Thoracic Surgery

Three different, distinct patterns of breathing and chest wall volume regulations were found in severe patients with COPD, interstitial pulmonary fibrosis (IPF), and cystic fibrosis (CF) adopted by the ventilatory pump to cope with chronic respiratory failure [44]. The same authors demonstrate that after lung transplantation (LTx), the chronic adaptations of the ventilatory pattern to advanced lung diseases are reversible, and that the main contributing factor is the lung itself rather than systemic effects of the disease. Another study performed in patients affected by cystic fibrosis treated with bilateral LTx demonstrated a rearrangement of the volumes of the different compartments, with a significant abdominal volume reduction, and lower rib cage increase, suggesting diaphragm repositioning [45].

Other studies employed OEP to assess the effects of laparoscopic surgery on chest wall kinematics and inspiratory muscle activity [46] and to study the effects of

Nuss surgical technique for pectus excavatum on chest wall function at rest and during exercise [47–49].

11.5.2.3 Neuromuscular Disorders

In Duchenne muscular dystrophy (DMD) patients, abdominal motion during spontaneous breathing in awake conditions and in supine position has been proven to be not only an important indicator of the degree of respiratory muscle impairment and disease progression but also an early indicator of nocturnal hypoxemia [50]. Inefficient cough in DMD, moreover, is associated with reduced operating lung and chest wall volume secondary to weakened inspiratory muscles. Abdominal contribution to tidal volume during spontaneous breathing has been shown to be a non-volitional and noninvasive index able to discriminate efficient and inefficient cough [51]. In adolescent and adult DMD patients who present either no sign or only mild nocturnal oxygen desaturation, a reduced abdominal contribution to inspiratory capacity is a specific marker of the onset of diaphragm weakness and should be considered to identify the correct timing for the institution of nocturnal NIV [52].

OEP, also, revealed mild initial modifications in the respiratory muscles in other muscular dystrophies, namely, limb-girdle muscular dystrophy, Becker muscular dystrophy, and facioscapulohumeral dystrophy, which could be helpful for functional and new therapeutic strategy evaluation [53].

11.5.2.4 Other Diseases

In a study performed on a group of patients with late-onset type II glycogenosis (Pompe disease), it has been shown that the abdominal percentage contribution to tidal volume in supine position well correlates with the postural change of forced vital capacity and therefore represents a noninvasive non-volitional index to detect diaphragmatic weakness in these patients [54]. Lanini et al. studied a group of hemiplegic patients due to a cerebrovascular accident [55]. The expansion of the paretic and healthy sides was similar during quiet breathing, but paretic displacement was higher during hypercapnic stimulation in most patients, suggesting that hemiparetic stroke produces asymmetric ventilation with an increase in carbon dioxide sensitivity and a decrease in voluntary ventilation on the paretic side. More recently, Lima et al. [56] have shown that incentive spirometry is able to promote an increased expansion in all compartments of the chest wall and to reduce the asymmetric expansion between right and left pulmonary rib cage, and, therefore, it should be considered as a tool for rehabilitation. Possible alterations in chest wall kinematics due to obesity have been recently investigated by Barcelar et al. [57]. Compared to controls, obese women are characterized by strongly altered increased abdominal volume variations. No differences were found between central and peripheral obese women suggesting that the amount of fat in the abdominal compartment, and not the peripheral, alters the respiratory system and determines restriction.

In osteogenesis imperfecta, an inherited connective tissue disorder characterized by bone fragility, multiple fractures, and significant chest wall deformities, the restrictive respiratory pattern is closely related to the severity of the disease and to the sternal deformities. Patients classified as type III patients show structural rib cage deformities (pectus carinatum) that alter respiratory muscles coordination, leading to chest wall and rib cage distortions (i.e., paradoxical inspiratory inward motion of the pulmonary rib cage, see Fig. 11.3) and an inefficient ventilator pattern [58].

11.5.3 OEP Studies in Intensive Care Patients, During Mechanical Ventilation and Anesthesia

As reported above, OEP has been introduced in the ICU and the method has been validated in patients during both pressure support ventilation (PSV) and continuous positive pressure ventilation (CPPV) [21]. Using OEP in the supine position, significant differences in the distribution of tidal volume in the different chest wall compartments between normal subjects and mechanically ventilated patients and between patients receiving CPPV and patients receiving PSV were observed. For spontaneously breathing subjects, distribution of chest wall volume changes is dictated by the mechanical characteristics of the respiratory system and the relative activity of the diaphragm and inspiratory rib cage muscles. For paralyzed CPPV patients, only the mechanical characteristics of the system are involved. Conversely, during PSV, a part of the breathing pattern is controlled by the patient, and the situation is more complex. The synchronization of respiratory muscle action and the resulting chest wall kinematics are valid indicator of the patient's adaptation to the ventilator.

In a study performed on nine patients with acute lung injury/acute respiratory distress syndrome [59], it was shown that at pressure support levels lower than 15 cmH_2O, all the following parameters increased: the pressure developed by the inspiratory muscles, the contribution of the rib cage compartment to the total tidal volume, the phase shift between the rib cage and abdominal compartments, the post-inspiratory action of the inspiratory rib cage muscles, and the expiratory muscle activity. PSV, therefore, should not be considered a "unique form" of ventilation, because its effects may be quite different depending on the pressure support level and pressure support levels greater than 10 cmH_2O are necessary to allow homogeneous recruitment of respiratory muscles, with resulting synchronous thoracoabdominal expansion.

OEP was also recently used to study the effects of anesthesia on chest wall motion during spontaneous breathing and positive pressure ventilation [60] in a group of subjects undergoing elective surgery requiring general anesthesia (Fig. 11.9). Chest wall volumes were continuously monitored by optoelectronic plethysmography during quiet breathing (QB) in the conscious state, induction of propofol anesthesia, spontaneous breathing during anesthesia (SB), pressure support ventilation (PSV), and pressure control ventilation (PCV) after muscle paralysis (Fig. 11.7). The total chest wall volume significantly decreased immediately after induction by equal reductions in the rib cage and abdominal volumes. During QB, rib cage volume displacement corresponded to 34.2 ± 5.3 % of the tidal volume.

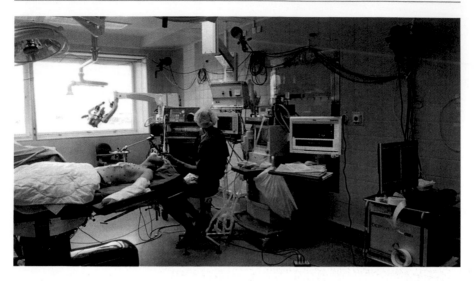

Fig. 11.9 OEP measurements at Uppsala University Hospital, Sweden, during the analysis of chest wall volume variations during induction of anesthesia

During SB, PSV, and PCV, this increased to 42.2 ± 4.9, 48.2 ± 3.6 and 46.3 ± 3.2 %, respectively, with a corresponding decrease in the abdominal contribution. Breathing was initiated by the rib cage muscles during SB. Propofol anesthesia decreases end-expiratory chest wall volume, with a more pronounced effect on the diaphragm than on the rib cage muscles, which initiate breathing after apnea.

More recently, OEP was used to compare different modes of jet ventilation (JV), including high-frequency jet ventilation (HFJV) that is today routinely used for airway surgery (e.g., laryngo-microscopic or bronchoscopic procedures) and that can be beneficial for thoracic surgery and during procedures requiring minimal respiratory excursion (e.g., radiofrequency ablation of small tumors in the lung or liver) [61]. In this situation, OEP is the only system that can estimate operating volume and ventilation by monitoring chest wall volume variations. In fact, when evaluating different HFJV techniques, tidal volume and minute ventilation are difficult to assess because HFJV is applied in open systems, and standard pneumotachography does not provide accurate values.

Conclusions

Optoelectronic plethysmography has the great advantage that it can measure breathing patterns in any condition (e.g., rest, exercise, phonation, sleep) where the chest wall can be visualized totally noninvasively. It is highly accurate in the measurement of total chest wall volume variations, allowing partitioning of the complex shape of the chest wall into different compartments. In addition to being noninvasive, it requires no connection to the patient. Furthermore, it can be used without a subject-specific calibration, because it provides a direct measurement of the volumes in a three-dimensional reference frame and the calibration is not based on particular respiratory maneuvers requiring subject cooperation.

All these features make the OEP not only a reliable system for basic physiological and pathophysiological studies but also an attractive tool for evaluating breathing under a wide variety of circumstances both in health and disease.

References

1. Gilbert R, Auchincloss JH Jr, Brodsky J, Boden W (1972) Changes in tidal volume, frequency, and ventilation induced by their measurement. J Appl Physiol 33(2):252–254
2. Tobin MJ (1986) Noninvasive evaluation of respiratory movement. In: Nochomovitz ML, Cherniack NS (eds) Noninvasive respiratory monitoring, vol 3, Contemporary issues in pulmonary disease. Churchill Livingstone, New York
3. Mead J, Peterson N, Grimby G, Mead J (1967) Pulmonary ventilation measured from body surface movements. Science 156:1383–1384
4. Chadha TS, Watson H, Birch S et al (1982) Validation of respiratory inductive plethysmography using different calibration procedures. Am Rev Respir Dis 125:644
5. Zimmerman PV, Connellan SJ, Middleton HC, Tabona MV, Goldman MD, Price N (1983) Postural changes in rib cage and abdominal volume-motion coefficients and their effect on the calibration of a respiratory-inductive plethysmograph. Am Rev Respir Dis 127:209–214
6. Sackner MA, Watson H, Belsito AS, Feinerman D, Suárez M, Gonzalez G, Bizousky F, Krieger B (1989) Calibration of respiratory inductance plethysmography during natural breathing. J Appl Physiol 66:410–420
7. Gramse V, De Groote A, Paiva M (2003) Novel concept for a noninvasive cardiopulmonary monitor for infants: a pair of pajamas with an integrated sensor module. Ann Biomed Eng 31(2):152–158
8. Pennock BE (1990) Rib cage and abdominal piezoelectric film belts to measure ventilatory airflow. J Clin Monit 6(4):276–283
9. Lafortuna CL, Passerini L (1995) A new instrument for the measurement of rib cage and abdomen circumference variation in respiration at rest and during exercise. Eur J Appl Physiol Occup Physiol 71(2–3):259–265
10. D'Angelo LT, Weber S, Honda Y, Thiel T, Narbonneau F, Luth TC (2008) A system for respiratory motion detection using optical fibers embedded into textiles. Conf Proc IEEE Eng Med Biol Soc 2008:3694–3697
11. Milledge JS, Stott FD (1977) Inductive plethysmography – a new respiratory transducer. J Physiol (Lond) 267:4
12. Peacock A, Gourlay A, Denison D (1985) Optical measurement of the change in trunk volume with breathing. Bull Eur Physiopathol Respir 21:125–129
13. Saumarez RC (1986) Automated optical measurements of human torso surface movements during breathing. J Appl Physiol 60(2):702–709
14. Chen H, Cheng Y, Liu D, Zhang X, Zhang J, Que C, Wang G, Fang J (2010) Color structured light system of chest wall motion measurement for respiratory volume evaluation. J Biomed Opt 15(2):026013
15. Cala SJ, Kenyon C, Ferrigno G, Carnevali P, Aliverti A, Pedotti A, Macklem PT, Rochester DF (1996) Chest wall and lung volume estimation by optical reflectance motion analysis. J Appl Physiol 81(6):2680–2689
16. Aliverti A, Dellacà R, Pelosi P, Chiumello D, Gattinoni L, Pedotti A (2001) Compartmental analysis of breathing in the supine and prone positions by Optoelectronic Plethysmography. Ann Biomed Eng 29:60–70
17. Aliverti A, Cala SJ, Duranti R, Ferrigno G, Kenyon CM, Pedotti A, Scano G, Sliwinski P, Macklem PT, Yan S (1997) Human respiratory muscle actions and control during exercise. J Appl Physiol 83(4):1256–1269
18. Kenyon CM, Cala SJ, Yan S, Aliverti A, Scano G, Duranti R, Pedotti A, Macklem PT (1997) Rib cage mechanics during quiet breathing and exercise in humans. J Appl Physiol 83(4):1242–1255

19. Ward ME, Ward JW, Macklem PT (1992) Analysis of chest wall motion using a two-compartment rib cage model. J Appl Physiol 72:1338–1347
20. Konno K, Mead J (1967) Measurement of the separate volume changes of rib cage and abdomen during breathing. J Appl Physiol 22:407–422
21. Aliverti A, Dellacà R, Pelosi P, Chiumello D, Pedotti A, Gattinoni L (2000) Opto-electronic plethysmography in intensive care patients. Am J Respir Crit Care Med 161:1546–1552
22. Dellaca' RL, Ventura ML, Zannin E, Natile M, Pedotti A, Tagliabue P (2010) Measurement of total and compartmental lung volume changes in newborns by optoelectronic plethysmography. Pediatr Res 67(1):11–16
23. Layton AM, Moran SL, Garber CE, Armstrong HF, Basner RC, Thomashow BM, Bartels MN (2013) Optoelectronic plethysmography compared to spirometry during maximal exercise. Respir Physiol Neurobiol 185(2):362–368
24. Boudarham J, Pradon D, Prigent H, Vaugier I, Barbot F, Letilly N, Falaize L, Orlikowski D, Petitjean M, Lofaso F (2013) Optoelectronic vital capacity measurement for restrictive diseases. Respir Care 58(4):633–638
25. Vieira DS, Hoffman M, Pereira DA, Britto RR, Parreira VF (2013) Optoelectronic plethysmography: intra-rater and inter-rater reliability in healthy subjects. Respir Physiol Neurobiol 189(3):473–476
26. Aliverti A, Bovio D, Fullin I, Dellacà RL, Lo Mauro A, Pedotti A, Macklem PT (2009) The abdominal circulatory pump. PLoS One 4(5):e5550
27. Aliverti A, Uva B, Laviola M, Bovio D, Lo Mauro A, Tarperi C, Colombo E, Loomas B, Pedotti A, Similowski T, Macklem PT (2010) Concomitant ventilatory and circulatory functions of the diaphragm and abdominal muscles. J Appl Physiol 109(5):1432–1440
28. Dellacà R, Aliverti A, Pelosi P, Carlesso E, Chiumello D, Pedotti A, Gattinoni L (2001) Estimation of end-expiratory lung volume variations by optoelectronic plethysmography (OEP). Crit Care Med 29(9):1807–1811
29. Vogiatzis I, Georgiadou O, Golemati S, Aliverti A, Kosmas E, Kastanakis E, Geladas N, Koutsoukou A, Nanas S, Zakynthinos S, Roussos C (2005) Patterns of dynamic hyperinflation during exercise and recovery in patients with severe chronic obstructive pulmonary disease. Thorax 60(9):723–729
30. Aliverti A, Iandelli I, Duranti R, Cala SJ, Kayser B, Kelly S, Misuri G, Pedotti A, Scano G, Sliwinski P, Yan S, Macklem PT (2002) Respiratory muscle dynamics and control during exercise with externally imposed expiratory flow limitation. J Appl Physiol 92(5):1953–1963
31. Iandelli I, Aliverti A, Kayser B, Dellacà R, Cala SJ, Duranti R, Kelly S, Scano G, Sliwinski P, Yan S, Macklem PT, Pedotti A (2002) Determinants of exercise performance in normal men with externally imposed expiratory flow limitation. J Appl Physiol 92(5):1943–1952
32. Sanna A, Bertoli F, Misuri G, Gigliotti F, Iandelli I, Mancini M, Duranti R, Ambrosino N, Scano G (1999) Chest wall kinematics and respiratory muscle action in walking healthy humans. J Appl Physiol 87(3):938–946
33. Smith JA, Aliverti A, Quaranta M, McGuinness K, Kelsall A, Earis J, Calverley PM (2012) Chest wall dynamics during voluntary and induced cough in healthy volunteers. J Physiol 590(Pt 3):563–574
34. Binazzi B, Lanini B, Bianchi R, Romagnoli I, Nerini M, Gigliotti F, Duranti R, Milic-Emili J, Scano G (2006) Breathing pattern and kinematics in normal subjects during speech, singing and loud whispering. Acta Physiol (Oxf) 186(3):233–246
35. Cossette I, Monaco P, Aliverti A, Macklem PT (2008) Chest wall dynamics and muscle recruitment during professional flute playing. Respir Physiol Neurobiol 160(2):187–195
36. Aliverti A, Stevenson N, Dellacà RL, Lo Mauro A, Pedotti A, Calverley PM (2004) Regional chest wall volumes during exercise in chronic obstructive pulmonary disease. Thorax 59(3):210–216
37. Aliverti A, Rodger K, Dellacà RL, Stevenson N, Lo Mauro A, Pedotti A, Calverley PM (2005) Effect of salbutamol on lung function and chest wall volumes at rest and during exercise in COPD. Thorax 60(11):916–924

38. Georgiadou O, Vogiatzis I, Stratakos G, Koutsoukou A, Golemati S, Aliverti A, Roussos C, Zakynthinos S (2007) Effects of rehabilitation on chest wall volume regulation during exercise in COPD patients. Eur Respir J 29(2):284–291

39. Aliverti A, Macklem PT (2001) How and why exercise is impaired in COPD. Respiration 68(3):229–239

40. Vogiatzis I, Athanasopoulos D, Habazettl H, Aliverti A, Louvaris Z, Cherouveim E, Wagner H, Roussos C, Wagner PD, Zakynthinos S (2010) Intercostal muscle blood flow limitation during exercise in chronic obstructive pulmonary disease. Am J Respir Crit Care Med 182(9):1105–1113

41. Louvaris Z, Zakynthinos S, Aliverti A, Habazettl H, Vasilopoulou M, Andrianopoulos V, Wagner H, Wagner P, Vogiatzis I (2012) Heliox increases quadriceps muscle oxygen delivery during exercise in COPD patients with and without dynamic hyperinflation. J Appl Physiol 113(7):1012–1023

42. Aliverti A, Quaranta M, Chakrabarti B, Albuquerque AL, Calverley PM (2009) Paradoxical movement of the lower ribcage at rest and during exercise in COPD patients. Eur Respir J 33(1):49–60

43. Priori R, Aliverti A, Albuquerque AL, Quaranta M, Albert P, Calverley PM (2013) The effect of posture on asynchronous chest wall movement in COPD. J Appl Physiol 114(8):1066–1075

44. Wilkens H, Weingard B, Lo Mauro A, Schena E, Pedotti A, Sybrecht GW, Aliverti A (2010) Breathing pattern and chest wall volumes during exercise in patients with cystic fibrosis, pulmonary fibrosis and COPD before and after lung transplantation. Thorax 65(9): 808–814

45. Nosotti M, Laviola M, Mariani S, Privitera E, Mendogni P, Nataloni IF, Aliverti A, Santambrogio L (2013) Variations of thoracoabdominal volumes after lung transplantation measured by opto-electronic plethysmography. Transplant Proc 45(3):1279–1281

46. Lunardi AC, Paisani Dde M, Tanaka C, Carvalho CR (2013) Impact of laparoscopic surgery on thoracoabdominal mechanics and inspiratory muscular activity. Respir Physiol Neurobiol 186(1):40–44

47. Acosta J, Bradley A, Raja V, Aliverti A, Badiyani S, Motta A, Moriconi S, Parker K, Rajesh P, Naidu B (2014) Exercise improvement after pectus excavatum repair is not related to chest wall function. Eur J Cardiothorac Surg 45:544–548

48. Binazzi B, Innocenti Bruni G, Gigliotti F, Coli C, Romagnoli I, Messineo A, Lo Piccolo R, Scano G (2012) Effects of the Nuss procedure on chest wall kinematics in adolescents with pectus excavatum. Respir Physiol Neurobiol 183(2):122–127

49. Redlinger RE Jr, Wootton A, Kelly RE, Nuss D, Goretsky M, Kuhn MA, Obermeyer RJ (2012) Optoelectronic plethysmography demonstrates abrogation of regional chest wall motion dysfunction in patients with pectus excavatum after Nuss repair. J Pediatr Surg 47(1):160–164

50. Lo Mauro A, D'Angelo MG, Romei M, Motta F, Colombo D, Comi GP, Pedotti A, Marchi E, Turconi AC, Bresolin N, Aliverti A (2010) Abdominal volume contribution to tidal volume as an early indicator of respiratory impairment in Duchenne muscular dystrophy. Eur Respir J 35(5):1118–1125

51. Lomauro A, Romei M, D'Angelo MG, Aliverti A (2014) Determinants of cough efficiency in Duchenne muscular dystrophy. Pediatr Pulmonol 49:357–365

52. Romei M, D'Angelo MG, LoMauro A, Gandossini S, Bonato S, Brighina E, Marchi E, Comi GP, Turconi AC, Pedotti A, Bresolin N, Aliverti A (2012) Low abdominal contribution to breathing as daytime predictor of nocturnal desaturation in adolescents and young adults with Duchenne Muscular Dystrophy. Respir Med 106(2):276–283

53. D'Angelo MG, Romei M, Lo Mauro A, Marchi E, Gandossini S, Bonato S, Comi GP, Magri F, Turconi AC, Pedotti A, Bresolin N, Aliverti A (2011) Respiratory pattern in an adult population of dystrophic patients. J Neurol Sci 306(1–2):54–61

54. Remiche G, Lo Mauro A, Tarsia P, Ronchi D, Bordoni A, Magri F, Comi GP, Aliverti A, D'Angelo MG (2013) Postural effects on lung and chest wall volumes in late onset type II glycogenosis patients. Respir Physiol Neurobiol 186(3):308–314

55. Lanini B, Bianchi R, Romagnoli I, Coli C, Binazzi B, Gigliotti F, Pizzi A, Grippo A, Scano G (2003) Chest wall kinematics in patients with hemiplegia. Am J Respir Crit Care Med 168(1):109–113
56. Lima IN, Fregonezi GA, Rodrigo M, Cabral EE, Aliverti A, Campos TF, Ferreira GM (2014) Acute effects of volume-oriented incentive spirometry on chest wall volumes in patients after stroke. Respir Care (in press)
57. Barcelar Jde M, Aliverti A, Melo TL, Dornelas CS, Lima CS, Reinaux CM, de Andrade AD (2013) Chest wall regional volumes in obese women. Respir Physiol Neurobiol 189(1): 167–173
58. LoMauro A, Pochintesta S, Romei M, D'Angelo MG, Pedotti A, Turconi AC, Aliverti A (2012) Rib cage deformities alter respiratory muscle action and chest wall function in patients with severe osteogenesis imperfecta. PLoS One 7(4):e35965
59. Aliverti A, Carlesso E, Dellacà R, Pelosi P, Chiumello D, Pedotti A, Gattinoni L (2006) Chest wall mechanics during pressure support ventilation. Crit Care 10(2):R54
60. Aliverti A, Kostic P, Lo Mauro A, Andersson-Olerud M, Quaranta M, Pedotti A, Hedenstierna G, Frykholm P (2011) Effects of propofol anaesthesia on thoraco-abdominal volume variations during spontaneous breathing and mechanical ventilation. Acta Anaesthesiol Scand 55(5):588–596
61. Leiter R, Aliverti A, Priori R, Staun P, Lo Mauro A, Larsson A, Frykholm P (2012) Comparison of superimposed high-frequency jet ventilation with conventional jet ventilation for laryngeal surgery. Br J Anaesth 108(4):690–697

Respiratory Muscle Blood Flow Measured by Near-Infrared Spectroscopy (NIRS) and Indocyanine Green Dye (ICG)

12

Zafeiris Louvaris, Spyros Zakynthinos, and Ioannis Vogiatzis

12.1 Introduction

The ability to measure respiratory muscle blood flow in humans has the potential to provide insight into a number of physiological and pathophysiological conditions. Along these lines an important question in exercise physiology and pathophysiology is how blood flow is distributed between respiratory and locomotor muscles during exercise. For addressing this fundamental issue, accurate measurement of respiratory muscle blood flow is important for understanding patterns of blood flow distribution during exercise in healthy individuals and those with chronic diseases.

Z. Louvaris
Department of Physical Education and Sports Sciences,
National and Kapodistrian University of Athens, Athens, Greece

1st Department of Critical Care Medicine and Pulmonary Services,
GP Livanos and M Simou Laboratories, Evangelismos Hospital, Medical School of Athens,
Athens, Greece

S. Zakynthinos
1st Department of Critical Care Medicine and Pulmonary Services,
GP Livanos and M Simou Laboratories, Evangelismos Hospital, Medical School of Athens,
Athens, Greece

I. Vogiatzis (✉)
Department of Physical Education and Sports Sciences,
National and Kapodistrian University of Athens, Athens, Greece

1st Department of Critical Care Medicine and Pulmonary Services,
GP Livanos and M Simou Laboratories, Evangelismos Hospital, Medical School of Athens,
Athens, Greece

Institute of Clinical Exercise and Health Sciences, University of the West of Scotland,
Scotland, UK

Thorax Foundation, 3str Ploutarhou 10675, Athens, Greece
e-mail: gianvog@phed.uoa.gr

A. Aliverti, A. Pedotti (eds.), *Mechanics of Breathing*,
DOI 10.1007/978-88-470-5647-3_12, © Springer-Verlag Italia 2014

Traditional techniques for measuring respiratory muscle blood flow in humans are capable of measuring instantaneously diaphragm blood flow by recording blood-drop count rates from the cannulated left inferior phrenic vein [1]. However, this method is not appropriate during exercise since it is highly invasive as it requires inferior phrenic vein catheterization as well as iatrogenic sedation. Moreover, measuring blood flow to the several respiratory muscles in humans during exercise is difficult owing to their complex anatomical arrangement, the extensive network of feed arteries and veins, and the large variations in muscular recruitment that occurs in the respiratory muscles with varying degrees of ventilation [2–5]. In addition, much of what we know about respiratory muscle blood flow during exercise or high ventilation rates stems mainly from animal investigations [2–8].

To overcome respiratory muscle blood flow measurement difficulties during exercise, a more versatile method was needed to quantify muscle blood flow in humans. Accordingly, the present chapter focuses on the studies that have employed a new method for measuring respiratory muscle blood flow by employing near-infrared spectroscopy (NIRS) in combination with the light-absorbing tracer indocyanine green dye (ICG). In addition, this chapter reports the latest physiological findings of this method with regard to respiratory muscle blood flow in healthy individuals and patients with chronic obstructive pulmonary disease (COPD).

12.2   Muscle Blood Flow Measurements by NIRS–ICG

Near-infrared spectroscopy (NIRS) is a noninvasive tool used to assess dynamic changes in tissue oxygenation. The NIRS technique has seen rapid development since its inception in the 1970s [5]. Furthermore, near-infrared light easily penetrates biological tissue and allows for detection of changes in specific chromophore concentrations in human tissue [9]. In addition, NIRS is advantageous because it is noninvasive, exhibits low movement artifacts, and provides good temporal and spatial resolution [10].

Numerous studies have used this method for examining the oxygenation profile in respiratory and locomotor muscles [11–15], brain [16–19], and connective tissues [20], in addition to the clinical assessment of circulatory and metabolic abnormalities [21–24].

A decade ago a technique combining NIRS with the light-absorbing tracer indocyanine green (ICG) was employed to measure blood flow by applying the Fick's principle [20]. Indocyanine green dye is a water-soluble tricarbocyanine, a light-absorbing dye with a peak absorption in human blood in the NIR range of 800 nm. It has been used routinely for measuring cardiac output as well as limb blood flow with the use of photodensitometry [25]. After intravascular injection, ICG is predominantly bound to albumin [26] and is metabolized rapidly by hepatic parenchymal cells making it ideal for repeated blood flow measurements.

By using NIRS–ICG technique, blood flow is calculated from the rate of tissue ICG accumulation over time measured by NIRS according to the Saperstein principle [27]. Accordingly, for any given time interval less than the time to reach peak tissue accumulation of the tracer, the tissue receives the same fraction of the ICG bolus as quantified in arterial blood. Two separate time points within the first half of the curve is used to calculate the flow, and the average value is taken to represent ICG accumulation. Therefore, the total blood flow is calculating using the following equation:

$$\text{Blood flow}\left(\text{ml}\cdot100\ \text{ml}\cdot\text{min}^{-1}\right)=\frac{k\cdot[\text{ICG}]_m\cdot t}{\int\limits_{o}^{t}[\text{ICG}]_a\,dt},$$

where k is a constant for the conversion of ICG in moles to grams per liter measured from in vitro blood phantoms, $[\text{ICG}]_m$ is the accumulation of ICG in muscles over time expressed in micromoles, and $\int_{o}^{t}[\text{ICG}]_a\,dt$ is the time integral of the arterial [ICG] expressed in milligrams per liter [27].

A schematic representation of the ICG tracer procedure for blood flow measurements with NIRS is shown in Fig. 12.1. After venous bolus injection, the ICG bolus circulates to the right heart and lungs and emerges into the arterial circulation. Arterial blood is withdrawn by a pump, and the ICG is recorded by photodensitometry, whereas downstream in the tissue microcirculation, ICG accumulation is detected by measuring light attenuation with NIRS [20].

12.3 Validation of NIRS–ICG Technique

The NIRS–ICG technique has been used and validated for measurements of respiratory and locomotor muscle blood flow during exercise against previously established methods in healthy humans and patients with chronic respiratory failure (i.e., dye dilution, ^{133}Xe washout, magnetic resonance imaging). The results indicate that this technique is indeed valid and accurate for quantifying both respiratory and locomotor muscle blood flow during exercise [14, 20, 28–30].

Specifically, Boushel and colleagues [20] using the NIRS–ICG technique quantified blood flow in the calf and the Achilles tendon region during plantar flexion in healthy subjects. They found a linear increase in tissue ICG accumulation in both the calf and the Achilles tendon region for a given ICG dose as workload increased. In addition, a good agreement was found between NIRS–ICG technique and ^{133}Xe washout and magnetic resonance imaging methods during exercise. Similarly, a study in healthy subjects by the same group of investigators [28] quantified the vastus lateralis and the vastus medialis muscle blood flow during dynamic knee extension exercise. The results revealed that in both locomotor muscles, blood flow increased linearly as workload increased while muscle blood flow decreased when muscle vasodilatation factors during exercise were inhibited, thereby indicating that beyond validity the NIRS–ICG technique is a sensitive method for quantifying locomotor muscle blood flow during exercise [28].

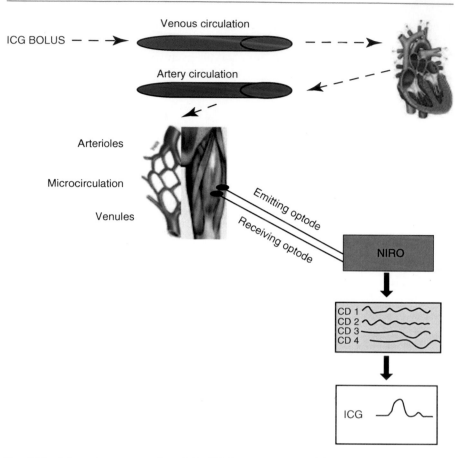

Fig. 12.1 Schematic representation of the NIRS measurements of indocyanine green (ICG) in tissue after a venous bolus infusion. *From top left*, an ICG bolus is injected into the venous circulation; it passes through the heart and lungs and into the arterial circulation and microcirculation. The NIRS optodes positioned over the tissue detect the ICG at several wavelengths, and by use of specific extinction coefficients in a matrix operation, the ICG curve is isolated. The circles represent the vessels from which the NIRS is detected

Guenette and colleagues [29] were the first to quantify respiratory muscle blood flow in healthy subjects during resting isocapnic hyperpnea at different fractions of maximum minute ventilation. In this study NIRS optodes were placed on the left seventh intercostal space including the internal and external intercostal muscles while authors simultaneously measured esophageal and gastric pressure in order to calculate the work of breathing and the transdiaphragmatic pressure. The results of the study demonstrated that as ventilation rose, respiratory muscle blood flow was highly correlated with the increase in cardiac output, the work of breathing, and transdiaphragmatic pressure, suggesting that the NIRS–ICG technique provides feasible and sensitive values of respiratory muscle blood flow in healthy humans.

In this context, Vogiatzis and colleagues [14, 30], using the same NIRS–ICG technique, simultaneously measured intercostal and quadriceps muscle blood flow in healthy subjects and patients with chronic obstructive pulmonary disease (COPD). The measurements were conducted during resting isocapnic hyperpnea and at several work intensities up to peak work rate during exercise on a bike. The results of the study demonstrated that in both healthy and COPD patients, intercostal muscle blood flow linearly increased with the work of breathing, minute ventilation, and cardiac output not only during resting hyperpnea but also during cycle exercise of increasing intensity.

The above results [14, 30] suggest that the NIRS–ICG technique for measuring respiratory muscle blood flow has a good signal integrity during body movement such as exercise while multiple NIRS channels allow simultaneous measurements of different muscle groups in addition to mapping of blood flow patterns within and between muscles.

12.4   Blood Flow Index (BFI) Derived by NIRS–ICG Technique

Although the NIRS–ICG technique itself is noninvasive, the respiratory muscle blood flow measurement requires arterial cannulation and continuous withdrawal of blood through a photodensitometer for several seconds after injection. Furthermore, one needs to consider that arterial cannulation is associated with the potential risks of bleeding, vascular perforation, vascular insufficiency, and injury to adjusted nerves [31]. Considering the above situation and the fact that the equipment for constant rate of blood withdrawal and measurements of ICG may not be available, the NIRS–ICG technique is not feasible in all conditions. For the above reasons, an alternative algorithm has been proposed to calculate tissue perfusion from the NIRS data, namely, the blood flow index (BFI) [32].

Specifically, the BFI is calculated by dividing the ICG peak concentration by the rise time from 10 to 90 % of peak (Fig. 12.2) [32]. In addition, the BFI is derived only from the transcutaneously measured NIRS–ICG curve and not from the arterial ICG curve. Thus, the only invasive component of this technique is venous cannulation for bolus injection of the ICG tracer. For that reason, the BFI is a relative measure of blood flow, as absolute flow cannot be determined unless arterial ICG concentration is measured.

BFI has traditionally been used for the assessment of cerebral blood flow [33–36]. Recently, this method has been validated in human skeletal muscles [32–37]. Furthermore, a retrospective analysis by Habazettl and colleagues [32] compared BFI values within the vastus lateralis and the 7th intercostal space against absolute muscle blood flow determined using NIRS–ICG technique during cycling exercise at different intensities. The results indicated a very good agreement between the BFI and NIRS–ICG technique measured in both respiratory and quadriceps muscles (Fig. 12.3). In addition, the study by Guenette and colleagues [37] extend the observation by Habazettl and colleagues [32] by determining whether BFI can be used to assess blood flow to respiratory muscles using a prospective experimental design.

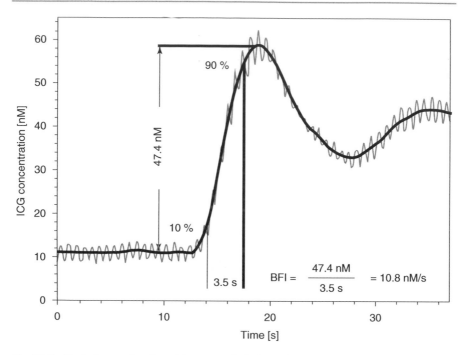

Fig. 12.2 Typical example of quadriceps muscle indocyanine green (ICG) concentration curve recorded by near-infrared spectroscopy (NIRS) during exercise at 30 % limit of tolerance. The original tracing (*gray line*) appears with marked oscillations (at a frequency of 84/min, 1.4 Hz) owing to muscle contraction and relaxation during cycling. Low-pass filtering with a cutoff frequency of 0.5 Hz produced the smoothed curve (*black line*) that was used for blood flow index (BFI) calculation. Data points at 10 and 90 % of ICG concentration peak are indicated, and an example of BFI calculation is given [32]

BFI from the intercostal and sternocleidomastoid muscles was measured during resting isocapnic hyperpnea across a wide range of ventilations with simultaneous measurements of electromyography and work of breathing. The results supported the findings of Habazettl and colleagues [32] as the BFI showed a strong correlation with the work of breathing and electromyography data for both aforementioned respiratory muscles. The aforementioned findings suggest that BFI closely reflects respiratory muscle blood flow across a wide range of exercise intensities and ventilations and provides a less invasive and less technically demanding alternative technique for measuring muscle perfusion in humans during exercise.

12.5   Respiratory Muscle Blood Flow by NIRS–ICG Technique in Healthy Subjects

Measurement of regional muscle blood flow (MBF) in humans is an important tool for exercise physiology studies aiming at investigating factors that limit exercise performance in healthy trained subjects.

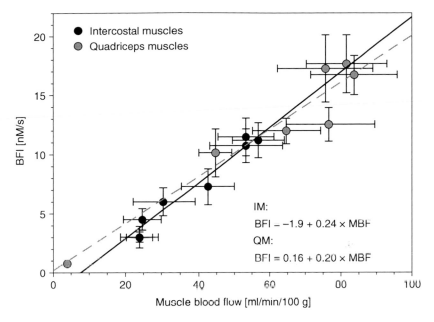

Fig. 12.3 Regression analyses of mean±SE BFI versus MBF for intercostal (*black symbols, black line*) and quadriceps (*gray symbols, gray line*) muscles, $r=0.98$ for intercostal, and $r=0.96$ for quadriceps muscles, respectively; $p<0.001$, for both muscle groups [32]

Based on this concept, limitations in exercise performance may occur because of the competition for blood flow between the locomotor and the respiratory muscles. Indeed during maximal exercise in fit subjects, competition for blood flow between the locomotor and the respiratory muscles exists, such that respiratory muscle blood flow may increase at the expense of blood flow to working limb muscles [38, 39]. Such a notion of blood flow redistribution from the locomotor to the respiratory muscles during exercise was originally evolved from studies in healthy humans showing reductions in limb blood flow with respiratory muscle loading and an increase in locomotor muscle blood flow with respiratory muscle unloading [38, 39]. However, these results must be interpreted cautiously as only limb and not respiratory muscle blood flow measurements were performed in those studies [38, 39].

In this context, the study by the group of Vogiatzis [30] investigated whether during maximal exercise in athletes there is an increase in blood flow in favor of the respiratory muscles at the expense of the exercising leg muscles. Authors performed simultaneous measurements of the intercostal and quadriceps femoris muscle blood flow using the NIRS–ICG technique during graded exercise up to maximal levels and during resting hyperpnea at the same levels of minute ventilation and work of breathing as during the different levels of exercise (Fig. 12.4). Authors reasoned that if intercostal muscle blood flow during maximal exercise was greater than that recorded during resting hyperpnea at the same work of breathing when legs were inactive, this would support the notion that the work of breathing normally experienced during maximal exercise causes redistribution of blood flow from the legs to the respiratory muscles [38–41]. The results showed that intercostal muscle blood flow and vascular conductance were lower during maximal exercise than during hyperpnea at the same work of breathing compared to that measured during maximal exercise. In addition, intercostal muscle blood flow during maximal exercise was lower than during submaximal exercise, whereas cardiac output, quadriceps muscle perfusion, and vascular conductance reached a plateau but did not significantly fall at heavy exercise. Collectively, these observations suggested that at maximal exercise, restriction of intercostal muscle blood flow along with the attainment of a plateau in cardiac output and quadriceps muscle perfusion represents the inability of the circulatory system to satisfy the energy demands of both locomotor and intercostal muscles (Fig. 12.4).

12.6   Respiratory Muscle Blood Flow by NIRS–ICG Technique in Patients with COPD

Expiratory flow limitation is present in a significant proportion of patients with COPD resulting in increased work of breathing and metabolic requirement of the respiratory muscles. This phenomenon has been alleged to aggravate the competition for blood flow between the locomotor and the respiratory muscles during exercise. In the study by Athanasopoulos and colleagues [42], the concept of blood flow redistribution from locomotor to respiratory muscles [38] was explored by exercising healthy subjects with and without expiratory flow limitation mimicking the symptoms and respiratory limitations experienced by patients with COPD. Direct and simultaneous measurements of both intercostal muscles and vastus lateralis muscle blood flow was employed by utilizing NIRS–ICG technique. Accordingly, the results showed that with expiratory muscle loading, intercostal muscle blood flow was greater and quadriceps muscle blood flow was lower compared to exercise without respiratory muscle loading [42].

However, a study from the same laboratory [14] challenged the concept of blood flow redistribution in favor of the respiratory muscles during grated incremental exercise in patients with COPD as it revealed that intercostal muscle blood flow was limited during high-intensity exercise, while quadriceps muscle perfusion was preserved (Fig. 12.5). This occured under conditions of attenuation in the increase in cardiac output that was interpreted as a representation of the inability of the circulatory system to satisfy the energy demands of both locomotor and respiratory muscles.

Interestingly, the increase in quadriceps muscle blood flow was insufficient to prevent the mismatch between oxygen delivery to and demand of the quadriceps muscles, as quadriceps local muscle oxygen saturation progressively decreased, ultimately making these muscles vulnerable to fatigue [14]. Why the results of the latter study in COPD [14] differ from those in healthy individuals [38, 42] artificially manipulating the work of breathing is a matter of discussion. Perhaps, in healthy subjects the procedure of manipulating the work of breathing causes abrupt adjustments in the regulation of systemic blood flow [38, 42] most likely forcing redistribution of blood flow from the locomotor to the respiratory muscles. In contrast, in COPD, the phenomenon of increased breathing work is chronic, and as such certain central and/or peripheral muscle adjustments in blood flow regulation may

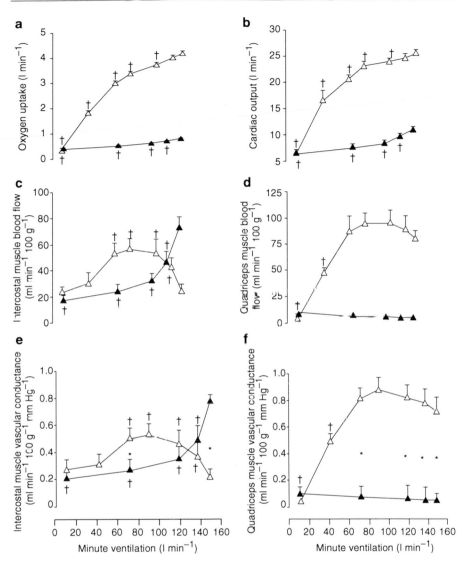

Fig. 12.4 Metabolic and haemodynamic responses during exercise and isocapnic resting hyperpnoea. Oxygen uptake (**a**), cardiac output (**b**), intercostal muscle blood flow (**c**), quadriceps muscle blood flow (**d**), intercostal muscle vascular conductance (**e**) and quadriceps muscle vascular conductance (**f**), at different levels of minute ventilation during exercise (*open triangles*) and isocapnic, resting hyperpnoea (*filled triangles*). Values are means±S.E.M. for 10 subjects. *Asterisks* denote significant differences between the two conditions at different fractions of WRpeak. *Crosses* denote significant differences compared to maximal ventilation, $P < 0.05$ [30]

have taken place to accommodate locomotor muscle energy supply relative to demand, ultimately giving preference to the locomotor muscles.

The findings questioning redistribution of blood flow in favor of the respiratory muscles [14] theoretically do not contrast those of respiratory muscle unloading in

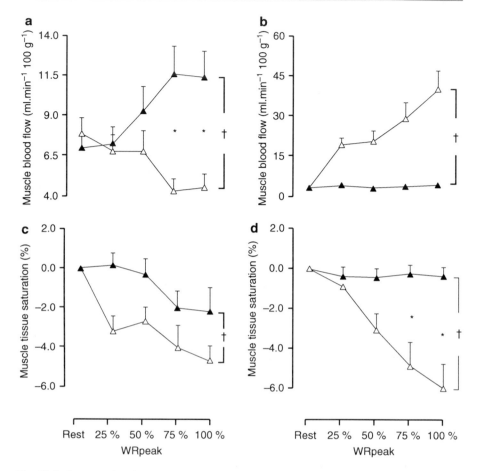

Fig. 12.5 Intercostal and quadriceps muscle blood flow and tissue oxygen saturation responses. (**a**) Intercostal muscle blood flow, (**b**) intercostal muscle oxygen saturation, (**c**) quadriceps muscle blood flow, and (**d**) quadriceps muscle oxygen saturation recorded at different fractions of peak work rate (WRpeak) during exercise (*open triangles*) and during isocapnic hyperpnea trials (*filled triangles*) that were sustained at levels of minute ventilation similar to those recorded during exercise. Values are means ± SEM for 10 subjects. *Asterisks* denote significant differences between the two conditions at different fractions of WRpeak. *Crosses* denote significant differences across the two trials [30]

COPD [43, 44] as lightening the work of breathing could potentially further increase blood flow and oxygen delivery to the quadriceps muscles and, thus, by minimizing the mismatch between tissue oxygen delivery and demand, improve exercise tolerance. However, a recent study [45] revealed that intercostal muscle blood flow does not decrease with heliox administration (aiming at unloading the respiratory muscles) during exercise ranging from submaximal to supramaximal levels, but in fact was increased during exercise along with an increase in quadriceps muscle blood flow. Based on such evidence, it was suggested that blood flow redistribution from the intercostal to locomotor muscles does not represent a mechanism of leg muscle hemodynamic improvement with heliox during exercise in COPD. Whether redistribution of blood flow from the diaphragm or the expiratory abdominal muscles could occur following heliox administration, still remains a plausible mechanism.

References

1. Aubier M, Murciano D, Menu Y, Boczkowski J, Mal H, Pariente R (1989) Dopamine effects on diaphragmatic strength during acute respiratory failure in chronic obstructive pulmonary disease. Ann Intern Med 110:17–23
2. Manohar M (1990) Inspiratory and expiratory muscle perfusion in maximally exercised ponies. J Appl Physiol 68:544–548
3. Manohar M (1988) Costal vs. crural diaphragmatic blood flow during submaximal and near-maximal exercise in ponies. J Appl Physiol 65:1514–1519
4. Robertson CH Jr, Foster GH, Johnson RL Jr (1977) The relationship of respiratory failure to the oxygen consumption of, lactate production by, and distribution of blood flow among respiratory muscles during increasing inspiratory resistance. J Clin Invest 59:31–42
5. Jobsis F (1977) Noninvasive, infrared monitoring of cerebral and myocardial oxygen sufficiency and circulatory parameters. Science 198:1264–1267
6. Johnson RL Jr, Hsia CC, Takeda S, Wait JL, Glenny RW (2002) Efficient design of the diaphragm: distribution of blood flow relative to mechanical advantage. J Appl Physiol 93: 925–930
7. Manohar M (1986) Blood flow to the respiratory and limb muscles and to abdominal organs during maximal exertion in ponies. J Physiol 377:25–35
8. Musch TI, Friedman DB, Pitetti KH, Haidet GC, Stray-Gundersen J, Mitchell JH, Ordway GA (1987) Regional distribution of blood flow of dogs during graded dynamic exercise. J Appl Physiol 63:2269–2277
9. Chance B, Dait M, Zhang C, Hamaoka T, Hong L (1992) Recovery from exercise-induced desaturation in the quadriceps muscles of elite competitive rowers. Am J Physiol Cell Physiol 262:766–775
10. Boushel R, Langberg H, Olesen J, Gonzales-Alonzo J, Bulow J, Kjaer M (2001) Monitoring tissue oxygen availability with near infrared spectroscopy (NIRS) in health and disease. Scand J Med Sci Sports 11:213–222
11. Boushel R, Pott F, Madsen P, Radegran G, Nowak M, Quistorff B, Secher N (1998) Muscle metabolism from near infrared spectroscopy during rhythmic handgrip in humans. Eur J Appl Physiol Occup Physiol 79:41–48
12. Hampson NB, Piantadosi CA (1988) Near infrared monitoring of human skeletal muscle oxygenation during forearm ischemia. J Appl Physiol 64:2449–2457
13. Chiappa GR, Queiroga F Jr, Meda E, Ferreira LF, Diefenthaeler F, Nunes M, Vaz MA, Machado MC, Nery LE, Neder JA (2009) Heliox improves oxygen delivery and utilization during dynamic exercise in patients with chronic obstructive pulmonary disease. Am J Respir Crit Care Med 179:1004–1010
14. Vogiatzis I, Athanasopoulos D, Habazettl H, Aliverti A, Louvaris Z, Cherouveim E, Wagner H, Roussos C, Wagner PD, Zakynthinos S (2010) Intercostal muscle blood flow limitation during exercise in chronic obstructive pulmonary disease. Am J Respir Crit Care Med 182: 1105–1113
15. Louvaris Z, Zakynthinos S, Aliverti A, Habazettl H, Vasilopoulou M, Andrianopoulos V, Wagner H, Wagner P, Vogiatzis I (2012) Heliox increases quadriceps muscle oxygen delivery during exercise in COPD patients with and without dynamic hyperinflation. J Appl Physiol 113:1012–1023

Assessment of Dyspnoea

13

Giorgio Scano, Giulia Innocenti-Bruni,
Loredana Stendardi, and Francesco Gigliotti

13.1   Introduction

Dyspnoea is a very common symptom in patients with respiratory disorders. It presents major challenges to the medical community, so that clinicians and scientists need to maintain continuous interest in the progress being made in overcoming this problem. In this chapter, we wish to contribute to keeping pneumologists abreast of considerable progress that has been made in recent years in understanding the symptoms and the mechanisms underpinning both obstructive and restrictive pulmonary disease.

Dyspnoea is characterised by a subjective experience of breathing discomfort that consists of qualitatively distinct sensations that vary in intensity [1]. The experience derives from interactions among multiple physiological, psychological, social and environmental factors and may induce secondary physiological and behavioural responses. This definition underlines the importance of the different qualities covered by the term dyspnoea, the involvement of integration of multiple sources of neural information about breathing and the physiological consequences.

The American Thoracic Society [2] has recently proposed that instruments or subsections of instruments (e.g. subscale) pertaining to dyspnoea should be

G. Scano (✉)
Department of Internal Medicine, Section of Clinical Immunology,
Allergology and Respiratory Disease, University of Florence,
Viale Morgagni 87, Florence 50134, Italy

Fondazione Don C. Gnocchi, Istituto di Ricerca e Cura a Carattere Scientifico,
Via di Scandicci snc, Florence 50143, Italy
e-mail: gscano@unifi.it

G. Innocenti–Bruni • L. Stendardi • F. Gigliotti
Fondazione Don C. Gnocchi, Istituto di Ricerca e Cura a Carattere Scientifico,
Via di Scandicci snc, Florence 50143, Italy
e-mail: g.innocentibruni@yahoo.it; giordan1969@alice.it; fgigliotti@dongnocchi.it

A. Aliverti, A. Pedotti (eds.), *Mechanics of Breathing*,
DOI 10.1007/978-88-470-5647-3_13, © Springer-Verlag Italia 2014

classified as pertaining to domains of *sensory–perceptual experience, affective distress or symptom/disease impact or burden*. Sensory–perceptual measures include *ratings of intensity and sensory quality*. Ratings of intensity involve one or more separate single-item scales such as the visual analogue scale (*VAS*), *Borg* ratings or numerical rating scales. Sensory quality involves cluster descriptors of the sensation (the language of dyspnoea). Measurement of affective distress may use single- or multiple-item scales. Affective distress deals with a perception of immediate unpleasantness or a cognitive–evaluative response to or judgement about the possible consequences of what is perceived. Impact measures (e.g. how breathing affects behaviour and beliefs) involve a multiple-item scale across multiple dimensions (functional performance or disability, quality of life, health status and psychological function). These measures, although very important, do not directly assess what breathing feels like. It is noteworthy that while the time frame for ratings may be the present (i.e. real-time ratings) or the immediate past (end of an experimental session), the time frame for impact measures is commonly either some relapsed interval or an unspecific interval.

13.2 Sensory–Perceptual Experience

13.2.1 Ratings of Intensity

13.2.1.1 Visual Analogue Scale

A visual analogue scale (VAS) or a category–ratio scale may be used to assess dyspnoea during an exercise test [3, 4]. With VAS the subject is instructed to provide a quantification of his/her dyspnoea placing a mark on a horizontal or vertical line, usually 100 mm in length, with or without descriptors like "*no breathlessness*" and "*intolerable breathlessness*" or significant images (positioned as anchors at the two extremes) [5].

13.2.1.2 Category–Ratio Scale

The modified 0–10 category–ratio Borg scale is the most widely used scale to rate dyspnoea during exercise testing [6]. This scale consists of a vertical line labelled 0–10 with nonlinear spacing of verbal descriptors of severity corresponding to specific numbers. The subject can choose the number or the verbal descriptor to reflect presumed ratio properties of sensation or symptom intensity.

The VAS and the Borg scale provide similar scores during incremental cardiopulmonary exercise testing in healthy subjects and in chronic obstructive pulmonary disease (*COPD*) patients [7]. The descriptors on the Borg scale permit comparisons among individuals based on the assumption that the verbal descriptors on the scale describe the same intensity for different subjects. Usually, both healthy individuals and patients with cardiorespiratory disease stop exercise at submaximal (at ratings between 5 and 8 on the Borg scale) intensities of dyspnoea and/or leg discomfort [3] independent of the peak power obtained [8]. Patients can also give ratings at specific times (iso-time) or workload (iso-workload) increment during the exercise test [3]. A numerical value or descriptor on the Borg scale may be used as a dyspnoea "target" (as opposed to a measured length in mm on the VAS) for prescribing and monitoring exercise training [3, 4].

13.2.2   The Language of Dyspnoea

The use of verbal descriptors of dyspnoea may contribute to the understanding of the mechanisms of dyspnoea and assist in identifying or predicting a specific diagnosis. Using the *descriptors of dyspnoea*, normal volunteers are able to distinguish between the kinds of dyspnoea induced by different stimuli, such as breath holding, carbon dioxide inhalation, exercise, resistive and elastic respiratory loads and constrained tidal volume [9]. These individuals find it easy to identify the discomfort associated with the different tasks and to select different phrases to describe their discomfort. Descriptors of dyspnoea are also readily obtained in symptomatic patients with different cardiorespiratory diseases. Standardised descriptors are grouped in discrete clusters with high discriminating value among diseases [9].

Multiplicity, uniqueness and sharing characterise the association of qualitative clusters of dyspnoea with different disease states: (1) The pathological conditions characterised by many clusters suggest that dyspnoea comprises more than one sensation; (2) each condition is characterised by a unique set of clusters, and (3) some clusters are shared by more than one condition, suggesting that similar pathways or receptors modify dyspnoea, respectively. There is no obvious relationship between the qualitative descriptors of dyspnoea and the quantitative intensity among the patient groups; a cluster may be shared by a disease with the highest and lowest intensity of dyspnoea. In contrast, diseases with the highest scores of dyspnoea may have different patterns of clusters. Thus, the quality of the sensation, not the quantity of intensity, differentiates the diseases [9]. Based on the hypothesis that various qualities of respiratory discomfort result from different pathophysiological abnormalities, language can help to define one or more of the abnormalities responsible for breathing discomfort.

The following is a list of clusters of dyspnoea most commonly selected by patients with respiratory disorders.

13.2.2.1   Chest Tightness
Chest tightness is frequently reported by asthmatic patients. During acute bronchoconstriction, chest tightness may arise from the stimulation of sensory receptors within the lungs mediated through vagal and autonomic pathways. Slowly adapting receptors are excited by the contraction of airway smooth muscles; rapidly adapting (irritant) receptors and C fibres may respond to the local inflammation of the airways [10].

13.2.2.2   Work/Effort
These descriptors characterise several clinical conditions [9]. Regardless of the specific disorder, work/effort intensifies during exercise. The increase in motor command to ventilatory muscles relayed by interneurons high in the central nervous system to the sensory cortex (corollary discharge) can be perceived as a sensation of effort [11, 12].

13.2.2.3 Inspiratory Difficulty

The central motor command output to the sensory cortex (the corollary discharge) is modulated by peripheral feedback from a host of respiratory mechanoreceptors that provide precise kinaesthetic information about inspiratory muscle displacement (muscle spindles), tension development (Golgi tendon organs), changes in respired volume and flow and airway calibre (vagal lung and airway mechanoreceptors) [13]. Reduced instantaneous peripheral feedback from the lung and chest wall is thought to account for the uncoupling between reduced lung volumes and a prevailing increase in respiratory drive [14–18].

Rapid Breathing

Rapid breathing characterises the exercise response in patients with interstitial lung disease [19]. Vagal afferents are potentially implicated. Chest compression and lung deflation can potentially reduce the input from stretch receptors with resultant tachypnoea and simultaneously increase the input of rapidly adapting vagal receptors, which increase respiratory drive and ventilation, thus contributing to dyspnoea [20].

13.2.2.4 Air Hunger

The hypothesis that dyspnoea is largely a sense of respiratory effort does not account for the findings that, at a comparable level of ventilation, dyspnoea is greater during hypercapnic hyperpnoea than exercise hyperpnoea [21]. Our current thinking is that air hunger arises from the perception of a corollary copy of brainstem motor output that is transmitted to the forebrain and is relieved by an increase in mechanoreceptor afferent traffic consequent to increased pulmonary minute ventilation. Thus, if arterial carbon dioxide tension ($PaCO_2$) is increased or arterial oxygen tension (PO_2) is decreased and breathing is not allowed to increase, the subject experiences air hunger. Likewise if $PaCO_2$ is held constant and tidal volume is decreased, the subject experiences air hunger [22, 23].

13.3   Clinical Applications of the Language of Dyspnoea

13.3.1 Chronic Obstructive Pulmonary Disease (COPD)

COPD patients when exercising report qualitative perceptions of work/effort and inspiratory difficulty. Neurophysiologically increased breathing effort is believed to reflect the awareness of increased motor command output to the respiratory muscles and increased central corollary discharge. Inspiratory difficulty is associated with *dynamic hyperinflation* and its negative mechanical effects, i.e. elastic load and threshold load and the disparity between inspiratory effort and ventilatory output [14–18]. The important consequence of dynamic hyperinflation is the severe mechanical constraint on tidal volume expansion [14–16]. It has recently been reported that regardless of the exercise, the tidal volume plateaus mark a point where an increase in dyspnoea is associated with change in the quality of the descriptors from work/effort to inspiratory difficulty. These data indicate that intensity and quality of dyspnoea may evolve separately [24]. Pulmonary rehabilitation pro-grammes positively affect exercise-induced dyspnoea by improving mechanical constraints in these patients [16, 25]. If the improvement in mechanical factors that underlie neuromuscular decoupling [15, 16, 25] partially forms the basis for reduced dyspnoea perception, a pulmonary rehabilitation programme designed to improve mechanical constraints might affect both intensity and quality of dyspnoea during submaximal exercise in patients with COPD. Bianchi et al. [18] have recently found that three language subgroup COPD patients exhibited similar lung function at base-line and similar rating of dyspnoea and ventilatory changes during exercise. The pulmonary *rehabilitation* programme shifted the dyspnoea/inspiratory reserve vol-ume (IRV) relationship (less Borg at any given IRV) to the right without modifying the set of descriptors in most patients. These data suggest that pulmonary rehabilita-tion allows patients to tolerate a greater amount of restrictive dynamic ventilatory defect by modifying the intensity, but not necessarily the quality, of dyspnoea.

13.3.2   Asthma

In patients with *asthma*, symptoms following methacholine (MCh) inhalation are similar to those experienced during spontaneous asthma [26, 27]. Mahler et al. reported that 50 % of patients with asthma choose the descriptions "my chest feels tight" or "my chest is constricted" to describe their dyspnoea [28]. These findings are in line with the clinical observation that chest tightness is the most probable manifestation of asthma. Assessments of the intensity of dyspnoea alone may not accurately reflect the level of persistent airway obstruction.

The global rating of dyspnoea, in conjunction with frequency–intensity rating of work/effort, may reflect the persistence of obstruction–inflammation of the airways more clearly than ratings of overall intensity of dyspnoea alone [29]. Thus, attention to the language of dyspnoea would alert healthcare providers to significant remain-ing airway obstruction, despite improvements in, or resolution of overall dyspnoea, when assessed by general rating of the intensity of breathing discomfort [29].

The many descriptors that characterise bronchial asthma indicate that different pathophysiological mechanisms are potentially in action, suggesting that it is possible to distinguish among them by utilising symptom discrimination [30]. The discrimina-tion analysis shows symptoms (chest tightness and *chest pain*) that are easily dis-criminated, whereas other symptoms (breathlessness and air hunger) are not. Symptoms that can be reliably discriminated imply different pathophysiological mechanisms, whereas symptoms that cannot be reliably discriminated imply similar pathophysiological mechanisms. In induced asthma, the initial sensation of chest tightness reflects the breathing discomfort resulting from mild bronchoconstriction [31]; with a more severe FEV_1 decrease and hyperinflation, the sensation of work or effort of breathing takes place, which may be due to the related inflammatory compo-nent of asthma and associated mechanical load on the ventilatory muscles [32]. Therefore, there appear to be two distinct sensations of dyspnoea. The first sensation to be relieved with β_2-agonist treatment is chest tightness, which probably arises from stimulation of pulmonary receptors secondary to bronchospasm. The second—"work/ effort"—is probably associated with both dynamic hyperinflation and more severe airway obstruction. There is no obvious link between qualitative descriptors and over- all intensity of dyspnoea during bronchoconstriction in patients with asthma. In a recent study [33], three language subgroups were defined during MCh inhalation: chest tightness, work/effort and both descriptors. Patients selected chest tightness to a greater extent (42.85 %) than work/effort (14.3 %) and both descriptors (26.5 %) to a lesser extent at the lowest level of bronchoconstriction (FEV_1 fall <10 %) as at 20 % fall in FEV_1. *Language* subgroups were equally distributed across perceiver sub- groups as assessed in terms of increase in Borg score at 20 % FEV_1 fall (PB20). These data indicate that PB20 and the language of dyspnoea independently contribute to defining the condition of the disease in patients with clinically stable asthma.

Based on the contrasting effects of airway obstruction and dynamic *hyperinfla- tion* on the language of dyspnoea during MCh inhalation [31], and the finding that in short exercise sessions an increase in lung volumes does not appear to be a crucial contributor to exercise limitation and dyspnoea intensity in severe asthma [34], it has recently been hypothesised that, regardless of the global score of intensity of dyspnoea, different descriptors may be selected by patients during short exercise sessions (CPET) and MCh [35]. According to the above hypothesis, obstruction/ hyperinflation and work rate are highly reliable predictors of Borg rating of dys- pnoea during and short CPET, respectively. Regardless of the global score of inten- sity of dyspnoea, different descriptors may be selected by patients during short CPET and MCh. Different qualitative dyspnoea sensations can help explain the underlying mechanisms of the symptom.

13.3.3   Restrictive Lung Disease

Patients with restrictive lung disease identify work/effort, unsatisfied inspiration, inspiratory difficulty and rapid and shallow breathing as appropriate descriptors [9, 19, 28]. These sensations have their physiological basis partially in an impaired ability to increase lung volume and displace the thorax appropriately in the setting of increased *ventilatory drive*. Patients display a parabolic or U-shaped relationship between tidal volume (V_T) and dyspnoea: a slight increase or decrease in V_T from the average resting value causes a marked increase in dyspnoea. The former is asso- ciated with greater respiratory work, whereas the latter is associated with increased dead space ventilation and *hypercapnia* [30]. The U-shaped curve relating difficulty of breathing to ventilation (V'_E) with the V'_E at the centre of the spontaneous breath- ing level [36, 37] probably describes the effects of two different sensations: the left limb describes air hunger, and the right limb describes work/effort [38].

13.3.4   Neuromuscular Disease

Impairment of neuromuscular coupling underlies the high scoring of dyspnoea in patients with neuromuscular disease. The association of muscle weakness and elas- tic load in neuromuscular disease is responsible for the modulation of normal central respiratory output into a shallow pattern of breathing [19]. Contrary to an early hypothesis that an increase in inspiratory motor output could translate into an increased perception of dyspnoea in patients with abnormalities in respiratory mechanics, this perception was unexpectedly blunted in stroke patients [39]. This is probably because of the abnormality in the mechanisms of the process of integration of the afferent sensation. If the increased inspiratory motor output does not transmit the corollary discharge to the sensory centre, an unchanged perception may result. Might this be due to functional abnormalities of the sensory cortex? The hypothesis that damage to the sensory cortex attenuates the effect of the corollary discharge, which could influence a patient's ability to perceive dyspnoea, may not be excluded [39].

Studies raise the possibility that neuromuscular disease [40], COPD [14, 15], ILD [19] and airway involvement in multisystem diseases [41] share common mechanisms underlying the discomfort associated with the act of breathing. A common underlying pathophysiological mechanism explains the similarity of clusters selected in different disorders [42].

13.3.5 Chronic Heart Failure

When patients with *chronic heart failure* were asked to describe their dyspnoea, they selected the following clusters: suffocating at rest, rapid breathing, air hunger [9] or work/effort during exercise [28]. It is not easy to explain the underlying pathophysiology due to the conflicting data reported on whether respiratory function contributes to exercise limitation in chronic heart failure patients. O'Donnell et al. [43] show that inspiratory pressure support decreases leg effort, probably by reducing the left ventricular afterload, increasing peripheral blood flow and improving local acid–base equilibrium, which reduces muscular afferents associated with the perception of "effort". Nonetheless, the observation of no evident effect on dyspnoea during the constant load exercise test suggests that factors other than mechanical loading contribute predominantly to dyspnoea. Verbal descriptors may help differentiate between patients with chronic heart failure and deconditioned patients who describe "heavy breathing" [44].

13.4 Affective Distress (Emotional, Affective Components of Dyspnoea)

Any assessment of dyspnoea must take into consideration the following question: "Are we trying to measure the intensity or quality of the sensation of respiratory discomfort or the emotional or behavioural response to the breathing discomfort?" [1]. Pivotal studies [45–47] have provided compelling evidence that sensory intensity and unpleasantness of pain are discrete dimensions since they can be independently manipulated in laboratory and clinical situations. They even appear to be subserved by separate neural pathways [45]. It has been postulated (but not definitely proven) that these structures might process the discrete components of dyspnoea [48, 49].

Further developments regarding the affective dimensions of pain have been divided into an initial stage (A1) of immediate unpleasantness or discomfort and a later stage (A2) of cognitively mediated emotional reactions such as depression, anxiety and fear that may lead to behavioural outcomes [47]. Early evidence suggests similar multidimensionality in the perception of both pain and dyspnoea. Healthy subjects breathing against increased inspiratory loads experience a stronger perception in unpleasantness than in intensity, indicating that the sensory and the affective dimensions of dyspnoea can be differentiated similarly from the perception of pain [50].

In patients with asthma, a high sensitivity seems favourable because it allows the early detection of deteriorating lung function and quick medication relief. A moderate degree of asthma-specific sensitivity (anxiety) is adaptive because it may be associated with enhanced perception of bronchoconstriction. In contrast, the absence of anxiety may lead to indifference and neglect of symptoms [51, 52].

A multidimensional model of dyspnoea subsuming sensory components (i.e. intensity and quality) and affective components has recently been proposed [53, 54]. Affective responses are a major stimulus for learning strategies to avoid biologically threatening sensations, thus motivating patients to seek treatment or alter their lifestyle to avoid dyspnoea. An exaggerated perception of dyspnoea, which may lead to excessive use of medical resources, may be an overresponse in the affective dimension. In this connection, it has been hypothesised that the affective dimension of dyspnoea (unpleasantness, emotional response) does not strictly depend on the intensity of the dyspnoea. The unpleasantness of dyspnoea can vary, independently of the perceived intensity, consistent with the prevailing model of pain that multiple dimensions of dyspnoea exist and can be measured [53, 54].

13.5   Symptom/Disease Impact

13.5.1 MRC Scale

Since 1959 the Medical Research Council (MRC) scale has been used extensively as a discriminative instrument based on the magnitude of task that provokes dyspnoea. The MRC scale is simple to administer and correlates with other dyspnoea scales and with scores of health status [3]. MRC and other similar scales focus only on one dimension that affects dyspnoea; the grades are quite broad so that it may be difficult to detect small but important changes with particular interventions [3].

13.5.2 BDI–TDI

The Baseline (BDI) and Transition (TDI) Dyspnea Indexes include two components—functional impairment and magnitude of effort—in addition to magnitude of the task that provoked breathing difficulty [3, 55]. The BDI is a discriminative instrument to measure dyspnoea at a single point in time, whereas the TDI was developed as an evaluative instrument to measure changes in dyspnoea from the baseline state. Ratings or scores for dyspnoea are obtained from an interviewer who selects a score for each of the three components based on the patient's answers using the specific criteria for the grades as described for the instruments. Translations in different languages are available including an Italian translation (G. Scano and K. Ferrari) [3].

13.5.2.1 CRDQ

Dyspnoea is one of the four components of a quality of life instrument, the Chronic Respiratory Disease Questionnaire (CRDQ) for patients with respiratory disease [56]. The individual patient is asked to select the five most important activities that cause dyspnoea over the past 2 weeks by recalling and then reading from a list of 26 activities. The severity of dyspnoea is graded by the patient who selects a score on a scale of 1–7 for each of the five activities. The overall score can then be divided by the number of activities (usually 5) selected by the patient. There is no correlation between the effort dyspnoea evaluated by the Borg scale and the dyspnoea category of the CRDQ [3].

13.5.2.2 Other Questionnaires

Other multidimensional questionnaires include the Oxygen Cost Diagram (OCD) [3] which is a VAS with 13 activities along a 100-mm line. The position of these activities along this vertical line corresponds approximately to their oxygen requirements. The patient is asked to indicate the level of activity at which he/she begins to experience dyspnoea. The OCD score is measured in millimetres. The shorter the distance, the greater the breathlessness. This measure is simple to use and has thus been used quite widely.

The *University of Cincinnati Dyspnea Questionnaire* (UCDQ) [57] was developed to measure the impact of dyspnoea during physical activity, speech and simultaneous speech and physical activity. The following items of the speech section of the UCDQ are reported to cause dyspnoea in patients with COPD [58]: conversation, raising the voice, phoning, speaking to a group, talking in a noisy place and singing. For patients with limited physical activities who use oral communication for most social activities, the assessment of dyspnoea during speech activities may provide relevant measurement criteria [58].

Conclusion

Although cultural, socio-economic, linguistic and educational backgrounds may influence the use of the language of dyspnoea, our ability to provide the best care possible to patients with dyspnoea depends upon our capacity to break down any communication barriers between physician and patients. As dyspnoea is a fundamental part of a patient's clinical history, physicians should become more fluent in the language of dyspnoea. Some questions still need to be addressed. Should the various aspects of dyspnoea identified by verbal descriptors be independently quantified? Should improvement of the physiological derangements modify the language of dyspnoea? Should reduction of dynamic hyperinflation modify the relevant descriptor(s)? These points need further investigation.

References

1. American Thoracic Society (1999) Dyspnea. Mechanisms, assessment and management: a consensus statement. Am J Respir Crit Care Med 159:321–340
2. Parshall MB, Schwartzstein RM, Adams L et al (2012) An Official American Thoracic Society Statement: update on the mechanisms, assessment, and management of dyspnea. Am J Respir Crit Care Med 185:435–452
3. Mahler DA, Jones PW, Guyatt GH (1998) Clinical measurement of dyspnea. In: Mahler DA (ed) Dyspnea. Marcel Dekker, New York, pp 149–198
4. Ambrosino N, Scano G (2001) Measurement and treatment of dyspnea. Respir Med 95:539–547
5. Gift AG (1989) Visual analogue scales: measurement of subjective phenomena. Nurs Res 38:286–288
6. Borg GAV (1982) Psychological bases of perceived exertion. Med Sci Sport Exerc 14:377–381
7. Muza SR, Silverman MT, Gilmore GC et al (1990) Comparison of scales used to quantitate the sense of effort to breathe in patients with chronic obstructive pulmonary disease. Am Rev Respir Dis 141:909–913
8. Killian KJ, LeBlanc P, Martin DH et al (1992) Exercise capacity and ventilatory, circulatory, and symptom limitation in patients with chronic airflow limitation. Am Rev Respir Dis 146:935–940
9. Simon PM, Schwartzstein RM, Weiss JW et al (1990) Distinguishable types of dyspnea in patients with shortness of breath. Am Rev Respir Dis 142:1009–1014
10. Paintal A (1973) Vagal receptors and their reflex effects. Physiol Rev 53:159–227
11. McCluskey DI (1981) Corollary discharges: motor commands and perception. In: Brookhart JM, Mountcastle VB (eds) The nervous system. Handbook of physiology, section 1. Bethesda: American Physiological Society. 2(2):1415–1447
12. Gandevia SC (1988) Neural mechanisms underlying the sensation of breathlessness: kinesthetic parallels between respiratory and limb muscles. Aust N Z J Med 18:83–91
13. Killian KJ, Campbell EJM (1995) Dyspnea. In: Roussos C (ed) The thorax part B. Dekker, New York, pp 1709–1747
14. O'Donnell DE, Bertley JC, Chau LL et al (1997) Qualitative aspects of exertional breathlessness in chronic airflow limitation: pathophysiologic mechanisms. Am J Respir Crit Care Med 155:109–115
15. O'Donnell DE, Revill SM, Webb AK (2001) Dynamic hyperinflation and exercise intolerance in chronic obstructive pulmonary disease. Am J Respir Crit Care Med 164:770–777
16. Gigliotti F, Coli C, Bianchi R et al (2003) Exercise training improves exertional dyspnea in patients with COPD: evidence of role of mechanical factors. Chest 123:1794–1802
17. Innocenti-Bruni G, Gigliotti F, Binazzi B, et al. (2012) Dyspnea, chest wall hyperinflation, and rib cage distortion in exercising patients with chronic obstructive pulmonary disease. Med Sci Sport Exerc 44:1049–1056
18. Bianchi R, Gigliotti F, Romagnoli I et al (2011) Impact of a rehabilitation program on dyspnea intensity and quality in patients with chronic obstructive pulmonary disease. Respiration 81:186–195
19. O'Donnell DE, Chau LKL, Webb AK (1998) Qualitative aspects of exertional dyspnea in patients with interstitial lung disease. J Appl Physiol 84:2000–2009
20. Adrian ED (1933) Afferent impulses in the vagus and their effect on respiration. J Physiol (Lond) 70:332–358
21. Chonan T, Mulholland MB, Leitner J et al (1990) Sensation of dyspnea during hypercapnia, exercise and voluntary hyperventilation. J Appl Physiol 68:2100–2106
22. Banzett RB, Lansing RW, Brown R, Topulos GP et al (1990) "Air hunger" arising from increased PCO_2 persists after complete neuromuscular block in humans. Respir Physiol 81:1–17

23. Banzett RB, Lansing RW, Reid MB et al (1989) "Air hunger" arising from increased PCO_2 in mechanically ventilated quadriplegics. Respir Physiol 76:53–68
24. Laveneziana P, Webb K, Ora J et al (2011) Evolution of dyspnea during exercise in COPD: impact of critical volume constraints. Am J Respir Crit Care Med 184:1367–1373
25. O'Donnell DE, McGuire M, Samis L et al (1995) The impact of exercise reconditioning on breathlessness in severe chronic airflow limitation. Am J Respir Crit Care Med 152:2005–2013
26. Binks AP, Moosavi SH, Banzett RB et al (2002) "Tightness" sensation of asthma does not arise from the work of breathing. Am J Respir Crit Care Med 165:78–82
27. Lougheed MD, Lam M, Forkert L et al (1993) Breathlessness during acute bronchoconstriction in asthma. Am Rev Respir Dis 148:452–459
28. Mahler DA, Harver A, Lentine T et al (1996) Descriptors of breathlessness in cardiorespiratory diseases. Am J Respir Crit Care Med 154:1357–1363
29. Moy ML, Latin ML, Harver A et al (1998) Language of dyspnea in assessment of patients with acute asthma treated with nebulized albuterol. Am J Respir Crit Care Med 158:749–753
30. Killian KJ, Watson R, Otis J et al (2000) Symptom perception during acute bronchoconstriction. Am J Respir Crit Care Med 162:490–496
31. Moy ML, Woodrow Weiss J, Sparrow D et al (2000) Quality of dyspnea in bronchoconstriction differs from external resistive loads. Am J Respir Crit Care Med 162:451–455
32. Gorini M, Iandelli I, Misuri G et al (1999) Chest wall hyperinflation during acute bronchoconstriction in asthma. Am J Respir Crit Care Med 160:808–816
33. Coli C, Picariello M, Stendardi L et al (2006) Is there a link between the qualitative descriptors and quantitative perception of dyspnea in asthma? Chest 130:436–441
34. Barreiro E, Gea J, Sanjuás C, Marcos R et al (2004) Dyspnea at rest and at the end of different exercises in patients with near-fatal asthma. Eur Respir J 24:219–225
35. Laveneziana P, Lotti P, Coli C et al (2006) Mechanisms of dyspnea and its language in patients with asthma. Eur Respir J 26:1–6
36. Brack T, Jubran A, Tobin M (2002) Dyspnea and decreased variability of breathing in patients with restrictive lung disease. Am J Respir Crit Care Med 165:1260–1264
37. Chonan T, Mulholland MB, Altose MD et al (1990) Effects of changes in level and pattern of breathing on the sensation of dyspnea. J Appl Physiol 69:1290–1295
38. Lansing RW, Im BS-H, Thwing JI et al (2000) The perception of respiratory work and effort can be independent of the perception of air hunger. Am J Respir Crit Care Med 162:1690–1696
39. Lanini B, Gigliotti F, Coli C et al (2002) Dissociation between respiratory effort and dyspnea in a subset of patients with stroke. Clin Sci 103:467–473
40. Lanini B, Misuri G, Gigliotti F et al (2001) Perception of dyspnea in patients with neuromuscular disease. Chest 120:402–408
41. Scano G, Seghieri G, Mancini M, Filippelli M et al (1999) Dyspnea, peripheral airway involvement and respiratory muscle effort in patients with type I diabetes mellitus under good metabolic control. Clin Sci 96:499–506
42. Scano G, Innocenti Bruni G, Stendardi L (2010) Do obstructive and restrictive lung disease share common underlying mechanisms of breathlessness? Respir Med 104:925–933
43. O'Donnell DE, D'Arsigny C, Raj S et al (1999) Ventilatory assistance improves exercise endurance in stable congestive heart failure. Am J Respir Crit Care Med 160:1804–1811
44. Schwartzstein RM (2002) The language of dyspnea. Eur Respir Rev 82:28–30
45. Price DD (1999) Psychological mechanism of pain and analgesia. IASP Press, Seattle
46. Rainville P, Duncan GH, Price DD et al (1997) Pain affect encoded in human anterior cingulate but not somatosensory cortex. Science 277:968–971
47. Price DD (2000) Psychological and neural mechanisms of the affective dimension of pain. Science 288:1769–1772
48. Banzett RB, Dempsey JA, O'Donnell DE et al (2000) Symptom perception and respiratory sensation in asthma. Am J Respir Crit Care Med 162:178–182

49. Peiffer C (2008) Dyspnea and emotion. What can we learn from functional brain imaging? Am J Respir Crit Care Med 177:937–938
50. Von Leupoldt A, Dahme B (2005) Cortical substrates for the perception of dyspnea. Chest 128:345–354
51. De Peuter S, Lemaigre V, Van Diest I et al (2007) Differentiation between the sensory and affective aspects of histamine-induced bronchoconstriction in asthma. Respir Med 101:925–932
52. De Peuter S, Van Diest I, Lemaigre V et al (2004) Dyspnea: the role of psychological processes. Clin Psychol Rev 24:557–581
53. Lansing RW, Gracely RH, Banzett RB (2009) The multiple dimensions of dyspnea: review and hypotheses. Respir Physiol Neurobiol 167:53–60
54. Banzett RB, Pedersen SH, Schwartzstein RM et al (2008) The affective dimension of laboratory dyspnea: air hunger is more unpleasant than work/effort. Am J Respir Crit Care Med 177:1384–1390
55. Mahler DA, Weinberg DH, Wells CK et al (1984) The measurement of dyspnea: contents, interobserver agreement, and physiologic correlates of two new clinical indexes. Chest 85:751–758
56. Guyatt GH, Berman LB, Townshend M et al (1987) A measure of quality of life for clinical trials in chronic lung disease. Thorax 42:773–778
57. Lee L, Friesen MA, Lambert IR et al (1998) Evaluation of dyspnea during physical and speech activities in patients with pulmonary disease. Chest 113:625–632
58. Binazzi B, Lanini B, Romagnoli I et al (2011) Dyspnea during speech in chronic obstructive pulmonary disease patients: effects of pulmonary rehabilitation. Respiration 81:379–385

Noninvasive Measures of Lung Structure and Ventilation Heterogeneity

14

Sylvia Verbanck and Manuel Paiva

14.1 Introduction

A major reason for the difficulty in understanding gas transport and mixing in the lung periphery is related to the impossibility to perform direct measurements of gas concentrations in the alveolar region without interfering with the mechanisms of transport. If the measurements are performed at the mouth, the gases are first inspired and convected to the lung periphery. During a breath cycle, they diffuse in a space with linear dimensions that are of the order of magnitude of the square root of the molecular diffusion coefficient. For air, this corresponds to a few millimeters. During expiration, the recorded concentration at the mouth gives an information about the last lung generations, where O_2 and N_2 have diffused. Part of this information is contained in the slope of the alveolar plateau of the single-breath (N_2) washout (SBW). Georg et al. [1] used gases of different diffusivities such as He and SF_6. Indeed, the different expiratory concentration profile of these gases carries information about the lung structure in a specific lung region. A renewed interest in SBW came also from the work of Cosio et al. [2] demonstrating correlations of SBW-derived indices, such as N_2 phase III slope and closing capacity, with morphological measures of peripheral lung lesion in smokers. A series of epidemiological studies followed, investigating the potential of these tests to predict a decline in forced expired volume in 1 s (FEV_1) in smokers, but with conflicting outcomes [3–6]. However, the interest in the SBW test increased with the results of a 13-year

S. Verbanck (✉)
Respiratory Division, Academic Hospital UZ Brussel, Vrije Universiteit Brussel,
Laarbeeklaan 101, Brussels, 1090, Belgium
e-mail: sylvia.verbanck@uzbrussel.be

M. Paiva
Chest Department, University Hospital Erasme, Université Libre de Bruxelles,
Route de Lennik 808, Brussels, 1070, Belgium
e-mail: mpaiva@ulb.ac.be

A. Aliverti, A. Pedotti (eds.), *Mechanics of Breathing*,
DOI 10.1007/978-88-470-5647-3_14, © Springer-Verlag Italia 2014

follow-up study [7] indicating that the N_2 phase III slope of the vital capacity SBW test was a key index in predicting the smoker developing overt COPD.

In the meanwhile, several groups had continued their investigations into the basic mechanisms of gas transport in, and its heterogeneous distribution over, the lungs. As reports of the actual geometrical configuration of the human lungs emerged [8–10], new models could be developed in an effort to simulate the SBW test. An essential feature of the anatomical basis for the lung models to be developed was that the lung was asymmetrical, in the conductive airway [8] as well as in the acinar airway segment [9, 10]. It was shown, for instance, how the interaction of convective and diffusive gas transport in the asymmetrical acinar air spaces could generate N_2 concentration differences that are reflected in a N_2 gradient in the alveolar phase III of an SBW exhalation [11]; in addition, this N_2 phase III gradient was expected to increase with increasing asymmetry. Although this is just one potential mechanism of ventilation heterogeneity, it illustrates how the delivery and recovery of gas concentrations can provide noninvasive indexes of ventilatory heterogeneity that are representative of lung structure, or its abnormality in the case of lung disease.

A different technique can be used as a tool to investigate pulmonary ventilation. It consists of aerosol inspiration and the analysis of particle concentration during the subsequent expiration. When aerosols are inspired as a bolus, the very low (Brownian) diffusion coefficient of the particles enables to target specific generations of the bronchial tree. For decades, fields of gas and particle transport in the lung proceeded in parallel, with very limited cross-fertilization. Despite being more difficult to generate and measure experimentally than gases, aerosols can be a very elegant tool to sample the structure in the lung periphery. We describe, at the end of this chapter, aerosol applications showing the complementarity of both approaches.

14.2 Gas Washout Tests

The washout technique basically consists of delivering to the lungs a gas mixture that is not originally present in the lungs and then characterizing the exhaled gas mixture as a function of exhaled volume. Figure 14.1 shows the concentration plot of N_2 as a function of exhaled volume after a vital capacity inhalation of 100 % O_2 (SBW test). One can clearly distinguish an initial phase where the inhaled gas is exhaled again without having been mixed with lung resident air (phase I), a transitional phase II, an alveolar phase III, and a final rise in phase IV. Depending on the subject under study, cardiogenic oscillations are superimposed on phases III and IV; yet, in most lung diseases which give rise to steeper phase III slopes, cardiogenic oscillations cannot be distinguished.

On the basis of experimental and modeling studies of gas transport in the human lungs, we can summarize the contributions to the phase III slope as follows:

- *Ventilation heterogeneity between upper and lower lung regions, generated by the weight of the lung on earth:* In normal lungs, the gravity-dependent contribution to the phase III slope has been investigated in studies involving different body positions [12, 13], in experiments aboard parabolic flights [14, 15], or

Fig. 14.1 Vital capacity SBW test in a healthy subject; exhaled N_2 concentration versus exhaled volume down to residual volume, showing phases I, II, III, and IV

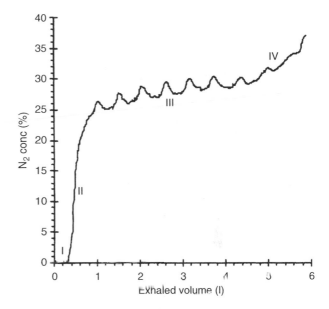

during Spacelab missions [16, 17], and depending also on the washout maneuver used, the gravity contribution to the N_2 phase III slope is seen not to exceed approximately one fifth; in fact, the largest contribution from gravity could be found in the phase III slope of a vital capacity SBW maneuver (as opposed to washout maneuvers covering the near-tidal volume range). Since certain disease patterns may be linked to distinct locations (e.g., in patients with predominant emphysema in upper lung zones), the effect of gravity can actually be exploited to investigate structure-function in these zones. Van Muylem et al. [18] proposed to place single-lung transplant patients in such a body posture that the SBW phase III could actually be linked to structure-function of the dependent and non-dependent lungs.

- *Ventilation heterogeneity between units within the acinus, which results from convective and diffusive gas transport competing in the structural asymmetry of the lung periphery:* Due to this so-called diffusion-convection interdependence [19], the smallest intra-acinar lung unit subtended by any pair of daughter branches shows the lowest N_2 concentration during inhalation; during subsequent exhalation, the differential convection from smaller and larger intra-acinar units and back diffusion of N_2 into the smaller of two units leads to a slope in the exhaled N_2 concentration versus volume trace. Over a wide range of structural asymmetries, interdependence predicts that the larger structural asymmetry leads to the greater N_2 phase III slope. In addition, the complex interaction of hundreds of parallel and serial branch points inside each acinus plays a key role [20, 21]. A model simulation study [22] has shown that not only the mean structural asymmetry at branch points of any given peripheral lung generation is a determinant of the phase III slope but also the heterogeneity in asymmetry among parallel branch points of that generation. For any given mean asymmetry, the larger parallel heterogeneity in asymmetry also leads to a steeper N_2 phase III slope. In fact, with simulations incorporating a realistic heterogeneity of intra-acinar asymmetry, the potential intra-acinar contribution to the N_2 phase III slope ranges 80–100 % [22] depending on the washout maneuver.

- *Ventilation heterogeneity between lung units, probably much smaller than the upper and lower lung regions, but larger than acini*, i.e., *at the level of lung units where convective gas transport dominates over diffusive gas transport:* This mechanism implies differences in specific ventilation (unit inspired volume per unit lung volume) and flow asynchrony between lung units upon emptying. This mechanism of ventilation heterogeneity can be generated by a heterogeneity in P-V characteristics of such lung units or a heterogeneity in airway resistance of the subtending airways; yet, in human subjects, no quantitative data on these properties at this scale exist. Also, heterogeneity in airway resistance or P-V characteristics should be such that the best ventilated lung unit is the one to empty preferentially early in expiration, in order to produce a positive contribution to the N_2 phase III slope. There are a huge number of branch points located in the conductive airways where such convection-dependent heterogeneity can occur. Maybe the number of possibilities can be limited by use of so-called integrated models such as the one offered by Tawhai et al. e.g., [23], with a very realistic appearance from a structural viewpoint. However, the way it simulates airway function is currently still burdened by oblique parameter fitting, which makes it almost impossible to determine where some highly unrealistic simulations, acknowledged by the authors, find their origin. Nevertheless, further development of such models, closely guided by the wealth of experimental washout data, should make it possible to quantitatively determine the confines within which this mechanism accounts for the phase III slope in normal man. While the net contribution to the N_2 phase III slope from this mechanism may actually be relatively modest during an SBW obtained from the normal lungs, its effect can be exaggerated in the diseased lung [24, 25] or in the asymptomatic lung after histamine bronchoprovocation [26].

- *Gas exchange:* The fact that the respiratory coefficient is <1 brings about volume shrinkage and hence a progressive concentration of all gases as the exhalation proceeds, leading to an amplification of the phase III slope for the lung resident gas N_2; in human lungs, its effect has been estimated at 10 % for a vital capacity SBW maneuver [27].

- *Airway closure:* When decomposing a vital capacity SBW, involving a continuous O_2 inhalation starting from residual volume, into separate washout experiments whereby 150 mL volumes of O_2 are inhaled at different lung volumes over the vital capacity range, it is possible to study the effect of ventilation heterogeneity at any given lung volume and relate it to the SBW phase III slope [28]. In this way, it has been shown that in the case of a vital capacity SBW test in normal subjects, the heterogeneous distribution of gas inhaled at lung volumes below FRC in fact produces a negative contribution to the N_2 phase III slope. Hence, exaggerated airway closure below FRC has an attenuating effect on phase III slope, while disease states, where airway closure also appears around and above

FRC, could yield a positive contribution to phase III slope. Hence, the actual contribution to N_2 phase III slope from airway closure is not straightforward.

The problem with these different mechanisms generating a N_2 phase III slope is that their relative contribution – positive or negative – may be hard to determine and is expected to vary, depending on the disease state of the lungs. Let us first reconsider the reason why tests of ventilation heterogeneity were thought of as a promising diagnostic tool:

- *For early detection of lung alterations:* It was expected that heterogeneity in structural change could reveal abnormality before a global change (e.g., overall airway narrowing) sets in to such an extent that spirometry becomes abnormal. An experimental demonstration of this potential was the observation that heart-lung transplant patients showed an abnormal SBW phase III slope with a median of 1 year before FEV_1 became abnormal to reflect a rejection episode [29].

- *For monitoring the lung periphery:* Experimental and theoretical work conducted over the years indicated that the phase III slope is in fact predominantly affected by peripheral air spaces, where resistance to flow is small and hence referred to as the "silent lung zone."

If it were possible to separate ventilation heterogeneity originating in the peripheral air spaces from that in the more proximal airways, this could bring about a sensitive diagnostic tool that is also more specific to structural alterations in a lung zone where spirometry performs poorly. In the mid-1980s, experimental work by Crawford et al. [30–33] emerged which displayed the potential of delivering such a tool, based on earlier modeling work [34]. Instead of having a subject perform one inhalation and exhalation (single-breath washout, SBW), the subject is asked to perform subsequent inhalations and exhalations (multiple-breath washout, MBW) such that by the nature of the mechanisms involved, their respective contributions to phase III slope will be accentuated as the MBW proceeds. Figure 14.2 shows how N_2 concentration continuously decreases during an MBW test, but also that each breath can be considered as an SBW curve where the N_2 phase III slope progressively increases relative to its mean expired N_2 concentration (insets of Fig. 14.2).

When the N_2 phase III slope of each expiration is normalized by its mean expired or end-expired N_2 concentration, the resulting normalized phase III slope (S) steadily increases as a function of breath number, even in a normal subject (Fig.14.3). For the sake of illustration, the exaggerated S increase in the same subject after histamine provocation is also shown, and for methodological reasons, S is represented as a function of lung turnover (TO, i.e., cumulative expired volume divided by FRC) instead of breath number [30].

While diffusion-convection interaction can indeed account for most of the S value of the first breath of an experimental MBW test [21], it is intrinsic to this mechanism that S only slightly increases as the MBW proceeds, and that after the first few breaths, a horizontal S asymptote is reached. An alternative mechanism to explain the increasing S as a function of breath number (or TO) beyond the first few breaths is the one where two units are ventilated to a different extent creating a concentration difference between them, which serves as the initial condition to the next inhalation. In any subsequent inhalation, concentration differences will become

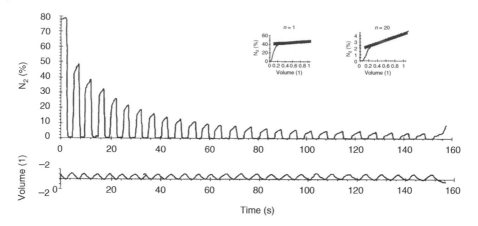

Fig. 14.2 MBW test obtained in a normal subject after histamine provocation to illustrate the rate of rise of the N_2 phase III slope with respect to the mean expired N_2 concentration as a function of breath number (n)

Fig. 14.3 Normalized slopes (S; mean ± SD) versus lung turnover (TO) obtained on a normal subject before (*closed circles*) and after (*open circles*) histamine

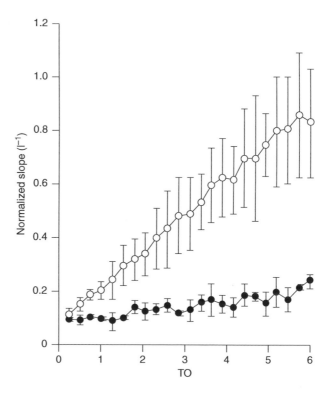

relatively greater, i.e., the concentration difference divided by the average concentration will progressively increase. This mechanism predicts an increasing S as a function of TO, however with an extrapolation to $S=0$ for $TO=0$ [34].

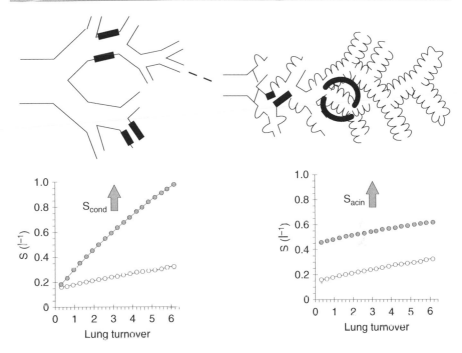

Fig. 14.4 Schematic representation of conductive and acinar structural alteration and its predicted effect on normalized phase III slopes (S) versus lung turnover (TO) and derived indices S_{cond} and S_{acin}

On basis of the above explanations, and without displaying the details here (these can be found in [35]), two indices of ventilation heterogeneity can be derived from the S versus TO curves as follows. The diffusion-convection interdependence mechanism (operational in the acinar lung zone) mainly affects the height of the S versus TO curve, but hardly contributes to the rate of S increase versus TO. Hence, the index of acinar ventilation heterogeneity (S_{acin}) is computed as the S value of the first breath minus a small contribution from the rate of S rise in the remainder of the MBW test ($S_{acin} = S(n=1) - TO(n=1) . S_{cond}$, where S_{cond} is given below). Convective ventilatory heterogeneity (operational in the conductive lung zone) mainly affects the increase of the S versus TO curve, but hardly contributes to the initial S value. Hence, the index of conductive ventilation heterogeneity (S_{cond}) corresponds to the regression slope of the S versus TO curve beyond the first few breaths (TO > 1.5). Figure 14.4 schematically displays S versus TO curves and the behavior of derived S_{acin} and S_{cond} in two schematic cases of acinar or conductive airway structural alterations. Whenever a patient displays an increased S_{cond}, this is thought to reflect an increased heterogeneity in airway lumen or in elastic properties of relatively large lung units subtended from the conductive airways. Whenever a patient displays an increased S_{acin}, this may be interpreted as result of a change in intra-acinar asymmetry either by cross-sectional heterogeneity or by changes in subtended volumes.

Two advantages of the MBW test are (1) that it involves near-tidal breathing above FRC which not only corresponds to lung volumes during natural breathing but also avoids the effect of airway closure at residual volume, and (2) that the S versus TO curves derived from the MBW are only poorly affected by the blurring effect of gravity [36]. Hence, the MBW indices can be almost entirely attributed to intrinsic structural and elastic properties of the lung, which renders this test particularly useful in the clinical context of the lung function laboratory. We summarize here the use of the normalized slope analysis of the MBW test in clinical applications, with Fig. 14.5 displaying average S_{acin} and S_{cond} values obtained from the same laboratory in either of the study groups described below. These results are then placed against other washout data from the literature.

14.2.1 Bronchoprovocation

For an average FEV_1 decrease of 26 % after a 2 mg cumulative dose of histamine, S_{cond} was shown to increase by 390 % with no significant change in S_{acin}, indicating that during provocation large ventilation heterogeneities occur and that the airways affected by the provocation process are situated proximal to the entrance of the acinar lung zone [26]. A methacholine provocation study showed a significant but small S_{acin} increase and a large S_{cond} increase [37]. The observed S_{cond} increase likely represents the inequality in response of parallel airways, superimposed on global airway narrowing. This could reflect density differences in muscarine receptors and/or cholinergic innervation between airways located at a given lung depth (i.e., airways of more or less the same lung generation) in addition to the reported proximal versus peripheral density differences along the bronchial tree [38]. Since the conductive airways (as reflected in S_{cond}) constitute the main source of ventilation heterogeneity during bronchoprovocation, and because this component is only poorly reflected in the SBW phase III slope, this could explain the moderate SBW phase III slope increases observed by others after provocation e.g., [39]. Although it is intrinsically impossible to determine the contribution from acinar and conductive air spaces by only studying the decline in mean expired concentration of an MBW test, several such reports in the case of bronchoprovocation [40, 41] did speculate on an important contribution from convection-dependent ventilation heterogeneity. A comparative study of two aspecific bronchoprovocation aerosols revealed an apparent paradox of a greater ventilation heterogeneity (largest S_{cond} increase) for the bronchoprovoking agent (methacholine) which induces the least deterioration of spirometry, at least in terms of FEV_1 [42]. It was suggested that the differential action of histamine and methacholine is confined to the conductive airways, where histamine likely causes greatest overall airway narrowing and methacholine induces largest parallel heterogeneity in airway narrowing, probably at the level of the large and small conductive airways, respectively. The observed ventilation heterogeneities predict a risk for dissociation between ventilation-perfusion mismatch and spirometry, particularly after methacholine challenge, as has been observed

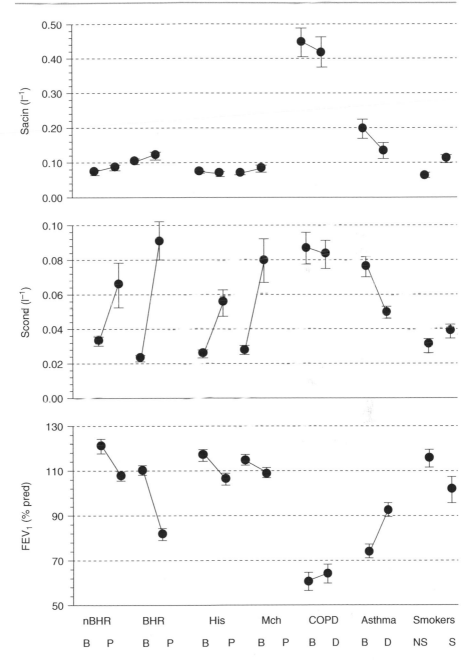

Fig. 14.5 Average values (±SE) of S_{acin} and S_{cond} and corresponding FEV_1 in normal subjects with bronchial hyperresponsiveness (*BHR*) or not (*nBHR*), in nBHR subjects provoked with histamine (*His*) or methacholine (*MCh*), in COPD and asthmatic patients, and in smokers (*S*) or never-smokers (*NS*); *B* baseline, *P* provocation, *D* dilatation

experimentally by others [43]. On the basis of SBW phase III slopes with different diffusivity gases, it has been suggested that adenosine 5'-monophosphate has an even more peripheral effect than methacholine [44].

14.2.2   COPD Patients

In a group of COPD patients with various degrees of airway obstruction (FEV_1/ $FVC = 52 \pm 11(SD)\%$) and transfer factor ($TL_{CO} = 77 \pm 25(SD)\%$), the relationship of S_{cond} and S_{acin} to standard lung function indices was evaluated by means of a principal component factor analysis [24], which linked correlated indices to independent factors accounting for 81 % of the total variance within the COPD group. S_{acin} was linked to the so-called acinar lung zone factor, comprising also diffusing capacity measurements. S_{cond} was linked to the so-called conductive lung zone factor, comprising also specific airway conductance and forced expiratory flows. The fact that S_{cond} and S_{acin} were linked to independent factors is a statistical confirmation of the hypothesis that S_{cond} and S_{acin} can reflect independent lung alterations, corresponding to different functional lung units. FEV_1/FVC was the only variable linked to both the conductive and the acinar lung zone factor, indicating a combined conductive and acinar contribution to airway obstruction in these COPD patients.

14.2.3   Asthmatics

Baseline S_{acin} values were found to be abnormal in asthmatics, despite normal diffusing capacity in this group [25]; these S_{acin} values were intermediate between those obtained in normal subjects and in COPD patients. Baseline S_{cond} was also abnormal in the asthmatics but similar to that obtained in the COPD patients. After salbutamol inhalations, significant changes in S_{cond} and S_{acin} were only observed in the asthmatics. These results indicate significant – but partially reversible – acinar airway impairment in asthmatics, as compared to the more severe baseline acinar airway impairment in COPD patients, none of which was reversible after salbutamol inhalation. The involvement of the peripheral airways in asthmatic patients in the baseline condition and after inhaled β_2-mimetic drugs has been a subject of considerable interest in the past, where the terminology "peripheral airways" actually covers a large range of airway generations depending on the measurement method used [45–47]. Ventilation distribution has also been previously investigated in asthmatics in terms of N_2 phase III slope of the SBW [47–51] or in terms of decaying concentration curves of the MBW [52], with a general observation of a diminished overall lung ventilation heterogeneity after inhalation of β_2-mimetic drugs. A modified single-breath washout maneuver employed by Cooper et al. [50] in asthmatic children started the O_2 inhalation from FRC rather than from residual volume, a maneuver which was indeed expected to better detect lung structural alterations [53]. Cooper et al. [50] found that the asthmatic patients with the steepest baseline N_2 phase III slopes were also the ones showing the largest decreases following isoproterenol inhalation, and that post-isoproterenol N_2 phase III slopes were still elevated with respect to normal values. Using the same SBW maneuver, Gustaffson et al. [51] studied the respective behavior of He and SF_6 phase III slopes to detect an intra-acinar contribution to ventilation distribution in asthma patients. Ventilation heterogeneity in the conductive airways (S_{cond}) has been identified as an independent contributor to airway hyperresponsiveness in asthma [54], and recent reports have also linked S_{cond} and S_{acin} to asthma control [55, 56].

14.2.4 Smokers

An early study in smokers with normal lung function found that S_{acin} was significantly larger than in never-smokers, while S_{cond} remained unaffected [57]. While being less abnormal than previously reported in COPD patients, S_{acin} did detect significant acinar airway alterations in these asymptomatic individuals. Previous reports of the decline in mean expired concentration of an MBW in smokers with relatively normal lung function had revealed an impaired ventilation distribution [58, 59], without however being able to indicate the location of structural alterations. An MBW study in larger cohorts of smokers with a range of smoking history (10–50 pack years) has since indicated structure-function alterations in the lung periphery around the acinar entrance affecting both S_{cond} and S_{acin}; in smokers with emphysema, S_{acin} was further enhanced [60]. In a subsequent smoking cessation study in smokers without airway obstruction [61], a transient S_{acin} decrease and a sustained S_{cond} decrease could be observed over the course of 1 year of smoking cessation. Previous ventilation distribution studies in smokers that made use of phase III slope analysis were essentially derived from the vital capacity SBW maneuver [1–5] where increased phase III slopes were often unduly referred to as an indication of peripheral alterations only.

Taken together, we can state that indices S_{acin} and S_{cond} can be used for the above-mentioned purposes: early detection of lung alterations and monitoring the lung periphery. For early detection purposes, it is important to realize that these indices also slightly vary with age in normal man, and reference values have now been produced [62]. For monitoring, potentially moving into advanced disease stages, care has to be taken that the basic assumptions for separating conductive and acinar effects are still met [35].

14.3 Aerosol Bolus Tests

Although gas bolus studies can give interesting information on lung volume dependence of ventilation distribution [28], they cannot be associated to specific locations in the bronchial tree. However, this becomes possible with aerosols, as illustrated in Fig. 14.6, because of the very low particle diffusivity. If we consider the symmetrical Weibel model of the lung, a particle bolus followed by a volumetric lung depth (VLD) inhalation of air corresponding to the volume of the first 2 generations would

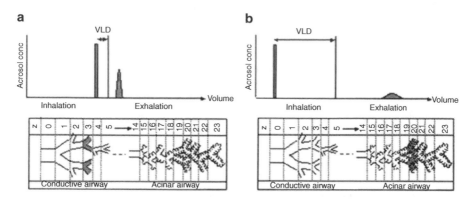

Fig. 14.6 Principle of the aerosol bolus dispersion test. An aerosol bolus is released at different instances during an inhalation, so as to deliver it to the proximal lung, corresponding to a low volumetric lung depth (*VLD*) (panel **a**) or to the peripheral lung and corresponding to a high volumetric lung depth (*VLD*) (panel **b**). Upon exhalation, the bolus is recovered and its dispersion (e.g., its standard deviation) is measured

bring the particles to generation 3 as represented in Fig. 14.6a. Alternatively, an aerosol bolus test with a VLD corresponding to the volume of the first 19 generations would deliver the particles to generation 20 (Fig. 14.6b). For a typical aerosol bolus test, a subject is instructed to inhale a given volume (e.g., 1,000 ml), and a valve system delivers a bolus (e.g., 75 ml) of aerosol at the desired instance of the aerosol-free inhalation. Upon exhalation, the non-deposited portion of the aerosol is recovered in the form of an aerosol bolus which is dispersed over at least twice the inhaled bolus volume.

Depending on the lung level at which the aerosol is inhaled, the aerosol bolus is seen to deposit more and to become more dispersed as it has traveled deeper into the lungs, even in normal subjects [63]. Moreover, it was postulated that in the case of lung structural alterations, particularly if these are heterogeneously distributed over the lungs, aerosol bolus dispersion would be increased. This hypothesis was confirmed experimentally in several lung diseases [64, 65]: in patients with cystic fibrosis [66], emphysema [67], and asthma [68] or in heart-lung transplant patients suffering a rejection period [69]. However, increased aerosol bolus dispersion was also observed in the case of asymptomatic smokers [70–72], suggesting its potential as a marker of lung alterations in the early stages of lung disease. Again, the key issue is how structural heterogeneity can affect aerosol bolus dispersion. Indeed, if a 75 ml aerosol bolus distributes over a complex structure, but recombines in a perfectly reversible fashion, the original aerosol bolus will be restored in its initial 75 ml volume. Heterogeneity in structural alterations that are perceived differently by the aerosol bolus during inspiration than during expiration is expected to introduce an irreversible component of aerosol bolus dispersion.

On the basis of the role of heterogeneity, some studies have indeed measured indices of gas ventilation distribution (SBW, MBW) alongside indices of aerosol distribution (aerosol bolus dispersion). Anderson et al. [71] found an increased N_2

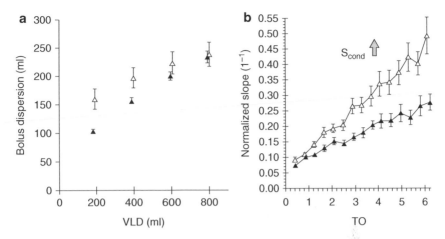

Fig. 14.7 Saline bolus tests (panel **a**) and multiple-breath washout tests (panel **b**) obtained on the same 10 subjects before and after histamine provocation (*closed and open symbols*, respectively). (Panel **a**) Aerosol bolus test: bolus dispersion (±SE) as a function of volumetric lung depth (*VLD*), indicating a structural alteration in the proximal lung. (Panel **b**) MBW test: normalized phase III slope (±SE) as a function of lung turnover, indicating a structural alteration in the conductive airways (S_{cond} increased; see also Fig. 14.4) after histamine

phase III slope of the vital capacity SBW in a smoker group which showed an increased dispersion of the most peripherally inhaled aerosol boluses. Also, in an effort to relate aerosol- and gas-related measures of convective ventilation heterogeneity, Brown et al. [73] found an association between bolus dispersion and ^{133}Xe washout-derived indices in cystic fibrosis patients. An essential issue which is sometimes overlooked in studies comparing gas and aerosol tests of ventilation distribution on the same subjects is the volume range spanned by the various testing procedures. For instance, a vital capacity single-breath washout – including airway closure – and an aerosol bolus test involving lung volumes well above residual volume are bound to only contain partly overlapping information, which may render comparisons disappointing.

Two studies [57, 74] have compared the specific patterns of aerosol bolus dispersion and gas washout (MBW) derived indices in two study groups with specific proximal or peripheral structural alterations. In one study, a group of 10 normal subjects underwent a histamine bronchoprovocation test, inducing a conductive airway alteration, as evidenced by an increased S_{cond} after histamine with respect to baseline. In the other study, 12 smokers were studied who differed from 12 never-smokers in terms of acinar airway alterations only as evidenced by an increased S_{acin} in the smokers versus the never-smokers. In the first group, an increased S_{cond} was paralleled by an increased aerosol bolus dispersion of the most shallowly inhaled aerosol boluses (Fig. 14.7). In the latter group, an increased S_{acin} was paralleled by an increased aerosol bolus dispersion of the most peripherally inhaled aerosol boluses (Fig. 14.8). Note that the lungs with the more peripheral structural alteration (Fig. 14.8) will only affect the dispersion of the most deeply inhaled boluses

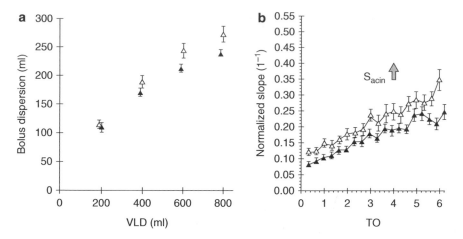

Fig. 14.8 Saline bolus tests (panel **a**) and multiple-breath washout tests (panel **b**) obtained on 12 never-smokers (*closed symbols*) and 12 smokers (*open symbols*). (Panel **a**) Aerosol bolus test: bolus dispersion (±SE) as a function of volumetric lung depth (*VLD*), indicating a structural alteration in the peripheral lung. (Panel **b**) MBW test: normalized phase III slope (±SE) as a function of lung turnover, indicating a structural alteration in the acinar airways (S_{acin} increased; see also Fig. 14.4) after histamine

(largest VLD). By contrast, the lungs with the more proximal structural alteration will affect primarily the most shallow boluses but will also affect the more peripherally inhaled boluses to some extent, since all boluses have to pass the most proximal structures [75] on their way to the lung periphery. Hence, in this case, the effect is most marked for lowest VLD and fades away toward the higher VLD.

Finally, a particularity of the tests shown in Figs. 14.7 and 14.8 was that the aerosol used for these bolus tests was isotonic saline and not the latex particles or oil droplets usually employed for these types of aerosol bolus studies. It was shown indeed that if only bolus dispersion – and not bolus deposition – is to be measured, saline aerosol boluses disperse to the same extent as a 1 μ latex aerosol bolus. Indeed, any potential size change that an isotonic aerosol bolus may undergo in the lungs appears to play a minor role in the dispersion of the bolus, and in fact, lung structure seems to be the major determinant of bolus dispersion. The possibility of using saline instead of latex or oil droplets to detect lung structural alterations may be more appealing for the clinical application of this technique. However, if, in addition to bolus dispersion, there is a need to quantify bolus deposition, for instance, to determine an effective airspace diameter [76], monodisperse aerosols are compulsory.

Conclusion

Depending on the patient population under study, one may consider using either gas- or aerosol-derived noninvasive probes of lung structural alterations. The choice of one technique over the other will essentially be made on basis of technical or practical issues. One practical consideration concerns inhaled volume, which should be around 1 L for a proper phase III slope analysis of the MBW test. This may be difficult to achieve in some patients, and in that case, a protocol with aerosol bolus tests that is limited to shallow inhaled boluses – involving lesser lung inflations – may still be meaningful, depending on the lung disease under study.

References

1. Georg J, Lassen NA, Mellemgaard K, Vinther A (1965) Diffusion in the gas phase of the lungs in normal and emphysematous subjects. Clin Sci 29:525–532
2. Cosio M, Ghezzo H, Hogg JC, Corbin R, Loveland M, Dosman J, Macklem PT (1978) The relations between structural changes in small airways and pulmonary-function tests. N Engl J Med 298:1277–1281
3. Dosman JA, Cotton DJ, Graham BL, Hall DL, Li R, Froh F, Barnett GD (1981) Sensitivity and specificity of early diagnostic tests of lung function in smokers. Chest 79:6–11
4. Olofsson J, Bake B, Svarsudd K, Skoogh BE (1986) The single breath N2 test predicts the rate of decline in FEV1. Eur J Respir Dis 69:46–56
5. Stanescu DC, Rodenstein DO, Hoeven C, Robert A (1987) "Sensitive tests" are poor predictors of the decline in forced expiratory volume in one second in middle-aged smokers. Am Rev Respir Dis 135:585–590
6. Buist AS, Vollmer WM, Johnson LR, McCamant LE (1988) Does the single-breath N2 test identify the smoker who will develop chronic airflow limitation? Am Rev Respir Dis 137:293–301
7. Stanescu D, Sanna A, Veriter C, Robert A (1998) Identification of smokers susceptible to development of chronic airflow limitation: a 13-year follow-up. Chest 114:416–425
8. Horsfield K, Cumming G (1968) Morphology of the bronchial tree in man. J Appl Physiol 24:373–383
9. Hansen JE, Ampaya EP (1975) Human air space shapes, sizes, areas, and volumes. J Appl Physiol 38:990–995
10. Haefeli-Bleuer B, Weibel ER (1988) Morphometry of the human pulmonary acinus. Anat Rec 220:401–414
11. Paiva M, Engel LA (1989) Gas mixing in the lung periphery. In: Chang HK, Paiva M (eds) Respiratory physiology: an analytical approach. Marcel Dekker, New York, p 245
12. Verhamme M, Roelandts J, De Roo M, Demedts M (1983) Gravity dependence of phases III, IV, and V in single-breath washout curves. J Appl Physiol 54:887–895
13. Rodríguez-Nieto MJ, Peces-Barba G, González Mangado N, Verbanck S, Paiva M (2001) Single-breath washouts in a rotating stretcher. J Appl Physiol 90:1415–1423
14. Lauzon AM, Prisk GK, Elliott AR, Verbanck S, Paiva M, West JB (1997) Paradoxical helium and sulfur hexafluoride single-breath washouts in short-term vs. sustained microgravity. J Appl Physiol 82:859–865
15. Michels DB, West J (1978) Distribution of pulmonary ventilation and perfusion during short periods of weightlessness. J Appl Physiol 45:987–998
16. Guy HJB, Prisk GK, Elliott AR, Deutschman RA III, West JB (1994) Inhomogeneity of pulmonary ventilation during sustained microgravity as determined by single-breath washouts. J Appl Physiol 76:1719–1729
17. Prisk GK, Guy HJB, Elliott AR, Paiva M, West JB (1995) Ventilatory inhomogeneity determined from multiple-breath washouts during sustained microgravity on Spacelab SLS-1. J Appl Physiol 78:597–607
18. Van Muylem A, Scillia P, Knoop C, Paiva M, Estenne M (2006) Single-breath test in lateral decubitus reflects function of single lungs grafted for emphysema. J Appl Physiol 100:834–838

19. Paiva M, Engel LA (1981) The anatomical basis for the sloping N2 plateau. Respir Physiol 44:325–337
20. Paiva M, Engel LA (1984) Model analysis of gas distribution within human lung acinus. J Appl Physiol 56:418–425
21. Verbanck S, Paiva M (1990) Model simulations of gas mixing and ventilation distribution in the human lung. J Appl Physiol 69:2269–2279
22. Dutrieue B, Van Holsbeek F, Verbanck S, Paiva M (2000) Model simulations of gas mixing and ventilation distribution in the human lung. J Appl Physiol 89:1859–1867
23. Mitchell JH, Hoffman EA, Tawhai MH (2012) Relating indices of inert gas washout to localised bronchoconstriction. Respir Physiol Neurobiol 183:224–233
24. Verbanck S, Schuermans D, Van Muylem A, Melot C, Noppen M, Vincken W, Paiva M (1998) Conductive and acinar lung-zone contributions to ventilation inhomogeneity in COPD. Am J Respir Crit Care Med 157:1573–1577
25. Verbanck S, Schuermans D, Noppen M, Paiva M, Vincken M (1999) Evidence of acinar airway involvement in asthma. Am J Respir Crit Care Med 159:1545–1550
26. Verbanck S, Schuermans D, Van Muylem A, Noppen M, Paiva M, Vincken W (1997) Ventilation distribution during histamine provocation. J Appl Physiol 83:1907–1916
27. Cormier Y, Bélanger J (1983) Quantification of the effect of gas exchange on the slope of phase III. Bull Eur Physiopathol Respir 19:13–16
28. Dutrieue B, Lauzon AM, Verbanck S, Elliott AR, Prisk GK, West JB, Paiva M (1999) Helium and sulfur hexafluoride bolus washin in short-term microgravity. J Appl Physiol 86:1594
29. Estenne M, Van Muylem A, Knoop C, Antoine M (2000) Detection of obliterative bronchiolitis after lung transplantation by indexes of ventilation distribution. Am J Respir Crit Care Med 162:1047–1051
30. Crawford ABH, Cotton DJ, Paiva M, Engel LA (1989) Effect of lung volume on ventilation distribution. J Appl Physiol 66:2502–2510
31. Crawford ABH, Makowska M, Engel LA (1987) Effect of bronchomotor tone on static mechanical properties of lung and ventilation distribution. J Appl Physiol 63:2278–2285
32. Crawford ABH, Makowska M, Kelly S, Engel LA (1986) Effect of breath holding on ventilation maldistribution during tidal breathing in normal subjects. J Appl Physiol 61:2108–2115
33. Crawford ABH, Makowska M, Paiva M, Engel LA (1985) Convection- and diffusion-dependent ventilation maldistribution in normal subjects. J Appl Physiol 59:838–846
34. Paiva M (1975) Two new pulmonary functional indexes suggested by a simple mathematical model. Respiration 32:389–403
35. Verbanck S, Paiva M (2011) Gas mixing in the airways and airspaces. Compr Physiol 1:835–882
36. Prisk GK, Elliott AR, Guy HJB, Verbanck S, Paiva M, West JB (1998) Multiple-breath washin of helium and sulfur hexafluoride in sustained microgravity. J Appl Physiol 84:244–252
37. King GG, Downie SR, Verbanck S, Thorpe CW, Berend N, Salome CM, Thompson B (2005) Effects of methacholine on small airway function measured by forced oscillation technique and multiple breath nitrogen washout in normal subjects. Respir Physiol Neurobiol 148:165–177
38. Mak JC, Barnes PJ (1994) Autonomic receptors in the upper and lower airways. In: Kaliner MA, Barnes PJ, Kunkell GH, Baranicek JN (eds) Neuropeptides in respiratory medicine. Marcel Dekker, New York, p 251
39. Scano G, Stendardi L, Bracamonte M, Decoster A, Sergysels R (1982) Site of action of inhaled histamine in asymptomatic asthmatic patients. Clin Allergy 12:281–288
40. Harris EA, Buchanan PR, Whitlock RML (1987) Human alveolar gas-mixing efficiency for gases of differing diffusivity in health and airflow limitation. Clin Sci 73:351–359
41. Langley F, Horsfield K, Burton G, Seed WA, Parker S, Cumming G (1988) Effect of inhaled methacholine on gas mixing efficiency. Clin Sci 74:187–192
42. Verbanck S, Schuermans D, Noppen M, Vincken W, Paiva M (2001) Methacholine versus histamine: paradoxical response of spirometry and ventilation distribution. J Appl Physiol 91:2587–2594

43. Rodriguez-Roisin R, Ferrer A, Navajas D, Agusti AGN, Wagner PD, Roca J (1991) Ventilation-perfusion mismatch after methacholine challenge in patients with mild bronchial asthma. Am Rev Respir Dis 144:88–94

44. Michils A, Elkrim Y, Haccuria A, Van Muylem A (2011) Adenosine 5'-monophosphate challenge elicits a more peripheral airway response than methacholine challenge. J Appl Physiol 110:1241–1247

45. Wagner EM, Liu MC, Weinmann GG, Permutt S, Bleecker ER (1990) Peripheral lung resistance in normal and asthmatic subjects. Am Rev Respir Dis 141:584

46. Yanai M, Ohrui T, Sekizawa K, Shimizu Y, Sasaki H, Takishima T (1991) Effective site of bronchodilation by antiasthma drugs in subjects with asthma. J Allergy Clin Immunol 87:1080–1087

47. Fairshter RD, Wilson AF (1980) Relationship between the site of airflow limitation and localization of the bronchodilator response in asthma. Am Rev Respir Dis 122:27–32

48. Olofsson J, Bake B, Skoogh BE (1986) Bronchomotor tone and the slope of phase III of the N2-test. Bull Eur Physiopathol Respir 22:489–494

49. Olofsson J, Bake B, Blomqvist N, Skoogh BE (1985) Effect of increasing bronchodilatation on the single breath nitrogen test. Bull Eur Physiopathol Respir 21:31–36

50. Cooper DM, Mellins RB, Mansell AL (1983) Ventilation distribution and density dependence of expiratory flow in asthmatic children. J Appl Physiol 54:1125–1130

51. Gustafsson PM, Ljungberg HK, Kjellman B (2003) Peripheral airway involvement in asthma assessed by single-breath SF6 and He washout. Eur Respir J 21:1033–1039

52. Lutchen KR, Habib RH, Dorkin HL, Wall MA (1990) Respiratory impedance and multibreath N2 washout in healthy, asthmatic, and cystic fibrosis subjects. J Appl Physiol 68: 2139–2149

53. Paiva M, Van Muylem A, Ravez P, Yernault JC (1986) Preinspiratory lung volume dependence of the slope of the alveolar plateau. Respir Physiol 63:327–338

54. Downie SR, Salome CM, Verbanck S, Thompson B, Berend N, King GG (2007) Ventilation heterogeneity is a major determinant of airway hyperresponsiveness in asthma, independent of airway inflammation. Thorax 62:684–689

55. Farah CS, King GG, Brown NJ, Downie SR, Kermode JA, Hardaker KM, Peters MJ, Berend N, Salome CM (2012) The role of the small airways in the clinical expression of asthma in adults. J Allergy Clin Immunol 129:381–387

56. Farah CS, King GG, Brown NJ, Peters MJ, Berend N, Salome CM (2012) Ventilation heterogeneity predicts asthma control in adults following inhaled corticosteroid dose titration. J Allergy Clin Immunol 130:61–68

57. Verbanck S, Schuermans D, Vincken W, Paiva M (2001) Saline Bolus dispersion versus ventilation maldistribution: I acinar airways alteration. J Appl Physiol 90:1754–1762

58. Fleming GM, Chester EH, Saniie B, Saidel GM (1980) Ventilation inhomogeneity using multibreath nitrogen washout: comparison of moment ratios and other indexes. Am Rev Respir Dis 121:789–794

59. Ericsson CH, Svartengren M, Mossberg B, Camner P (1993) Bronchial reactivity, lung function, and serum immunoglobulin E in smoking-discordant monozygotic twins. Am Rev Respir Dis 147:296–300

60. Verbanck S, Schuermans D, Meysman M, Paiva M, Vincken W (2004) Noninvasive assessment of airway alterations in smokers: the small airways revisited. Am J Respir Crit Care Med 170:414–419

61. Verbanck S, Schuermans D, Paiva M, Meysman M, Vincken W (2006) Small airway function improvement after smoking cessation in smokers without airway obstruction. Am J Respir Crit Care Med 174:853–857

62. Verbanck S, Thompson BR, Schuermans D, Kalsi H, Biddiscombe M, Stuart-Andrews C, Hanon S, Van Muylem A, Paiva M, Vincken W, Usmani O (2012) Ventilation heterogeneity in the acinar and conductive zones of the normal ageing lung. Thorax 67:789–795

63. Heyder J, Blanchard JD, Feldman HA, Brain JD (1988) Convective mixing in human respiratory tract: estimates with aerosol boli. J Appl Physiol 64:1273–1278

64. Anderson PJ, Dolovich M (1994) Aerosols as diagnostic tools. J Aerosol Med 7:77–88
65. Blanchard JD (1996) Aerosol bolus dispersion and aerosol-derived airway morphometry: assessment of lung pathology and response to therapy, Part 1. J Aerosol Med 9:183–205
66. Anderson PJ, Blanchard JD, Brain JD, Feldman HA, McNamara JJ, Heyder J (1989) Effect of cystic fibrosis on inhaled aerosol boluses. Am Rev Respir Dis 140:1317–1324
67. Kohlhaufl M, Brand P, Rock C, Radons T, Scheuch G, Meyer T, Schulz H, Pfeifer KJ, Haussinger K, Heyder J (1999) Noninvasive diagnosis of emphysema. Aerosol morphometry and aerosol bolus dispersion in comparison to HRCT. Am J Respir Crit Care Med 160:913–918
68. Schultz H, Schultz A, Brand P, Tuch T, von Mutius E, Erdl R, Reinhardt D, Heyder J (1995) Aerosol bolus dispersion and effective airway diameters in mildly asthmatic children. Eur Respir J 8:566–573
69. Brand P, App EM, Meyer T, Kur F, Muller C, Dienemann H, Reichart B, Fruhmann G, Heyder J (1998) Aerosol bolus dispersion in patients with bronchiolitis obliterans after heart-lung and double-lung transplantation. The Munich Lung Transplantation Group. J Aerosol Med 11:41–53
70. McCawley M, Lippmann M (1988) Development of an aerosol dispersion test to detect early changes in lung function. Am Ind Hyg Assoc J 49:357–366
71. Anderson PJ, Hardy KG, Gann LP, Cole R, Hiller FC (1994) Detection of small airway dysfunction in asymptomatic smokers using aerosol bolus behavior. Am J Respir Crit Care Med 150:995–1001
72. Brand P, Tuch T, Manuwald O, Bischof W, Heinrich J, Wichmann HE, Beinert T, Heyder J (1994) Detection of early lung impairment with aerosol bolus dispersion. Eur Respir J 7:1830–1838
73. Brown JS, Gerrity TR, Bennett WD (1998) Effect of ventilation distribution on aerosol bolus dispersion and recovery. J Appl Physiol 85:2112–2117
74. Verbanck S, Schuermans D, Paiva M, Vincken W (2001) Saline aerosol bolus dispersion. II. The effect of conductive airway alteration. J Appl Physiol 90:1763–1769
75. Jayaraju ST, Paiva M, Brouns M, Lacor C, Verbanck S (2008) Contribution of upper airway geometry to convective mixing. J Appl Physiol 105:1733–1740
76. Shaker SB, Maltbaek N, Brand P, Haeussermann S, Dirksen A (2005) Quantitative computed tomography and aerosol morphometry in COPD and alpha1-antitrypsin deficiency. Eur Respir J 25:23–30

Computed Tomography (CT)–Based Analysis of Regional Lung Ventilation

15

Andrea Aliverti, Francesca Pennati, and Caterina Salito

15.1 Regional Ventilation: First Studies with Radioactive Gases and Preliminary Findings

Classical studies on regional ventilation with lobar spirometry [1, 2] and radioactive gases [3, 4] demonstrated regional differences in the distribution of ventilation, preferentially toward the lower lung zones. The first quantitative results are reported by West and Dollery [3], measuring the removal rate of oxygen15-labeled carbon dioxide after a single breath of the radioactive gas by external counting, and by Ball et al. [4], who measured regional ventilation by xenon scintigraphy by relating the lung count rate after a single breath to that after isotope equilibration throughout the lung. These preliminary findings have demonstrated that the lower portion of the lung is better ventilated and receives a much greater fraction of the total pulmonary blood flow and that the middle and lower portions of the lung are better ventilated on the left than on the right during deep inspiration. Subsequent works from Milic-Emili and coworkers [5, 6] attributed this behavior to the combined effect of the gradient of pleural pressure and the static volume-pressure relation of the lung. They have demonstrated that there is a vertical gradient of pleural pressure which causes nondependent portion of the lung to be relatively more expanded than the dependent. Moreover, these more distended units at the top of the lung are on a flatter part of their pressure-volume curve than the smaller units at the bottom; thus, equal pressure increments produce smaller volume increments at the top than at the bottom of the lung (Fig. 15.1).

A. Aliverti, PhD (✉) • F. Pennati • C. Salito
Dipartimento di Elettronica, Informazione e Bioingegneria, Politecnico di Milano,
P.zza L. da Vinci, 32, Milano 20133, Italy
e-mail: andrea.aliverti@polimi.it

A. Aliverti, A. Pedotti (eds.), *Mechanics of Breathing*,
DOI 10.1007/978-88-470-5647-3_15, © Springer-Verlag Italia 2014

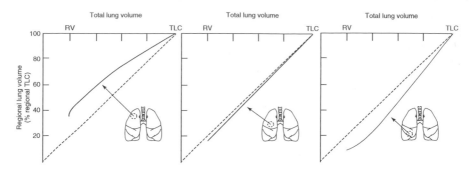

Fig. 15.1 Regional lung volume (expressed as percentage of TLCr) with respect to overall lung volume (expressed as percentage of TLC). From left to right, increasing distance from the top of the lung (apex) to the base

Multiple investigations followed these preliminary findings, and multiple imaging techniques have been developed for investigating regional ventilation. This chapter reviews the development of computed tomography in imaging regional lung ventilation.

15.2   Computed Tomography Imaging: Basic Principles

Computed tomography (CT) is currently the main imaging modality for diagnosing lung diseases. High-resolution CT scanners generate a three-dimensional view of the imaged organs with submillimeter resolution in axial sections. CT provides detailed information regarding the lung parenchyma and can delineate structures down to the level of the secondary pulmonary lobule, the smallest structure in the lung. It is particularly useful for image-based diagnosis since alteration of the lung anatomy, caused by a disease, can be clearly seen in a thin-slice CT image [7].

15.2.1 The Evolution of CT

CT was introduced in the early 1970s and has revolutionized not only diagnostic radiology but also the whole field of medicine. The introduction of spiral CT in the early 1990s constituted a fundamental evolutionary step in the development and ongoing refinement of CT imaging techniques. Until then, the examination volume had to be covered by subsequent axial scans in a "step-and-shoot" mode. Axial scanning required long examination times because of the interscan delays necessary to move the table incrementally from one scan position to the next, and it was prone to misregistration of anatomic details (e.g., pulmonary nodules) because of the potential movement of relevant anatomic structures between two scans (e.g., by patient motion, breathing, or swallowing). The most important advancement in these CT scanners has been the implementation of X-ray detectors that are physically separated in the z-axis direction and enable simultaneous acquisition of multiple slices of the patient's anatomy. Key benefits of multidetector computed tomography (MDCT) systems are faster scan speed, improved through-plane resolution, and better utilization of the available X-ray tube power. MDCT also expanded into new clinical areas, such as CT angiography of the coronary arteries with the addition of ECG gating capability [8, 9]. An 8-slice CT system, introduced in 2000, enabled shorter examination times but no improved spatial resolution (thinnest collimation 8×1.25 mm). In 2001, 16-slice CT systems became commercially available, with collimations of 16×0.5, 16×0.625, or 16×0.75 mm and faster gantry rotation (down to 0.42 s and later 0.375 s) [10]. In 2004, all major CT manufacturers introduced MDCT systems with simultaneous acquisition of 64 slices at 0.5, 0.6, or 0.625 mm collimated slice width and further reduced rotation times (down to 0.33 s). GE, Philips, and Toshiba aimed at increasing volume coverage speed by using detectors with 64 rows, in this way providing 64 collimated 0.5 or 0.625 mm slices with a total z-coverage of 32 or 40 mm. Siemens used 32 physical detector rows in combination with a z-flying focal spot to simultaneously acquire 64 overlapping 0.6 mm slices with a total z-coverage of 19.2 mm, with the goal of pitch-independent increase of through-plane resolution and reduction of spiral artifacts [11]. With 64-slice CT systems, CT scans with isotropic submillimeter resolution became feasible even for extended anatomic ranges. In 2007, an MDCT system with 128 simultaneously acquired slices was introduced based on a detector with 64×0.6 mm collimation and double z-sampling by means of a z-flying focal spot. Recently, simultaneous acquisition of 256 slices has become available, with a CT system equipped with a 128-row detector (0.625 mm collimated slice width) and z-flying focal spot. Clinical experience with 64-, 128-, or 256-slice CT indicates that the performance level of MDCT has reached a level of saturation, and mere adding of even more detector rows will not by itself translate into increased clinical benefit [10].

The applied dose is ultimately the limiting factor for the improvement of image quality and increase in isotropic resolution. In order to make best diagnostic use of the applied dose, sophisticated dynamic dose adaptation techniques to patient size and geometry have been developed. A recent study [12] showed that the use of additional tin filtration in the high-energy X-ray beam of a dual-source CT system provided several benefits for dual-energy CT applications, including a similar or lower radiation dose compared with the conventional single energy CT, increased dual-energy contrast, and improved image quality of dual-energy material-specific (e.g., virtual noncontrast) images. Moreover, the virtual noncontrast imaging of dual-energy CT has a potential to reduce the radiation dose by omitting precontrast scanning [13].

15.2.2 Radiation Dose

The increasing use of CT has sparked concern over the effects of radiation dose on patients, particularly for those who had repeated CT scans. The effective dose [14] from a CT scan on average is ~10 mSv [15]. The health risks, mainly cancer induction and mortality, from this level of radiation dose have been considered in detail by an expert Committee of the National Research Council of the National Academies of the USA and published as BEIR VII Phase 2 report [16].

Various measures are used to describe the radiation dose delivered by CT scanning, the most relevant being absorbed dose, effective dose, and CT dose index (or CTDI). The absorbed dose is the energy absorbed per unit of mass and is measured in grays (Gy). One gray equals 1 J of radiation energy absorbed per kilogram. The organ dose (or the distribution of dose in the organ) largely determines the level of risk to that organ from the radiation. The effective dose, expressed in sieverts (Sv), is used for dose distributions that are not homogeneous (which is always the case with CT); it is designed to be proportional to a generic estimate of the overall harm to the patient caused by the radiation exposure. The effective dose allows for a rough comparison between different CT scenarios but provides only an approximate estimate of the true risk. For risk estimation, the organ dose is the preferred quantity. Organ doses can be calculated or measured in anthropomorphic phantoms [17]. Historically, CT doses have generally been (and still are) measured for a single slice in standard cylindrical acrylic phantoms [18]; the resulting quantity, the CT dose index, although useful for quality control, is not directly related to the organ dose or risk [19]. The radiation doses to particular organs from any given CT study depend on a number of factors. The most important are the number of scans, the tube current and scanning time in milliampseconds (mAs), the size of the patient, the axial scan range, the scan pitch (the degree of overlap between adjacent CT slices), the tube voltage in the kilovolt peaks (kVp), and the specific design of the scanner being used. Many of these factors are under the control of the radiologist or radiology technician. Ideally, they should be tailored to the type of study being performed and to the size of the particular patient, a practice that is increasing but is by no means universal [20].

Efforts and measures to reduce noise can be initiated by the examiner by critically considering the indication and the choice of scanning protocols and parameters for any CT examination and by the manufacturer during the development of dose-efficient systems, together with special technical measures and methods. Patient dose has to be kept "as low as reasonably achievable" (ALARA principle), as postulated by the International Commission on Radiological Protection [21].

15.2.3 CT Images of the Lung

Image gray scale is measured in Hounsfield units (HU), an arbitrary linear scale defined as zero for water and approximately −1,000 for air, that results convenient for lung imaging as the density of any lung volume may be considered as a combination of air, at −1,000 HU, and "tissue" (cells, blood, collagen, water), at 0 HU. As the lung volume increases, gas volume increases while tissue remains constant. Thus, the overall lung density decreases as the lung expands. Changes in CT density provide accurate measurements of regional and global lung air and tissue volume as well as an indication of the heterogeneity of lung expansion.

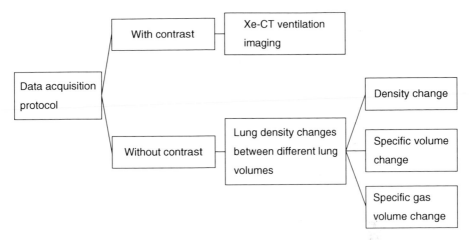

Fig. 15.2 CT based ventilation imaging

These principles are at the basis of functional pulmonary measurements. Tracer techniques for ventilation using a radio-dense gas have the advantage that the accumulation of tracer gas during regular breathing should follow the same gas transport principles as respiratory gases. Density-based methods and registration-based techniques require the assumption that the decrease in CT density due to region expansion is caused by only gas influx (Fig. 15.2).

15.3 Xenon-CT Ventilation Imaging

The use of xenon as a contrast agent for ventilation imaging was pioneered by Gur et al. [22], but only recently it has been updated, refined, and validated as a research tool in animal experiments [23–26]. Xenon is a nonradioactive gas with higher radio-density than air, resulting in a linear CT density increase with increasing gas concentration. Two Xe-enhanced computed tomography (Xe-CT) techniques for imaging regional ventilation have been developed: single-breath and multi-breath technique. The single-breath technique [23] is performed by asking the subject to take a single breath of a high Xe concentration mixture and comparing Xe-enhanced with unenhanced images. Regional ventilation is directly assessed by the Xe enhancement. Multi-breath technique measures regional pulmonary ventilation from the wash-in and wash-out rates of the Xe gas, as measured in serial CT scans (Fig. 15.3).

The temporal changes in CT density enhancement produced during the wash-in and wash-out phases in any region can be exponentially fitted, providing a time constant equal to the inverse of the local ventilation per unit volume, i.e., specific ventilation in the hypothesis of a single-compartment model (Fig. 15.3).

The quantification of Xe-CT is affected by the variable CT attenuation of the lung parenchyma of the scanned subject due to different lung volumes on sequential images, thus restricting the first studies to animal model [22–26]. Xenon-enhanced

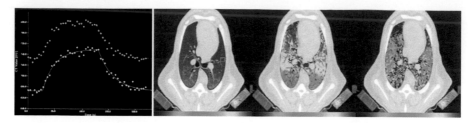

Fig. 15.3 Xe-CT with density-time curve for two ROIs of a mechanically ventilated sheep (*left*) and map of regional air content (% air, *middle*) and specific ventilation (sec^{-1}, *right*) (Modified from Simon [31])

dual-energy CT has been introduced by Chae et al. [27] to overcome this limitation, as the Xe component can be calculated from the dual-energy CT on the basis of the material decomposition theory without additional unenhanced acquisition. With this approach clinical studies have been performed, indicating dual-energy Xe-CT as a promising tool for detecting abnormal pulmonary ventilation [27–30].

The use of Xe-CT has a number of limitations. The anesthetic properties of xenon, that limit its use in humans to a maximum concentration around 30–35 % [31, 32], limit the maximum CT density enhancement achievable. Xenon is moderately soluble in blood and tissue, and this has been proposed to affect background density level and alveolar accumulation rates [26]. Nevertheless, Hoag et al. [33] demonstrated that Xe uptake has no significant impact on the measured lung density-time curve. Another important limitation is that Xe-CT is time and radiation intensive. Each study requires 20 up to 70 repeated respiratory-gated axial images at each location, with repeated scans for volumetric coverage [31].

15.4   Lung Aeration and Recruitment

Over the past 20 years, many experimental and clinical studies have described the different CT morphological patterns of acute lung injury (ALI). The pioneering CT studies of Gattinoni and coworkers [34–36] have demonstrated that ALI is characterized by significant regional differences in lung aeration and alveolar recruitment with tidal volume and positive end-expiratory pressure, and that these regional differences determine the local response to different ventilation strategies.

On the basis of the basic CT principles and assuming lung-specific weight equal to 1, the volume of gas in any lung region of interest can be related to regional density as

$$\frac{volume_{gas}}{volume_{gas} + volume_{tissue}} = \frac{meanHU}{HU_{gas} - HU_{water}}$$

where $volume_{gas}$ and $volume_{tissue}$ are, respectively, the volume of gas and tissue within the region of interest, meanHU is the mean density value of the region, and

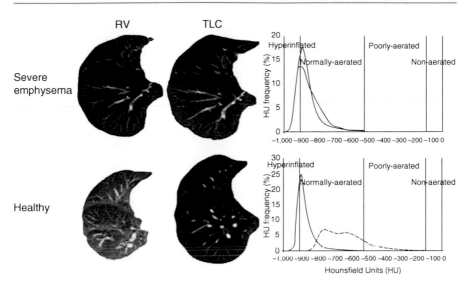

Fig. 15.4 The lung compartments, as defined by Hounsfield units, in severe emphysema (*top*) and in normal condition (*bottom*) for the right lung at RV (*dashed line*) and TLC (*solid line*)

HU_{gas} and HU_{water} are, respectively, the density value of gas ($-1,000$ HU) and water (0 HU).

From this simple relation, gas volume, tissue volume, and weight and the ratio gas/tissue are derived [35–37]:

$$Volume_{gas\_ROI} = volume_{ROI} \left(meanHU_{ROI} / -1,000 \right)$$

$$Tissue\_weight_{ROI} = volume_{ROI} \left(1 - \left(meanHU_{ROI} / -1,000 \right) \right)$$

Gattinoni et al. [38] proposed to divide the lung in different compartments according to their degree of aeration, from unaerated (from 0 to -100 HU) to poorly aerated (from -101 to -500 HU), normally aerated (from -501 to -900 HU), and hyperinflated (from -901 to $-1,000$ HU) (Fig. 15.4). Taking CT scans under different conditions, it is therefore possible to determine the alveolar recruitment and ventilation distribution. Alveolar recruitment, defined as the amount of gas entering unaerated tissue when the applied airway pressure increases, is estimated as the unaerated tissue change, expressed in grams, under different ventilatory conditions [38]. The distribution of ventilation is obtained as the alveolar inflation change between end inspiration and end expiration [39].

More recently, Dougherty et al. [40, 41] introduced a new method for mapping regional aeration within the lung: by applying deformable image registration at CT images acquired in breath-hold at residual volume and total lung capacity in patients with severe emphysema. Deformable image registration consists in finding the spatial mapping between corresponding voxels in two images. Therefore, the quantitative change of each voxel across different states of inflation can be determined by

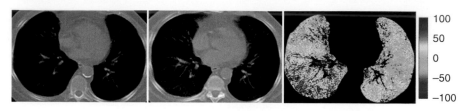

Fig. 15.5 Thoracic CT at total lung capacity (TLC, *left*), residual volume (RV, *middle*), and map of Hounsfield units difference (*right*) computed as $HU_{RV} - HU_{TLC}$ after registering RV onto TLC

image subtraction, and the resulting difference map can be used to visualize and quantify regional pulmonary air trapping [40, 41] (Fig. 15.5).

15.5   Specific Volume Change

Simon [42] proposed to quantify regional mechanical properties of the lung from CT density changes between pairs of breath-hold CT images. In the hypothesis that volume change occurs only because of the addition of fresh gas into the lung with inspiration, regional specific compliance (sC; compliance per unit volume) can be measured from CT images acquired at two different pressures, from the changes in local fraction of air content (F) with changes in inflation pressure (ΔP) as

$$sC = (F_2 - F_1) / (F_1 (1 - F_2) \Delta P)$$

Specific compliance measured between 0 and 15 cm H_2O airway pressures has shown good agreement to Xe-CT in two anesthetized mechanically ventilated dogs [42]. Thus, it has been proposed as a surrogate for regional ventilation, introducing the term specific volume change (sVol; change in volume divided by initial gas volume) [31]. Using the relationship between CT density (HU) and air fraction (F), specific volume change can be calculated from the density change as

$$sVol = 1,000(HU_2 - HU_1) / (HU_1 [HU_2 + 1,000])$$

However, this relationship is nonlinear and dependent on both initial region density and the magnitude of the density change. As shown in Fig. 15.6, there can be large differences in sVol for the same ROI density change depending on initial region density, illustrating why CT density change is a poor correlate for regional ventilation [42].

Guerrero et al. [43, 44] pioneered the use of sVol maps from four-dimensional CT in lung tumor patients in order to optimize the radiation therapy treatment planning, avoiding well-ventilated pulmonary regions which could reduce treatment-related complications (Fig. 15.7). The main advantage of 4D-CT functional imaging in lung tumor patients is that it requires no additional dose or extra cost to the patient as 4D-CT is routinely acquired through thoracic radiotherapy treatment planning. We would like to clarify some terminological inaccuracy arising from

Fig. 15.6 Specific volume change as a function of Hounsfield units difference at different initial densities

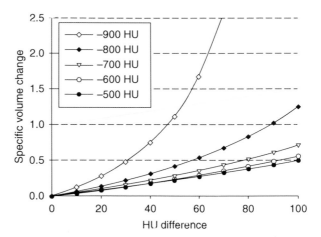

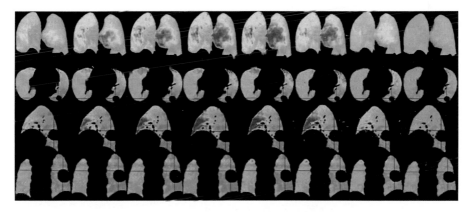

Fig. 15.7 The 4D-CT ventilation image set of a patient with lung tumor from end expiration up to end inspiration and again to end expiration (from *left* to *right*). Each image was paired with the maximum expiration phase to compute the change in specific volume change with respect to the maximum expiration. Volume-rendering (*first row*), transversal (*second row*), sagittal (*third row*), and frontal views (*fourth row*) are reported

Guerrero et al. [44], where the term "specific ventilation" was associated to specific volume change, which was introduced as a surrogate for regional ventilation [31]. Since then, several studies [45–48] developed in the field of radiotherapy reported the term "ventilation images" referring to maps of specific volume change obtained from 4D-CT lung images. Maps of specific volume change were compared to Xe-CT ventilation images in an anesthetized sheep [49] and to single-photon emission tomography (SPECT) ventilation images in lung tumor patients [45]. Results demonstrated high Dice similarity coefficient in regions with matched perfusion-ventilation defects but an overall low similarity and a low correlation coefficient between the two imaging techniques [45]. Yamamoto et al. [46] investigated specific volume change in patients with emphysema by correlating specific volume change defects with the disease. Further studies quantified the dosimetric impact of

Fig. 15.8 The frequency distribution of the CT voxels expressed as gas volume per gram of tissue at TLC. The solid line represents the healthy subjects; the dashed line represents the group with severe emphysema. These two distributions are different from each other ($p < 0.001$)

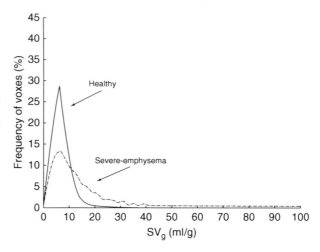

4D-CT functional imaging on treatment planning to avoid well-ventilated lung regions during radiation therapy [47]. Vinogradskiy et al. [48] used functional maps calculated from weekly 4D-CT data to study ventilation change throughout the radiation therapy.

15.6 Specific Gas Volume

Specific volume of gas (SV_g) is defined as volume of gas per gram of tissue (ml/g) and is derived pixel by pixel from CT images of lung density by converting the HU value to a measure of specific volume, which is a more physiologically meaningful measure [50–52]. SV_g can be calculated pixel by pixel as

$$SV_g = \text{specific volume}_{(tissue\&gas)} - \text{specific volume}_{(tissue)}$$

where specific volume (expressed in ml/g) is the inverse of density (g/ml).

The specific volume of the lung (tissue and gas) is measured from the CT as

$$SV_{(tissue\&gas)}(ml/g) = \frac{1,024}{HU(mg/ml) + 1,024}$$

where the specific volume of tissue was assumed to be equal to $1/1.065 = 0.939$ ml/g [53].

This method was first introduced by Coxson et al. [51, 54] in studies assessing regional lung volumes from CT scans. Figure 15.8 shows the frequency distribution for the quantity of gas per gram of tissue, at TLC, present in each CT voxel in a group of healthy subjects ($N = 10$) and in a group of patients with severe emphysema ($N = 10$).

The healthy lung shows a symmetrical distribution with mean, median, and mode values closely similar. The severe emphysema group has a flattened distribution that is markedly shifted and skewed to the right.

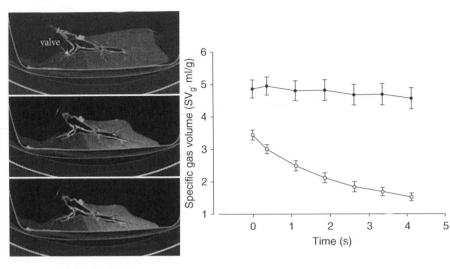

Fig. 15.9 (**a**) Dynamic CT scans of a longitudinal slice during 4.5 s of exhalation in a pig lung (three representative images from *top* to *bottom*, 2.25 s between images). The presence of trapped gas is clearly visible and stable in the obstructed lobe (upper lobe) in which the obstruction was created by inserting the one-way endobronchial exit valve (clearly visible in the upper lobar bronchus). (**b**) Graph of time-evolving SV_g of the obstructed and the unobstructed lobe (Modified from Salito et al. [52])

In recent studies performed on an animal model of airway obstruction [52] and in the emphysematous lungs in vivo [55], Salito et al. showed that CT-determined $SV_{g,r}$ is sensitive to the extent of regional trapped gas (Fig. 15.9).

Therefore, SV_g can be used to evaluate the extent of gas trapping on a regional base. SV_g is expected to change smoothly as a function of lung volumes. Total specific gas volume of the lung (SV_g) represents an average of all regional specific gas volume ($SV_{g,r}$). A reasonable hypothesis is that in the emphysematous lung, if there are regions where $SV_{g,r}$ varies little with lung volume (V) so that the slope of a plot of $\Delta SV_{g,r}$ versus overall ΔV is smaller than that for both lungs, there must be other regions where $\Delta SV_{g,r}/\Delta V$ is steeper indicating a greater than average decrease in $SV_{g,r}$ with decreasing V. In a normal lung there is no gas trapping above closing volume so that the spread of values of $\Delta SV_{g,r}/\Delta V$ should be small, whereas in emphysema the considerably larger set of slopes can potentially be used as a measure of inhomogeneous emptying (Fig. 15.10).

SV_g can be calculated for regions of interest, corresponding to different bronchopulmonary segments. This was done in healthy volunteers and emphysematous patients in whom CT images were taken at high and low lung volumes. Figure 15.11 shows two examples, one relative to a representative healthy subject and one showing the data of a patient with severe emphysema. In the healthy lung all bronchopulmonary segments show similar $\Delta SV_g/\Delta V$ slopes, while in emphysema the distribution of slopes is larger with more lung regions having low values of $\Delta SV_g.r/\Delta V$ and other with higher values. The former can be considered as regions in which gas trapping is more pronounced and therefore more feasible for interventions aimed to reduce volume.

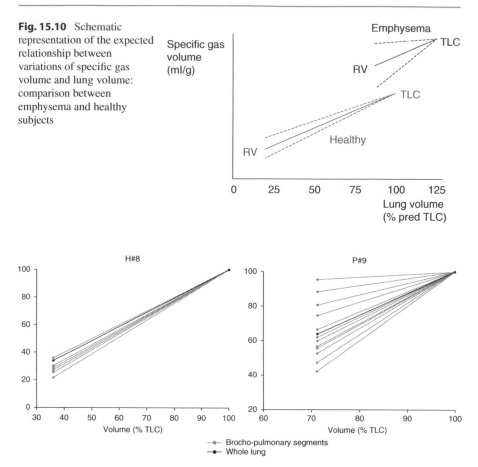

Fig. 15.10 Schematic representation of the expected relationship between variations of specific gas volume and lung volume: comparison between emphysema and healthy subjects

Fig. 15.11 Specific gas volume (SV_g, expressed as % $SV_{g,TLC}$) as function of the lung volume (expressed as %TLC volume) in a representative healthy subject (*left*) and in one patient with emphysema (*right*). *Gray lines*: segments connecting SV_g and volume values at TLC and RV in all bronchopulmonary segments. *Black lines*: segments connecting SV_g and volume values at TLC and RV in the whole lung

Recently, Aliverti et al. [56] introduced image registration to map regional lung function in terms of density and SV_g changes between different lung volumes in health and emphysema (Fig. 15.12) and showed that ΔSV_g is more homogeneously distributed within the lungs with no significant gravity dependence. Therefore, ΔSV_g maps, rather than ΔHU and sVol maps, have the advantage of minimizing the dependence of ventilation distribution on gravity. In other words, any heterogeneity has to be interpreted as the result of phenomena other than gravity, i.e., the disease.

These findings have clinical and physiological implications, not only in the assessment of the patient in the different stages of the disease but also to detect regional alterations in the lung function (e.g., gas trapping or collateral ventilation).

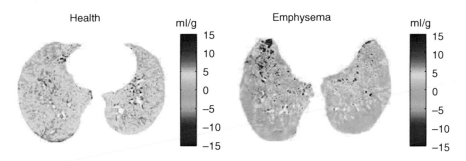

Fig. 15.12 Maps of specific gas volume change computed between total lung capacity and residual volume expressed in ml/g at the top diaphragm level of a representative healthy volunteer (*left*) and a representative patient with severe emphysema (*right*)

Such possibility would be extremely useful for planning and guiding interventions of bronchoscopic lung volume reduction surgery.

References

1. Martin CJ, Young AC (1956) Lobar ventilation in man. Am Rev Tuberc 73(3):330
2. Mattson SB, Carlens E (1955) Lobar ventilation and oxygen uptake in man; influence of body position. J Thorac Surg 30(6):676
3. West JB, Dollery CT (1960) Distribution of blood flow and ventilation-perfusion ratio in the lung, measured with radioactive CO2. J Appl Physiol 15(3):405–410
4. Ball WC, Stewart PB, Newsham LGS, Bates DV (1962) Regional pulmonary function studied with xenon133. J Clin Invest 41(3):519
5. Milic-Emili J, Henderson JA, Dolovich MB et al (1966) Regional distribution of inspired gas in the lung. J Appl Physiol 21:749–759
6. Bryan AC, Milic-Emili J, Pengelly D (1966) Effect of gravity on the distribution of pulmonary ventilation. J Appl Physiol 21:778–784
7. Webb RW, Muller N, Naidich DP (2009) High-resolution CT of the lung, 4th edn. Lippincott Williams & Wilkins
8. Kachelriess M, Ulzheimer S, Kalender W (2000) ECG-correlated image reconstruction from subsecond multi-slice spiral CT scans of the heart. Med Phys 27:1881–1902
9. Ohnesorge B, Flohr T, Becker C et al (2000) Cardiac imaging by means of electro—cardiographically gated multisection spiral CT—initial experience. Radiology 217:564–571
10. Flohr T (2013) CT systems. Curr Radiol Rep 1(1):52–63
11. Flohr TG, Stierstorfer K, Ulzheimer S et al (2005) Image reconstruction and image quality evaluation for a 64-slice CT scanner with zflying focal spot. Med Phys 32(8):2536–2547
12. Primak AN, Giraldo JC, Eusemann CD, Schmidt B, Kantor B, Fletcher JG, McCollough CH (2010) Dual-source dual-energy CT with additional tin filtration: dose and image quality evaluation in phantoms and in vivo. AJR Am J Roentgenol 195(5):1164–1174
13. Chae EJ, Song JW, Seo JB, Krauss B, Jang YM, Song KS (2008) Clinical utility of dual-energy CT in the evaluation of solitary pulmonary nodules: initial experience. Radiology 249(2):671–681
14. International Commission on Radiological Protection (2007) The 2007 Recommendations of the International Commission on Radiological Protection. ICRP publication 103. Ann ICRP 37(2–4):1–332

15. Fazel R, Krumholz HM, Wang Y et al (2009) Exposure to low-dose ionizing radiation from medical imaging procedures. N Engl J Med 361(9):849–857
16. Committee to Assess Health Risks From Exposure to Low Levels of Ionizing, Radiation National Research Council of the National Academies (2006) Health risks from exposure to low levels of ionizing radiation: BEIR VII phase 2. National Academies Press, Washington, DC
17. Groves AM, Owen KE, Courtney HM et al (2004) 16-Detector multislice CT: dosimetry estimation by TLD measurement compared with Monte Carlo simulation. Br J Radiol 77:662–665
18. McNitt-Gray MF (2002) AAPM/RSNA physics tutorial for residents – topics in CT: radiation dose in CT. Radiographics 22:1541–1553
19. Brenner DJ (2006) It is time to retire the computed tomography dose index (CTDI) for CT quality assurance and dose optimization. Med Phys 33:1189–1191
20. Paterson A, Frush DP, Donnelly LF (2001) Helical CT of the body: are settings adjusted for pediatric patients? AJR Am J Roentgenol 176:297–301
21. Kalender WA (2011) Computed tomography. Wiley, New York
22. Gur D, Drayer BP, Borovetz HS et al (1979) Dynamic computed tomography of the lung: regional ventilation measurements. J Comput Assist Tomogr 3:749–753
23. Tajik JK, Tran BQ, Hoffman EA (1996) Xenon enhanced CT imaging of local pulmonary ventilation. Proc SPIE 2709:40–54
24. Marcucci C, Nyhan D, Simon BA (2001) Distribution of pulmonary ventilation using Xe-enhanced computed tomography in prone and supine dogs. J Appl Physiol 90:421–430
25. Kreck TC, Krueger MA, Altemeier WA et al (2001) Determination of regional ventilation and perfusion in the lung using xenon and computed tomography. J Appl Physiol 91(4): 1741–1749
26. Chon D, Simon BA, Beck KC et al (2005) Differences in regional wash-in and wash-out time constants for xenon-CT ventilation studies. Respir Physiol Neurobiol 148(1–2):65–83
27. Chae EJ, Seo JB, Goo HW, Kim N, Song KS et al (2008) Xenon ventilation CT with a dual-energy technique of dual-source CT: initial experience. Radiology 248(2):615–624
28. Chae EJ, Seo JB, Lee J et al (2010) Xenon ventilation imaging using dual-energy computed tomography in asthmatics: initial experience. Invest Radiol 45(6):354–361
29. Park EA, Goo JM, Park SJ et al (2010) Chronic obstructive pulmonary disease: quantitative and visual ventilation pattern analysis at xenon ventilation CT performed by using a dual-energy technique. Radiology 256(3):985–997
30. Thieme SF, Hoegl S, Nikolaou K et al (2010) Pulmonary ventilation and perfusion imaging with dual-energy CT. Eur Radiol 20(12):2882–2889
31. Simon BA (2005) Regional ventilation and lung mechanics using X-ray CT. Acad Radiol 12(11):1414–1422
32. Lachmann B, Armbruster S, Schairer W et al (1990) Safety and efficacy of xenon in routine use as an inhalational anaesthetic. Lancet 335:1413–1415
33. Hoag JB, Fuld M, Brown RH, Simon BA (2007) Recirculation of inhaled xenon does not alter lung CT density. Acad Radiol 14(1):81–84
34. Gattinoni L, Mascheroni D, Torresin A et al (1986) Morphological response to positive end-expiratory pressure in acute respiratory failure: computerized tomography study. Intensive Care Med 12:137–142
35. Gattinoni L, Pesenti A, Torresin A et al (1986) Adult respiratory distress syndrome profiles by computed tomography. J Thorac Imaging 1:25–30
36. Gattinoni L, Pesenti A, Bombino M et al (1988) Relationships between lung computed tomographic density, gas exchange and PEEP in acute respiratory failure. Anesthesiology 69: 824–832
37. Gattinoni L, Pelosi P, Pesenti A, Brazzi L, Vitale G, Moretto A, Crespi A, Tagliabue M (1991) CT scan in ARDS: clinical and physiopathological insights. Acta Anasthesiol Scand 95: 87–94

38. Gattinoni L, Pesenti A, Avalli L, Rossi F, Bombino M (1987) Pressure-volume curve of total respiratory system in acute respiratory failure. Computed tomographic scan study. Am Rev Respir Dis 136:730–736

39. Pelosi P, Crotti S, Brazzi L, Gattinoni L (1996) Computed tomography in adult respiratory distress syndrome: what has it taught us? Eur Respir J 9(5):1055–1062

40. Dougherty L, Asmuth JC, Gefter WB (2003) Alignment of CT lung volumes with an optical flow method. Acad Radiol 10:249–254

41. Dougherty L, Torigian DA, Affusso JD et al (2006) Use of an optical flow method for the analysis of serial CT lung images. Acad Radiol 13:14–23

42. Simon BA (2000) Non-invasive imaging of regional lung function using x-ray computed tomography. J Clin Monit Comput 16:433–442

43. Guerrero T, Sanders K, Noyola-Martinez J, Castillo E, Zhang Y, Thapia R, Guerra R, BorgheroY KR (2005) Quantification of regional ventilation from treatment planning CT. Int J Radiat Oncol Biol Phys 62:630–634

44. Guerrero T, Sanders K, Castillo E et al (2006) Dynamic ventilation imaging from four-dimensional computed tomography. Phys Med Biol 51:777–791

45. Castillo R, Castillo E, Martinez J et al (2010) Ventilation from four-dimensional computed tomography: density versus jacobian methods. Phys Med Biol 55:4661–4685

46. Yamamoto T, Kabus S, Klinder T et al (2011) Investigation of four-dimensional computed tomography-based pulmonary ventilation imaging in patients with emphysematous lung regions. Phys Med Biol 56:2279–2298

47. Yaremko BP, Guerrero T, Noyola-Martinez J et al (2007) Reduction of normal lung irradiation in locally advanced non-small-cell lung cancer patients, using ventilation images for functional avoidance. Int J Radiat Oncol Biol Phys 68:562–571

48. Vinogradskiy YY, Castillo R, Castillo E, Chandler A, Martel MK, Guerrero T (2012) Use of weekly 4DCT-based ventilation maps to quantify changes in lung function for patients undergoing radiation therapy. Med Phys 39(1):289–298

49. Fuld MK, Easley RB, Saba OI, Chon D, Reinhardt JM, Hoffman EA, Simon BA (2008) CT-measured regional specific volume change reflects regional ventilation in supine sheep. J Appl Physiol 104(4):1177–1184

50. Hogg JC, Nepszy S (1969) Regional lung volume and pleural pressure gradient estimated from lung density in dogs. J Appl Physiol 27(2):198–203

51. Coxson HO, Mayo JR, Behzad H, Moore BJ, Verburgt LM, Staples CA, Paré PD, Hogg JC (1995) Measurement of lung expansion with computed tomography and comparison with quantitative histology. J Appl Physiol 79(5):1525–1530

52. Salito C, Aliverti A, Gierada DS, Deslée G, Pierce RA, Macklem PT, Woods JC (2009) Quantification of trapped gas with CT and 3 He MR imaging in a porcine model of isolated airway obstruction. Radiology 253(2):380–389

53. Hedlund LW, Vock P, Effmann EL (1983) Evaluating lung density by computed tomography. Semin Respir Crit Care Med 5:76–87

54. Coxson HO, Rogers RM, Whittall KP, D'yachkova Y, Paré PD, Sciurba FC, Hogg JC (1999) A quantification of the lung surface area in emphysema using computed tomography. Am J Respir Crit Care Med 159(3):851–856

55. Salito C, Woods JC, Aliverti A (2011) Influence of CT reconstruction settings on extremely low attenuation values for specific gas volume calculation in severe emphysema. Acad Radiol 18(10):1277–1284

56. Aliverti A, Pennati F, Salito C, Woods JC (2013) Regional lung function and heterogeneity of specific gas volume in healthy and emphysematous subjects. Eur Respir J 41(5):1179–1188

Functional Imaging of Airway Distensibility

16

Nicola Scichilone and Robert H. Brown

16.1 Background

Airways in healthy subjects dilate with each inspiration. This cyclic process is even more evident during sighing and deep inspirations to full lung inflation. This physiological function of the respiratory system is essential in distending airway smooth muscle and maintaining airway patency. Deep inspirations can reverse contracted airways, and this has been termed "deep inspiration-induced bronchodilation." It is believed that deep inspirations also provide a powerful mechanism of airway protection from subsequent bronchospastic stimuli. This has been termed "deep inspiration-induced bronchoprotection," and the loss of this function appears to be associated with the occurrence of airway hyperresponsiveness [1].

It is reasonable to hypothesize that deep lung inflations exert their beneficial effects through radial traction that is applied on the airway wall. Radial traction is generated by a network of alveolar attachments around the airway walls. Structural alterations of the airway wall (e.g., airway wall thickening) or the lung parenchyma (e.g., destruction of alveolar attachments) could impair the effectiveness of the distending forces, so that a deep inspiration would not be capable of generating enough force to stretch narrowed airways or reopen closed airways. In this context, it is possible that obstructive lung diseases may also lead to impairment of the beneficial effects of lung inflation.

N. Scichilone, MD
Dipartimento di Biomedicina e Medicina Interna e Specialistica, Sezione di Pneumologia, University of Palermo, Via Trabucco 180, Palermo 90146, Italy
e-mail: nicola.scichilone@unipa.it

R.H. Brown, MD, MPH (✉)
Departments of Anesthesiology and Critical Care Medicine, Medicine, Division of Pulmonary Medicine, Radiology, and Environmental Health Sciences, Johns Hopkins University, 615 North Wolfe Street, Baltimore, MD 21205, USA
e-mail: rbrown@jhsph.edu

A. Aliverti, A. Pedotti (eds.), *Mechanics of Breathing*,
DOI 10.1007/978-88-470-5647-3_16, © Springer-Verlag Italia 2014

As mentioned above, one possible mechanism for limited airway distention could be changes in the structure of the airway wall. The airway mucosa is incompressible, so as the airway smooth muscle contracts, the mucosa buckles and folds [2]. The basement membrane is a thin layer of specialized extracellular matrix between the epithelium and the stroma, which both supplies mechanical support to the airway and also influences epithelial cell-specific function [3]. The thickened appearance of the basement membrane in asthma results from a marked increase in type III collagen and fibronectin [3, 4]. Histological studies of the airways have assumed that the epithelial basement membrane is not distensible [5]. Therefore, the basement membrane is a limiting structure for airway distention [5, 6].

In asthma, epithelial cell damage and inflammation may be associated with wound repair processes in the airways. Wound repair is characterized by the appearance of extracellular matrix components, such as tenascin, which is expressed in healing wounds [7]. A study by Laitinen et al. [8] found tenascin either absent or present only as a thin interrupted line located beneath the epithelium, in control subjects. In contrast, the basement membrane layer of every patient with asthma showed strong immunoreactivity for tenascin as a broad continuous band [8]. Recently, James et al. [9] also showed there was an increase in the extracellular matrix in both fatal and nonfatal asthma cases.

Another component of the airway wall is the airway smooth muscle. Increases in the amount of airway smooth muscle, as a result of either hypertrophy or hyperplasia, may lead not only to increased contractility but also to decreased distensibility. James et al. [9] showed that hypertrophy of the airway smooth muscle cells occurred in the large airways in both fatal and nonfatal asthma, while airway smooth muscle hyperplasia occurred in the large and small airways only in the fatal cases they examined.

An alternative mechanism that is implicated in the impairment of the beneficial effect of lung inflations is the reduction in the distending forces. In 1960, Permutt and Martin demonstrated that, in healthy humans, lung elastic recoil became significantly depressed with increasing age [10]. In individuals with COPD, lung elastic recoil has been demonstrated to diminish as a function of the degree of emphysema [11, 12], primarily because of the disruption of the alveolar attachments that are responsible for the "stretching effect." For stretch to be exerted on the airway wall, the anatomic and functional interdependence between the lung parenchyma and the airways need to be intact. In COPD, alveolar attachments on airway walls are progressively destroyed and this is expected to impact on the ability of lung inflation by deep inspiration to stretch the airways. In fact, we have previously reported a correlation between loss of alveolar attachments and reduction in the beneficial effects of deep inspiration [13]. On the basis of all these observations, we reasoned that, in subjects with COPD, the ability of deep inspiration to dilate the airways is impaired, thus contributing to the occurrence and/or the severity of chronic respiratory symptoms. Indeed, using a modified bronchoprovocation methacholine test [1], we demonstrated that the bronchodilatory effect of deep inspirations is largely impaired in individuals with even mild COPD [14], as opposed to age-matched controls, and it decreased with the increasing severity of the disease [15]. Thus, it would seem that the deep inspiration defect in COPD is due to the loss of airway-parenchyma interdependence resulting from the emphysematous changes that are associated with this condition.

16.2 HRCT Functional Imaging

Conventional pulmonary function measurements are unable to assess airway stiffness, based on changes in airway size with lung inflation (distensibility). However, high-resolution computed tomography (HRCT) is unique in that it can be used to measure airway distensibility in animals [6, 16, 17] and in humans [18–22]. HRCT is a direct, noninvasive radiological technique that can accurately and reliably measure airway luminal area and airway wall thickness in human airways in vivo [23–25]. HRCT uses thin slices, high spatial frequency reconstruction algorithms, a small field of view, and increased kilovoltage and milliamperage to resolve structures as small as 200 µm [26]. HRCT is capable of excellent spatial resolution and provides anatomic detail of pulmonary structures.

Our laboratory was the first to demonstrate the utility of HRCT to study airway reactivity [23]. We have subsequently demonstrated that HRCT is uniquely capable of addressing questions about airway responsiveness in vivo that are not answerable by other techniques [6, 16, 27, 28]. HRCT can make repeated airway luminal and airway wall thickness measurements of multiple individual airways at different lung volumes in vivo. A body of evidence has accumulated to confirm the relationship between airway wall thickness, as assessed by HRCT, and the features of airway responsiveness in patients with stable asthma, with and without inhaled steroid treatment [29–38].

We can use HRCT to measure airway wall thickness in multiple airways (second to eight generation airways) in healthy subjects and in subjects with obstructed airways, both before and after interventions (Fig. 16.1). In addition, lung parenchymal density on the HRCT scans, expressed by lung attenuation parameters, can provide an estimate of parenchymal damage, which can also contribute to our understanding of the pathophysiological mechanisms of impaired airway distension.

16.3 Airway Distensibility

Although many investigators have studied the relationship between HRCT findings, such as airway wall thickness, and airflow limitation, or airway remodeling in patients with asthma and COPD, the HRCT-assessed dynamic behavior of the airways can provide unique information. The magnitude of the increase in the airway luminal area with a deep inspiration from functional residual capacity (FRC) to total lung capacity (TLC) represents airway distensibility and is expressed as a percentage (% distensibility). This methodology has been extensively used and validated in our studies. We previously demonstrated that canine airways do not expand isotropically with the lung [6]. When airways were completely relaxed, airway size

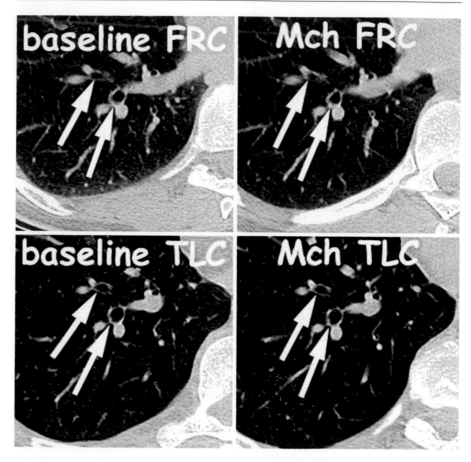

Fig. 16.1 Matched HRCT scans from one individual at baseline (*left column*) and after challenge with aerosolized methacholine (Mch, *right column*). Images were acquired at low lung volume (FRC, *upper row*) and at high lung volume (TLC, *lower row*). The *arrows* show the same airways matched under all conditions (Reprinted from Brown et al. [18]. With permission from American Thoracic Society. Copyright © 2012 American Thoracic Society)

reached a plateau at very low transpulmonary pressure (Ptp), and further increases in Ptp caused negligible changes. This is consistent with histological studies of the airways that presume that the epithelial basement membrane is not distensible. Therefore, changes in the composition of the airway wall can lead to thickening and shortening of the basement membrane and limit the distensibility of the airway.

Another possible mechanism for limited distention of the airways is changes in smooth muscle tone that stiffen the airways. We previously demonstrated in dogs [6], in sheep [16], and in humans [18] that when the airways had tone, not only was their baseline size reduced, but their distensibility was also decreased [6, 17, 18]. Furthermore, in asthma, intrinsic mechanisms may be the cause of stiffer airways. Skloot et al. showed that excessive airway narrowing in asthma may be caused by an intrinsic impairment of the ability of lung inflation to stretch airway smooth muscle [39].

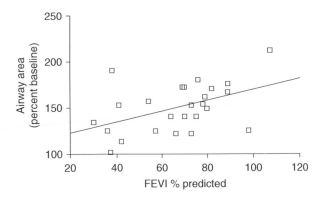

Fig. 16.2 The relationship between bronchodilation and airflow obstruction. There was a significant correlation between the airflow obstruction, as measured by the FEV₁ and the ability to bronchodilate the airways as measured by the change in airway area after maximum airway smooth muscle relaxation as a percent of baseline ($p=0.02$, $r^2=0.22$)

Moreover, an intrinsic airway abnormality that prevents dilation with lung inflation may become clinically apparent only after a certain degree or duration of airway constriction that occurs in individuals with chronic unresponsive obstruction [40].

Using HRCT, we measured the change in airway size (16–42 airways per subject, 2.2–17.4 mm in diameter) after complete airway smooth muscle relaxation compared to baseline. HRCT scans were performed at FRC at baseline and after complete airway smooth muscle relaxation with nebulized albuterol. Figure 16.2 demonstrates the relationship between chronic airflow obstruction and the component that is reversible with airway smooth muscle relaxation. Again, we observed an inverse correlation between the chronic airflow obstruction and the beta-adrenergic-responsive airway smooth muscle ($p=0.02$, $r^2=0.22$). The asthmatic subjects with the greatest airflow obstruction showed the lowest response to beta-adrenergic bronchodilation (Fig. 16.2). Since the airways in all the asthmatics did not bronchodilate to the same degree, factors other than airway smooth muscle tone must be involved in the chronic airway obstruction observed in moderate and severe asthma.

The mechanism by which intrapulmonary airways are stretched by inspiration is largely attributable to the increased radial traction on the airways exerted by the surrounding lung parenchyma [41–43]. It has been proposed that edema in the airway wall or in the peribronchial space could decrease the interdependence between the airway and the parenchyma, resulting in decreased radial forces acting on the smooth muscle with lung inflation [44, 45]. We demonstrated in dogs [28, 46] and sheep [16, 17] that substantial airway wall edema, up to a 50 % increase in airway wall area, can be elicited in the airway. Moreover, even this significant amount of airway edema did not affect airway distensibility [17]. Therefore, it is less likely that airway edema is a primary cause of unresponsive asthma.

Of course, remodeling changes in the airways, such as those observed in asthma and COPD, could stiffen the airways, thus opposing the distending forces of a deep

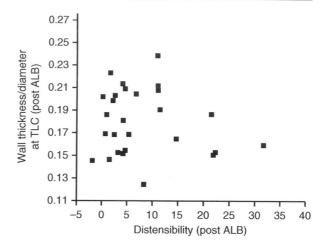

Fig. 16.3 Effect of airway wall thickness on airway distensibility. We found no significant correlation between airway wall thickness as a fraction of airway diameter after complete relaxation with albuterol (*ALB*) and airway distensibility after complete relaxation with ALB in individuals with asthma ($r^2=0.21$, $p=0.06$)

inspiratory maneuver. This could explain, for example, the reduced ability to stretch the airways that accounts for the loss of bronchodilation in severe asthma. Recently, James et al. have shown there is airway smooth muscle hypertrophy in the large airways in both fatal and nonfatal asthma and airway smooth muscle hyperplasia in the large and small airways in fatal asthma [9]. However, recent findings [47] and unpublished observations from our group showed that, even while the airway walls were thicker, this increased thickness did not appear to impede airway distensibility (Fig. 16.3). We infer that the inflammation-induced remodeling processes in chronic asthma, which can increase the airway wall thickness, do not appear to change the basic passive force-tension dynamics in vivo and, thus, do not appear to make airways more resistant to imposed stretch by deep inspiration.

16.4 Magnitude of Distensibility

The bronchodilator effects of a DI have been shown to be impaired in individuals with asthmatics and with COPD, compared to healthy subjects. Since the ability to generate high transpulmonary pressures (Ptp) at TLC depends on both lung properties and voluntary effort, we wondered how the response of the airways to DIs might be altered if the maneuver were performed at less than maximal inflation. To examine the effects on subsequent airway caliber of varying Ptp during the DI maneuver, we studied five anesthetized and ventilated dogs during Mch infusion and measured changes in airway size after DIs of increasing magnitude over the subsequent 5-min period using HRCT. Our results showed that the magnitude of the Ptp was extremely important, leading to a qualitative change in the airway response. A large DI (45 cm H_2O) caused subsequent airway dilation, while smaller DIs ($\leq$35 cm H_2O) caused bronchoconstriction [48] (Fig. 16.4). Furthermore, the duration of the DI also affected the subsequent airway caliber. In another study in anesthetized and

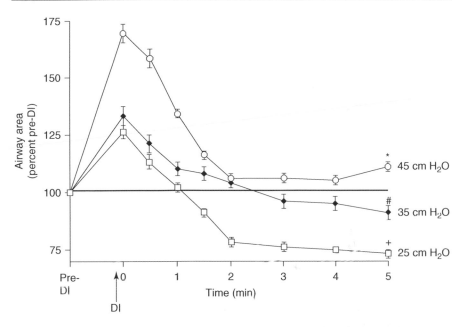

Fig. 16.4 Percent change in mean airway area immediately after a DI to a peak inflation pressure of 25 cm H_2O (*squares*), 35 cm H_2O (*diamonds*), and 45 cm H_2O (*circles*). For the larger DI (45 cm H_2O), the airway size remained above the baseline airway area for the entire measurement period (*$p < 0.0001$). In contrast, for the smaller (35 and 25 cm H_2O) DIs, the airways actively contracted to a smaller area than that of the pre-DI baseline. At 5 min, the airway area was 91 ± 3 % for the 35 cm H_2O DI (#$p < 0.0001$) and 73 ± 1 % for the 25 cm H_2O DI (+$p < 0.0001$) of pre-DI airway area (From Brown and Mitzner [48])

ventilated dogs during Mch infusion, we measured changes in airway size after DIs of the same magnitude with increasing duration over the subsequent 5-min period using HRCT. Our results showed that the duration of the DI was also important, leading to a qualitative change in the airway response. A long DI (30–60 s) caused subsequent airway dilation, while shorter DIs (5–10 s) caused bronchoconstriction [49]. To examine the potential mechanisms for these differences in airway caliber after DIs, we investigated the role of nitric oxide (NO) on DI-induced bronchodilation and subsequent airway caliber response in a canine model. In anesthetized and ventilated dogs during Mch infusion, we measured changes in airway size after a small (25 cm H_2O) and a large (45 cm H_2O) DI, before and after administering *NG-nitro-l-arginine* methyl ester to block NO synthesis over the subsequent 5-min period using HRCT. Our results showed that, consistent with the findings mentioned above, a DI to a higher pressure resulted in airway dilation, while a DI to a lower pressure lead to airway narrowing. When *N*G-nitro-L-arginine methyl ester was administered, both the large and small DIs resulted in subsequent airway constriction. These results support the idea that nitric oxide may be a potential bronchoprotective agent in the airways [50].

16.5   Airway Distensibility in Asthma

The effects of a DI in individuals with asthma differ from those observed in healthy subjects. It has been postulated that the beneficial effect of lung inflation is mediated by airway stretch. One hypothesis to explain the defects in the function of lung inflation in asthma is that a DI may be unable to sufficiently stretch the airways. This may result from attenuation of the tethering forces between the airways and the surrounding parenchyma. We used HRCT to examine the ability of a deep inspiration to distend the airways of mild asthmatics ($n=10$), compared to healthy subjects ($n=9$), at baseline and after increasing airway tone with Mch. We found that both at baseline and after the induction of smooth muscle tone with Mch, a DI distended the airways of healthy and asthmatic subjects to a similar extent, indicating that abnormal interdependence between the lung parenchyma and the airways was unlikely to play a major role in the loss or in the attenuation of the beneficial effect of lung inflation that characterizes asthma [18] (Fig. 16.5). Furthermore, we observed that after constriction had already been induced by Mch, following a deep inspiration, bronchodilation occurred in the healthy subjects, but further bronchoconstriction occurred in the asthmatics [18] (Fig. 16.6). Our findings suggest that an abnormal excitation/contraction mechanism in the airway smooth muscle of mild asthmatic subjects counteracts the bronchodilatory effect of a DI. These results suggest that the mechanism for reduced bronchodilation after deep inspirations in mild asthmatics may be intrinsic to the airway smooth muscle. This has been confirmed by the different dynamic responses of airways and lung parenchyma to lung inflations. When considering the effects of a deep inspiration, an implicit assumption is that all of the airways are distending in concert with the lung. If the contracted airways had slower dynamic responses than the lung parenchyma, then the timing of the deep inspiratory maneuver could affect the airway response. Using

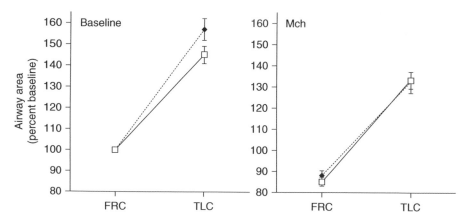

Fig. 16.5 The increase in airway area with a deep inspiration (distensibility) in the nine healthy (*open square, solid line*) and in the ten asthmatic (*closed diamond, dashed line*) subjects at baseline (*left*) and after bronchoconstriction with aerosol methacholine (*right*). There was no difference in distensibility between the healthy and the asthmatic subjects either at baseline ($p > 0.05$) or after methacholine administration ($p > 0.05$)

HRCT, we studied how well-matched the dynamic response of airways was to that of the lung parenchyma in dogs. Our results clearly demonstrated that airways contracted with Mch dilate at about a four times slower rate compared to the lung parenchyma during rapid lung inflation and deflation [51] (Fig. 16.7a, b). This effect may play a role in the unique response of asthmatic subjects to deep inspiration.

As a next step, we examined the distensibility of the airways of individuals with asthma with chronically abnormal airflow obstruction. We measured the ability of asthmatics with varying degrees of baseline airway obstruction to distend their airways with a deep inspiration. We showed that the reduced ability to distend the airways with lung inflation related to the extent of air trapping and airway smooth muscle tone [47].

There can be many causes of increased airflow obstruction in asthma. One likely cause in asthmatic subjects is increased airway smooth muscle tone as mentioned above. To examine other components in the airways that may lead to airway remodeling and decreased distensibility, we measured airway distensibility after complete relaxation with the beta-adrenergic bronchodilator, albuterol. As with the airway distensibility at baseline, we observed a correlation between the baseline airway obstruction and the ability to distend the relaxed airways in the asthmatic subjects ($p=0.02$, $r^2=0.21$). Thus, even after complete airway smooth muscle relaxation in the asthmatic subjects, greater baseline chronic airflow obstruction was associated with lower airway distensibility. These results support the hypothesis that the inability of airways to distend with a DI is due not only to increased airway smooth muscle tone but also to increased nondistensible components in the airway wall.

We found that airway bronchodilation and airway distensibility were related to disease severity in individuals with asthma, and that complete relaxation of the airway smooth muscle did not entirely relieve the chronic obstruction. Moreover, measurement of airway distensibility may give insight into the pathophysiology, progression of disease, and response to therapy in asthmatic patients.

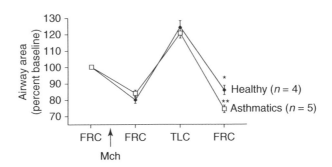

Fig. 16.6 The change in airway area with a deep inspiration (distensibility) in the four healthy (*closed diamond, dashed line*) and in five asthmatic (*open square, solid line*) subjects after bronchoconstriction with aerosol methacholine, a subsequent DI, and on return to FRC. There was a significant increase in airway luminal area after the DI in the healthy subjects compared to FRC after methacholine ($p=0.03$). In contrast, there was a significant decrease in airway luminal area after the DI in the asthmatic subjects compared to FRC after methacholine ($p<0.0001$)

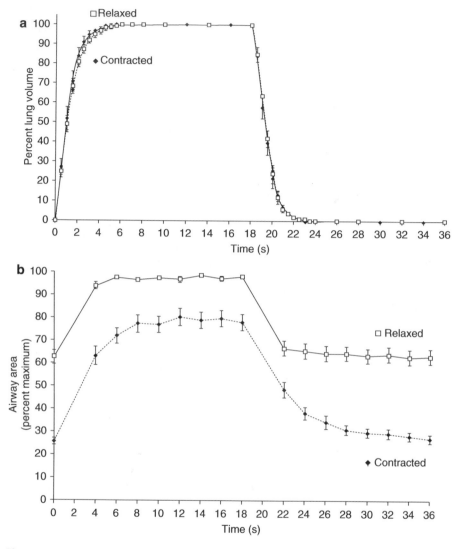

Fig. 16.7 (a) Percent changes in lung volume with a step increase and decrease in airway pressure averaged over the six dogs. In each animal, the 100 % value is taken as the value after 20 s at an airway pressure of 37 cm H$_2$O. The absolute mean ($\pm$ SEM) FRC and TLC in atropine-relaxed lungs was 1,190 ml $\pm$ 130 and 2,759 ml $\pm$ 380, respectively. During the Mch challenge, the absolute FRC and TLC were 1,149 ml $\pm$ 122 and 2,552 ml $\pm$ 265, and these were not significantly different from the values with atropine. The mean values for inspiratory capacity with atropine and Mch were 1,388 ml $\pm$ 230 and 1,347 ml $\pm$ 217, respectively (Reprinted with permission of the American Thoracic Society. Copyright © 2012 American Thoracic Society. Brown and Mitzner [51]). (b) Changes in mean airway area averaged across all dogs, expressed as a percent of maximal area. The maximal area for each airway was taken to be the airway area after 20 s at an airway pressure of 37 cm H$_2$O in animals that were given atropine (Reprinted from Brown and Mitzner [51]. With permission from American Thoracic Society. Copyright © 2012 American Thoracic Society)

16.6   Airway Distensibility in COPD

In previous studies, we demonstrated that the ability of a series of DIs to dilate constricted airways was largely attenuated or completely lost in individuals with COPD [14]. This was not surprising, given the hypothesized underlying mechanism of the loss of parenchymal tethering. Indeed, COPD is characterized by structural, mostly nonreversible, changes in the airways (e.g., airway wall thickening) and the surrounding parenchyma (e.g., destruction of alveolar attachments), which may oppose the distending forces to various extents.

We have shown that the bronchodilatory ability of deep inspiration was lost in mild COPD [14], and we speculated that the absence of deep inspiration-induced bronchodilation would contribute to the development and severity of chronic respiratory symptoms in COPD. By inducing bronchoconstriction in a standardized protocol that assessed the effects of deep inspirations, we measured the ability of deep inspiration maneuvers to reduce the degree of bronchoconstriction. We found that the bronchodilatory effect of lung inflation was profoundly impaired in individuals with mild COPD [14]. In addition, the reduced ability to dilate constricted airways was associated with the reduction in diffusing capacity of the lung for carbon monoxide (DLCO), suggesting that the primary mechanism responsible for the lack of the beneficial effect of DI on airways lies in the structural alterations of the parenchyma. We reasoned that because of the alveolar wall destruction, the loss of airway-parenchyma interdependence (mechanical decoupling between airways and parenchyma) resulted in diminished airway wall and airway smooth muscle stretch, thus impairing a primary step in the mechanism of bronchodilation by deep inspiration.

To further explore this phenomenon, we extended the use of HRCT to this population, with the aim of assessing the degree of airway distensibility at baseline conditions. In our study [15], we provided evidence of a relationship between airway distensibility in individuals with COPD, as measured by HRCT, and the Global Initiative for Chronic Obstructive Lung Disease (GOLD) classification as well as between distensibility and various aspects of baseline lung function, including those reflective of airflow limitation and those reflective of hyperinflation. Indeed, our findings clearly demonstrated that the severity of COPD was associated with reduced airway distensibility by deep inspiration (Fig. 16.8). The magnitude of the effect of airway distensibility was also related to indices of airway obstruction, likely associated with structural changes in the airways, such as increased airway smooth muscle tone and airway remodeling. In addition, we found a significant inverse relationship between airway distensibility and hyperinflation, as measured by RV/TLC, suggesting that the increase in lung volume could be one of the factors that affects this process. This is important in COPD, where lung hyperinflation is a pivotal functional abnormality. Static hyperinflation results from the loss of elastic recoil and is attributable to the emphysematous damage to the lung parenchyma. Recently, Diaz and colleagues [52] demonstrated that airway distensibility by lung inflation was largely attenuated in subjects with an emphysema-predominant phenotype as opposed to those with airway-predominant alterations (intrinsic narrowing of the airways due to inflammation and fibrosis).

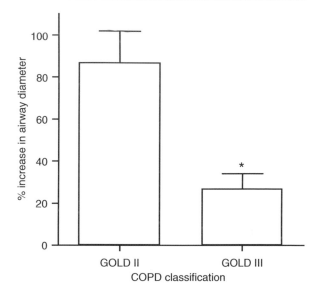

Fig. 16.8 The extent of airway distensibility as measured by the percent increase in airway area with lung inflation was associated with the severity of COPD. Individuals with COPD GOLD stage III had lower airway luminal distensibility than individuals with COPD GOLD stage II (*$p = 0.003$)

To further explore the factors that affect the magnitude of deep inspiration-induced airway distensibility with HRCT, we tested the degree of distensibility in subjects with asthma and COPD who had a comparable degree of bronchial obstruction. Two sets of scans were obtained, one at functional residual capacity (FRC) and the other at total lung capacity (TLC). The change in airway diameter, as measured by airway distensibility, was the main outcome. Airway wall thickness and lung density were measured to evaluate which radiological abnormalities could potentially affect the airway distensibility. Lung function variables were also obtained. In 12 asthmatics and 8 subjects with COPD, a total of 701 airways were analyzed. No significant difference between the two groups were detected when airway distensibility was calculated for either all airways (Fig. 16.9) or by airway size for the small ($p = 0.27$), the medium ($p = 0.94$), and the large ($p = 0.40$) airways. These results suggest that the lack of airway distensibility is the main cause of persistent airflow limitation, regardless of the etiology of the obstructive lung disease. However, the major determinants of airway distensibility were different for the two groups. In the asthmatic group, the dynamic ability to alter lung volume was the main factor that affected airway distensibility, while, in the subjects with COPD, the static lung volumes influenced the degree of airway distensibility.

Thus, it seems that in asthma and COPD, functional alterations can be defined not only by the degree of bronchial obstruction but also by the magnitude of the distensibility of the airways to deep inspirations. Functional imaging of airway distensibility can contribute to a better understanding of the mechanisms of action of deep inspirations and, consequently, to the understanding of the disease processes in asthma and COPD. Future studies could explore the role of functional imaging in the monitoring of the severity of the disease and the response to treatment.

Fig. 16.9 The degree of
airway distensibility in
individuals with asthmatic
($n=12$) and COPD ($n=8$)
with similar magnitude of
airway obstruction. There
was no difference in airway
distensibility between the
groups $p>0.05$

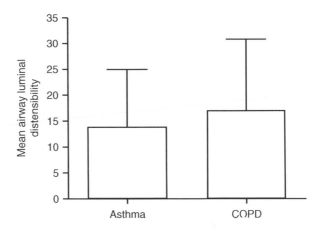

Bibliography

1. Scichilone N, Permutt S, Togias A (2001) The lack of the bronchoprotective and not the bronchodilatory ability of deep inspiration is associated with airway hyperresponsiveness. Am J Respir Crit Care Med 163(2):413–419
2. Lambert RK, Codd SL, Alley MR, Pack RJ (1994) Physical determinants of bronchial mucosal folding. J Appl Physiol 77(3):1206–1216
3. Merker HJ (1994) Morphology of the basement membrane. Microsc Res Tech 28(2):95–124
4. McCarter JH, Vazquez JJ (1966) The bronchial basement membrane in asthma. Arch Pathol 82(4):328–335
5. James AL, Hogg JC, Dunn LA, Pare PD (1988) The use of the internal perimeter to compare airway size and to calculate smooth muscle shortening. Am Rev Respir Dis 138(1):136–139
6. Brown RH, Mitzner W (1996) Effect of lung inflation and airway muscle tone on airway diameter in vivo. J Appl Physiol 80(5):1581–1588
7. Raghow R (1994) The role of extracellular matrix in postinflammatory wound healing and fibrosis. FASEB J 8(11):823–831
8. Laitinen A, Altraja A, Kampe M, Linden M, Virtanen I, Laitinen LA (1997) Tenascin is increased in airway basement membrane of asthmatics and decreased by an inhaled steroid. Am J Respir Crit Care Med 156(3 Pt 1):951–958
9. James AL, Elliot JG, Jones RL, Carroll ML, Mauad T, Bai TR et al (2012) Airway smooth muscle hypertrophy and hyperplasia in asthma. Am J Respir Crit Care Med 185(10): 1058–1064
10. Permutt S, Martin HB (1960) Static pressure-volume characteristics of lungs in normal males. J Appl Physiol 15:819–825
11. Baldi S, Miniati M, Bellina CR, Battolla L, Catapano G, Begliomini E et al (2001) Relationship between extent of pulmonary emphysema by high-resolution computed tomography and lung elastic recoil in patients with chronic obstructive pulmonary disease. Am J Respir Crit Care Med 164(4):585–589
12. Silvers GW, Petty TL, Stanford RE (1980) Elastic recoil changes in early emphysema. Thorax 35(7):490–495
13. Scichilone N, Bruno A, Marchese R, Vignola AM, Togias A, Bellia V (2005) Association between reduced bronchodilatory effect of deep inspiration and loss of alveolar attachments. Respir Res 6:55
14. Scichilone N, Marchese R, Catalano F, Vignola AM, Togias A, Bellia V (2004) Bronchodilatory effect of deep inspiration is absent in subjects with mild COPD. Chest 125(6):2029–2035

15. Scichilone N, La Sala A, Bellia M, Fallano K, Togias A, Brown RH et al (2008) The airway response to deep inspirations decreases with COPD severity and is associated with airway distensibility assessed by computed tomography. J Appl Physiol 105(3):832–838

16. Brown RH, Mitzner W, Bulut Y, Wagner EM (1997) Effect of lung inflation in vivo on airways with smooth muscle tone or edema. J Appl Physiol 82(2):491–499

17. Brown RH, Mitzner W, Wagner EM (1997) Interaction between airway edema and lung inflation on responsiveness of individual airways in vivo. J Appl Physiol 83(2):366–370

18. Brown RH, Scichilone N, Mudge B, Diemer FB, Permutt S, Togias A (2001) High-resolution computed tomographic evaluation of airway distensibility and the effects of lung inflation on airway caliber in healthy subjects and individuals with asthma. Am J Respir Crit Care Med 163(4):994–1001

19. Brown RH, Herold C, Zerhouni EA, Mitzner W (1994) Spontaneous airways constrict during breath holding studied by high-resolution computed tomography. Chest 106(3):920–924

20. de Jong PA, Muller NL, Pare PD, Coxson HO (2005) Computed tomographic imaging of the airways: relationship to structure and function. Eur Respir J 26(1):140–152

21. Grenier P, Cordeau MP, Beigelman C (1993) High-resolution computed tomography of the airways. J Thorac Imaging 8(3):213–229

22. Paganin F, Vignola AM, Seneterre E, Bruel JM, Chanez P, Bousquet J (1995) Heterogeneity of airways obstruction in asthmatic patients using high-resolution computed tomography. Chest 107(3 Suppl):145S–146S

23. Brown RH, Herold CJ, Hirshman CA, Zerhouni EA, Mitzner W (1991) In vivo measurements of airway reactivity using high-resolution computed tomography. Am Rev Respir Dis 144(1): 208–212

24. Amirav I, Kramer SS, Grunstein MM, Hoffman EA (1993) Assessment of methacholine-induced airway constriction by ultrafast high-resolution computed tomography. J Appl Physiol 75(5):2239–2250

25. Wood SA, Zerhouni EA, Hoford JD, Hoffman EA, Mitzner W (1995) Measurement of three-dimensional lung tree structures by using computed tomography. J Appl Physiol 79(5):1687–1697

26. Zerhouni EA, Naidich DP, Stitik FP, Khouri NF, Siegelman SS (1985) Computed tomography of the pulmonary parenchyma. Part 2: Interstitial disease. J Thorac Imaging 1(1):54–64

27. Brown RH, Herold CJ, Hirshman CA, Zerhouni EA, Mitzner W (1993) Individual airway constrictor response heterogeneity to histamine assessed by high-resolution computed tomography. J Appl Physiol 74(6):2615–2620

28. Brown RH, Zerhouni EA, Mitzner W (1995) Visualization of airway obstruction in vivo during pulmonary vascular engorgement and edema. J Appl Physiol 78(3):1070–1078

29. Awadh N, Muller NL, Park CS, Abboud RT, FitzGerald JM (1998) Airway wall thickness in patients with near fatal asthma and control groups: assessment with high resolution computed tomographic scanning. Thorax 53(4):248–253

30. Boulet L, Belanger M, Carrier G (1995) Airway responsiveness and bronchial-wall thickness in asthma with or without fixed airflow obstruction. Am J Respir Crit Care Med 152(3): 865–871

31. Chen FH, Chen ZG, Chen H, Ji JZ, Chen YF, Peng BX et al (2006) Correlation of reticular basement membrane thickness and airway wall remolding in asthma patients. Zhonghua Yi Xue Za Zhi 86(7):468–471

32. Gono H, Fujimoto K, Kawakami S, Kubo K (2003) Evaluation of airway wall thickness and air trapping by HRCT in asymptomatic asthma. Eur Respir J 22(6):965–971

33. Gorska K, Krenke R, Kosciuch J, Przybylowski T, Domagala-Kulawik J, Hildebrand K et al (2007) The relationship between markers of airway inflammation and thickness of the basement membrane in patients with asthma. Pneumonol Alergol Pol 75(4):363–369

34. Kosciuch J, Krenke R, Gorska K, Zukowska M, Maskey-Warzechowska M, Chazan R (2009) Relationship between airway wall thickness assessed by high-resolution computed tomography and lung function in patients with asthma and chronic obstructive pulmonary disease. J Physiol Pharmacol 60(Suppl 5):71–76

35. Kurashima K, Kanauchi T, Hoshi T, Takaku Y, Ishiguro T, Takayanagi N et al (2008) Effect of early versus late intervention with inhaled corticosteroids on airway wall thickness in patients with asthma. Respirology 13(7):1008–1013

36. Little SA, Sproule MW, Cowan MD, Macleod KJ, Robertson M, Love JG et al (2002) High resolution computed tomographic assessment of airway wall thickness in chronic asthma: reproducibility and relationship with lung function and severity. Thorax 57(3):247–253

37. Niimi A, Matsumoto H, Amitani R, Nakano Y, Mishima M, Minakuchi M et al (2000) Airway wall thickness in asthma assessed by computed tomography. Relation to clinical indices. Am J Respir Crit Care Med 162:1518–1523

38. Niimi A, Matsumoto H, Takemura M, Ueda T, Chin K, Mishima M (2003) Relationship of airway wall thickness to airway sensitivity and airway reactivity in asthma. Am J Respir Crit Care Med 168(8):983–988

39. Skloot G, Permutt S, Togias A (1995) Airway hyperresponsiveness in asthma: a problem of limited smooth muscle relaxation with inspiration. J Clin Invest 96(5):2393–2403

40. Lim TK, Pride NB, Ingram RH Jr (1987) Effects of volume history during spontaneous and acutely induced air-flow obstruction in asthma. Am Rev Respir Dis 135(3):591–596

41. Gunst SJ, Warner DO, Wilson TA, Hyatt RE (1988) Parenchymal interdependence and airway response to methacholine in excised dog lobes. J Appl Physiol 65(6):2490–2497

42. Lai-Fook SJ, Hyatt RE, Rodarte JR (1978) Effect of parenchymal shear modulus and lung volume on bronchial pressure-diameter behavior. J Appl Physiol 44(6):859–868

43. Mead J, Takishima T, Leith D (1970) Stress distribution in lungs: a model of pulmonary elasticity. J Appl Physiol 28(5):596–608

44. Lai-Fook SJ, Beck KC, Sutcliffe AM, Donaldson JT (1984) Effect of edema and height on bronchial diameter and shape in excised dog lung. Respir Physiol 55(2):223–237

45. Macklem PT (1989) Mechanical factors determining maximum bronchoconstriction. Eur Respir J Suppl 6:516s–519s

46. Brown RH, Zerhouni EA, Mitzner W (1995) Airway edema potentiates airway reactivity. J Appl Physiol 79(4):1242–1248

47. Pyrgos G, Scichilone N, Togias A, Brown RH (2011) Bronchodilation response to deep inspirations in asthma is dependent on airway distensibility and air trapping. J Appl Physiol 110(2):472–479

48. Brown RH, Mitzner W (2001) Airway response to deep inspiration: role of inflation pressure. J Appl Physiol 91(6):2574–2578

49. Brown RH, Mitzner W (2003) Duration of deep inspiration and subsequent airway constriction in vivo. J Asthma 40(2):119–124

50. Brown RH, Mitzner W (2003) Airway response to deep inspiration: role of nitric oxide. Eur Respir J 22(1):57–61

51. Brown RH, Mitzner W (2000) Delayed distension of contracted airways with lung inflation in vivo. Am J Respir Crit Care Med 162(6):2113–2116

52. Diaz AA, Come CE, Ross JC, San Jose Estepar R, Han MK, Loring SH et al (2012) Association between airway caliber changes with lung inflation and emphysema assessed by volumetric CT scan in subjects with COPD. Chest 141(3):736–744

Function and Microstructure by Hyperpolarized Gas MRI

17

Jason C. Woods, Dmitriy A. Yablonskiy,
and Mark S. Conradi

17.1 Background

The ability to regionally assess lung function and/or microstructure has both scientific and diagnostic advantages. For example, it is not well understood why many lung diseases are spatially heterogeneous and how alveolar microstructure and regional ventilation or gas exchange change with disease onset and progression. Imaging assessment of such pulmonary function would elucidate specific physiological aspects of normal lungs in health and disease and has the potential as a biomarker for the development and assessment of new treatments, especially those that may regionally target the most-diseased bronchopulmonary segments. X-ray CT has had extraordinary success as a diagnostic tool for many pulmonary abnormalities, with the greatest advantage being its simplicity as a spatially resolved densitometer. However, X-ray CT does not easily allow regional assessment of either function or microstructure. Lung MRI with ^1H has very low signal-to-noise ratio compared to CT due to multiple air-tissue interfaces in lung parenchyma that

J.C. Woods, PhD (✉)
Center for Pulmonary Imaging Research, Pulmonary Medicine & Radiology,
Cincinnati Children's Hospital Medical Center, 3333 Burnet Ave,
Cincinnati, OH 45229, USA

Department of Physics, Washington University,
One Brookings Drive, St Louis, MO 63130, USA
e-mail: jason.woods@cchmc.org

D.A. Yablonskiy
Department of Radiology, Washington University,
510 S. Kingshighway, St Louis, MO 63108, USA
e-mail: yablonskiyd@wustl.edu

M.S. Conradi
Department of Physics, Washington University,
One Brookings Drive, St Louis, MO 63130, USA
e-mail: msc@wuphys.wustl.edu

A. Aliverti, A. Pedotti (eds.), *Mechanics of Breathing*,
DOI 10.1007/978-88-470-5647-3_17, © Springer-Verlag Italia 2014

17.2.4 Applications of Ventilation Imaging to Disease

Since many lung diseases, including asthma, COPD, and cystic fibrosis (CF), result in nonuniform distribution of inhaled gas, ventilation imaging is applicable to many diseases. Here, we briefly discuss a few applications of ventilation imaging for COPD, which is the focus of our research.

COPD spans the continuum between emphysema (loss of elastic recoil and destruction of alveolar tissue) and chronic bronchitis (small airways inflammation and excessive mucous). Diffusion MRI of hyperpolarized gas has become a gold standard for research characterizing COPD, especially for the quantification of emphysema (see later sections of this review).

Simple, static ventilation images can be used to identify large portions of the lungs with poor ventilation in patients with COPD [42]. The image in Fig. 17.1 from a patient with severe COPD reveals a very nonuniform distribution of the inhaled bolus of ^{3}He gas upon breath hold compared to that of a healthy subject. The ventilation pattern of asthmatic lungs, an example of which is also shown in Fig. 17.1, has been studied in some detail by ^{3}He MRI [39, 44] and often demonstrates wedge-shaped defects that often are persistent with time [45]. Ventilation images in asthmatic patients after methacholine challenge reveal larger defects, as expected, which resolve upon full bronchodilation [46]. The effects of bronchodilators upon ventilation defects in COPD also have been reported [47, 48], as have ventilation abnormalities in CF and bronchiolitis obliterans [42, 49–51]. In some cases, the size of the defects in severe disease comprises most of the lung, which is in keeping with the low pulmonary function of these patients [52]. In fact, the volume percentage of these defects correlates well with pulmonary function [53], giving rise to the idea of regional pulmonary function measures. One additional quantitative measure of ventilation that has emerged is fractional ventilation, which facilitates the gathering of regional information on "new" gas supplied by each breath [43].

Time-resolved imaging can reveal real-time ventilation dynamics that are not captured by static imaging. A dynamic imaging study via radial-projection MRI presents images of one COPD patient and one patient with severe asthma (see Figure 6b in [37]). A pronounced mottled appearance early in the inhalation becomes smoother at later times, thus demonstrating that dynamic imaging may be

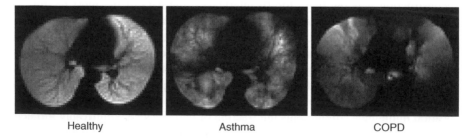

Healthy   Asthma   COPD

Fig. 17.1 Axial slices of ^{3}He static ventilation MRI in a healthy volunteer, patient with severe asthma, and patient with severe COPD

more sensitive to regional nonuniformities, alveolar recruitment, and/or collateral ventilation than static breath-hold imaging. [3]He gas trapping is clearly evident in a patient with mild-to-moderate asthma as a region of enhanced [3]He signal amplitude upon exhalation (see Figure 7 in [39]). These results indicate that images of the highest resolution are not required to display many or most of the changes in disease, which is positive for the field since lower-resolution images require substantially less (or less-polarized) hyperpolarized gas [54].

17.3   Diffusion Lung Imaging

17.3.1   Diffusion Background

Diffusion MRI with hyperpolarized gases is based on measurements of diffusion of hyperpolarized gas (either [3]He or [129]Xe) introduced into the lung airspaces during inhalation. The simplest MR measurement of diffusion is the Stejskal-Tanner pulsed field gradient (PFG) experiment [55] in which a free-induction decay MR signal is acted upon by two opposite-polarity gradient pulses (Fig. 17.2), the so-called diffusion-sensitizing gradients. This method is restricted by MRI signal T_2^* decay (on the order of 20–30 ms) and can be used only to study short-range diffusion. Measurements of the [3]He diffusion coefficient at longer diffusion times (seconds) proposed by Owers-Bradley et al. [56] (see also [57–61]) allow exploring the "connectivity" of acinar airways and alveoli, thus providing information on airway and alveolar wall integrity (i.e., holes through the walls) and collateral ventilation pathways [59, 60].

In the presence of gradient pulses, nuclear spins suffer a net phase shift proportional to their displacement during the diffusion time, Δ, resulting in decreased signal amplitude. In the case of unrestricted diffusion, the MR signal S decays as $S = S_0 \exp(-bD_0)$. Here, S_0 is the MR signal intensity in the absence of

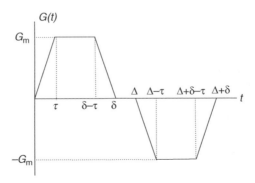

Fig. 17.2 Diffusion-sensitizing pulse gradient waveform employed in diffusion MRI with hyperpolarized gases at short diffusion times. In this diagram G_m is the gradient lobe amplitude, Δ is the spacing between the leading edges of the positive and negative lobes (the diffusion time), δ is the full duration of each lobe, and τ is a ramp-up and ramp-down time

diffusion-sensitizing gradients, and the b-value is determined by the gradient wave-form shape [62, 63]. For the gradient pulses in Fig. 17.2, the corresponding b-value calculation is

$$b = \left(\gamma G_m\right)^2 \left[\delta^2 \left(\Delta - \frac{\delta}{3}\right) + \tau \left(\delta^2 - 2\Delta\delta + \Delta\tau - \frac{7}{6}\delta\tau + \frac{8}{15}\tau^2\right)\right] \quad (17.1)$$

In the presence of barriers such as alveolar walls and walls of lung airways, the diffusive motion is restricted and the MR signal decay is often described in terms of the ADC using:

$$S = S_0 \exp\left(-b \cdot ADC\right) \quad (17.2)$$

Contrary to the free diffusion case where ADC is equal to D_0 and depends only on the molecular diffusion properties, the ADC for restricted diffusion evaluated from Eq. 17.2 also depends on the tissue structure and on the timing details of the gradient waveform shape and gradient strength.

17.3.2 ADC Measurements in Lungs

ADC measurements are usually done with two b-values to cover a substantial part of the lungs in a single breath hold. Initial reports [63–66] have demonstrated that ADC of hyperpolarized ^{3}He gas in the lungs dramatically increases in emphysema (compared to normal lungs), suggesting the potential use of this technique as a diagnostic tool for clinical applications. Examples of ventilation images (MRI-measured distribution of ^{3}He gas inhaled by a subject) and ^{3}He gas ADC maps of normal human lungs and lungs with severe emphysema are shown in Fig. 17.3.

The remarkable differences in the ADC values between healthy (0.17 cm^2/s) and diseased (0.52 cm^2/s) lung indicate that diffusion imaging of the lung with hyperpolarized ^{3}He could provide a very sensitive tool for clinical evaluation of emphysema. Indeed, Fig. 17.4 demonstrates the correlation between ADC and either mean alveolar internal area (AIA) in rats with elastase induced emphysema [68], mean chord length (MCL) in elastase-induced emphysematous rabbit lungs [69], mean linear intercept (L_m) in healthy and emphysematous human lungs with data obtained at different diffusion times [70], or mean linear intercept (L_m) in healthy human lungs and lungs with severe emphysema [71].

In addition to the correlation with histology as seen in Fig. 17.3, ADC in healthy subjects has been correlated with lung inflation level [72], subjects' age [72–74], and spirometric indices [66]. Although most of these studies were based on ^{3}He gas measurements, several authors also have reported measurements of ^{129}Xe-based ADC in healthy and emphysematous lungs [69, 75–80]. Kirby et al. [78] demonstrated a significant correlation between ^{3}He ADC and ^{129}Xe ADC as well as between

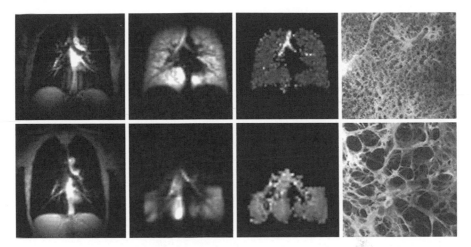

Fig. 17.3 Images of normal and emphysematous human lungs. Left to right: proton MRI, ³He ventilation maps, ³He gas ADC maps, and histological slices (the latter adapted from West [67]). *First row*: normal lungs. *Second row*: emphysematous lungs. ADC in a normal lung is rather homogeneous, except for large airways (trachea and its first branches), and is ~0.17 cm²/s. In the emphysematous lungs, ³He gas penetrates only into ventilated regions (lower portion of the lung in this case) and has an ADC ~3× larger (~0.55 cm²/s) than the ADC in the normal lung

ADCs and CT measurements. In healthy lungs, ³He ADC and ¹²⁹Xe ADC were found to be ~0.20 cm²/s and ~0.055 cm²/s, respectively. In lungs with COPD, the corresponding values are ~0.55–0.6 cm²/s and ~0.07–0.09 cm²/s. In another study, the mean ¹²⁹Xe ADC in healthy volunteers was reported to be ~0.04 cm²/s [77]. Such a difference in ¹²⁹Xe ADC could be explained by different experimental conditions, including concentration of ¹²⁹Xe in gas mixtures.

17.4 In Vivo Lung Morphometry: Evaluation of Lung Microstructure by Diffusion Measurements

A fundamental question needs to be answered to advance diffusion measurements to research and clinical practice. What aspects of lung microstructure are being measured by ³He or ¹²⁹Xe ADC? To obtain quantitative information on lung microstructure at the acinar level, geometrical parameters describing the lung microstructure should be related to the parameters extracted from MR measurements independent of pulse sequence parameters and/or gas concentration. Obviously, such a complicated structure as the lung cannot be analyzed without some simplifications and assumptions. To date, numerous models for lung microstructure have been explored to simulate diffusion-attenuated MRI signal using the Monte Carlo approach or finite difference methods. A modified Weibel model [81, 82] has been used [1, 63, 83–85]. Other examples include a porous media approach proposed by Mair et al. [86, 87], a cylindrical model with semi-spherical alveolar shape and

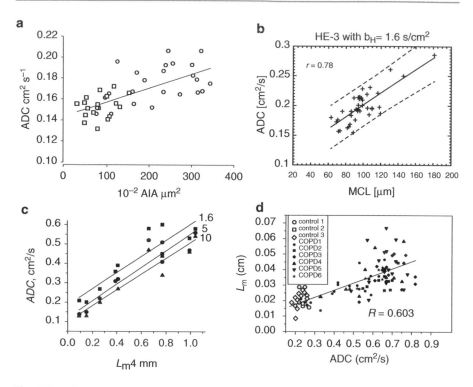

Fig. 17.4 Correlation between ADC and (**a**) mean alveolar internal area (*AIA*) in rats with elastase-induced emphysema [68]; (**b**) mean chord length (*MCL*) in elastase-induced emphysematous rabbit lungs [69]; (**c**) mean linear intercept L_m in healthy and emphysematous human lungs with data obtained at different diffusion times (in ms, shown by number by the lines) (■) −1.6 ms; (•) −5 ms; (▲) −10 ms) [70]; (**d**) mean linear intercept L_m in healthy human lungs and lungs with severe emphysema [71]

two-dimensional grape-like structures used by Fichele et al. [88], the Kitaoka et al. model (three-dimensional labyrinth filling a cubic volume [89]) used by Grebenkov [90], and tree-like branching structures used by Verbanck et al. [91, 92], Perez-Sanchez et al. [93], Conradi et al. [94], and Bartel et al. [60]. Models based on morphological images or high-resolution X-ray tomography were used by Miller et al. [95] and Tsuda et al. [96]. A geometrical model utilizing Voronoi meshing techniques [97] was simulated by Plotkowiak et al. [98]. All of these publications provide important insights into gas diffusion properties in lung airways, and some of them were discussed in detail by Plotkowiak et al. [98].

For any of these approaches to become a useful research and clinical tool in studying lungs in health and disease, they need to provide a solution of the *inverse* problem—evaluation of lung geometrical parameters from specially designed MRI experiments. Currently there is only one such approach, in vivo lung morphometry [1, 63, 83–85]. The theory behind this approach captures the salient features of gas diffusion in lung airways *in the millisecond diffusion time range* and its microscopically

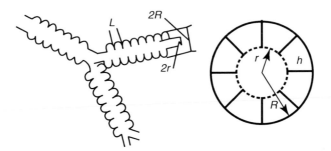

Fig. 17.5 *Left panel*: schematic structure of two levels of acinar airways. Open spheres represent alveoli forming an alveolar sleeve around each cylindrical airway. *Right panel*: cross section of the acinar airway model [1] with two main parameters—external radius, R, and internal radius, r. The other parameters, the depth of alveolar sleeve, h, and the alveolar length, L, are $h = R - r$, $L = 2R$ $\sin(\pi/8) = 0.765R$ (8-alveolar model)

anisotropic but macroscopically isotropic nature. In vivo lung morphometry is based on the well-established lung model developed by Weibel and colleagues [81, 82], in which the lung acinar airways (where 90 % of gas resides) are treated as cylindrical passages covered with alveolar sleeves (see schematic structure, Fig. 17.5). Anisotropic diffusion in a single acinar airway is described by two distinct diffusion coefficients, parallel or perpendicular to the airway axis. While diffusion in each airway is anisotropic, it is practically *isotropic on a macroscopic scale* since each imaging voxel contains a multitude of acinar airways with a nearly isotropic distribution of directions. This fundamental property of gas diffusion in lung acinar airways, confirmed by experimental measurements in humans [1, 63, 99, 100], canines [101], mice [23, 102], and rats [103, 104] using hyperpolarized ^{3}He gas, was recently confirmed using hyperpolarized ^{129}Xe gas in both humans [100] and rats [80].

The experimental and theoretical framework for ^{3}He lung morphometry in humans was worked out by deriving a set of empirical equations based on computer Monte Carlo simulations of gas diffusion in acinar airways connecting the multi-*b* diffusion MR signal to lung geometrical parameters (main radius of acinar airways, R, and depth of alveolar sleeve, h) for a specific diffusion time interval Δ of 1.6–1.8 ms [1, 83]. It is important to emphasize that the diffusion time Δ used for the lung morphometry technique is a crucial parameter, and only a specified diffusion time interval should be used in experiments. This diffusion time is selected such that diffusing gas atoms are expected to diffuse away from single alveoli but remain mostly in the same alveolar duct or sac throughout the duration of the bipolar diffusion-sensitizing gradient pulse (i.e., a short diffusion time, but not too short). For ^{3}He, this restricts the diffusion time Δ in human lungs to about 2 ms [1, 84] and for ^{129}Xe, with its smaller free diffusivity, to about 15 ms [85]. In small animal lungs, where the alveolar ducts and sacs are shorter, the diffusion time Δ should be much shorter, a fraction of a millisecond [23, 85, 102, 104]. This constraint recognizes acinar airways (respiratory broncheoli, alveolar ducts, and alveolar sacs) as the elementary geometrical units contributing to the gas diffusion MR signal. Also, under these conditions, effects of the branching structure of acinar airways play little role in diffusion MR signal formation [84].

Theoretical parameters used in this approach also allow calculation of standard lung morphological parameters analogous to those extracted from direct histological measurements, such as alveolar surface area, S_a, lung volume per alveolus, V_a, alveolar number density, N_v, which is the number of alveoli per unit lung volume, and the mean linear intercept, L_m, hence the term "in vivo lung morphometry" [1]:

$$S_a = \frac{\pi}{4} R \cdot L + \frac{\pi}{4} h \cdot (2R - h) + 2h \cdot L; \quad V_a = \frac{\pi}{8} R^2 L;$$

$$L = 2R \sin \frac{\pi}{8}; \quad N_v = \frac{1}{V_a}; \quad S/V = S_a / V_a = 4 / L_m \quad (17.3)$$

The MRI-based measurements of lung morphometric parameters were validated in explanted human lungs against direct invasive morphometric measurements [1], which is the current gold standard. The results demonstrate images of L_m in healthy lungs and lungs with different levels of emphysema (mild, moderate, and severe) and an excellent agreement between direct histological and ^{3}He-based measurements of L_m (Fig. 17.6). It should be noted that the MRI experiment provides for much higher statistical power since the data are collected from thousands of voxels as compared to very few regions (20–40) from histological cores.

Osmanagic et al. [102] employed the lung morphometry technique with hyperpolarized ^{3}He diffusion MR to study explanted lungs in mice. The MR protocol and empirical relationships relating diffusion measurements to geometrical parameters of lung acinar airways were adjusted to accommodate the substantially smaller acinar airway length in mice and acquire data with much shorter diffusion times as compared to humans. These measurements yielded mean values of lung

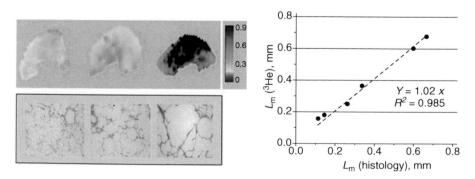

Fig. 17.6 *Left panel, upper row:* examples of the L_m (in mm) maps obtained from normal human lung (*left*) and lungs with different stages of emphysema (mild, *middle;* and severe, *right*). *Left panel, lower row:* examples of histological slices obtained from the same lungs as shown above. *Right panel:* plot of mean linear intercept obtained by means of lung morphometry with hyperpolarized ^{3}He diffusion MRI vs. direct measurement (Adapted from Yablonskiy et al. [1])

surface-to-volume ratio of 670 cm^{-1}, alveolar density of 3,200 per mm^3, alveolar depth of 55 μm, and mean chord length of 62 μm, all consistent with various results from the literature obtained by stereological analysis of mouse lungs [105–113]. The technique was further implemented by Wang et al. [23] for in vivo lung imaging in mice with results indicating agreement between in vivo morphometry via ^{3}He MRI and microscopic morphometry after sacrifice.

Quirk et al. [99] used the in vivo ^{3}He lung morphometry technique to quantitatively characterize early emphysematous changes in lung microstructure of current and former smokers. Thirty subjects with over 30 pack-year histories and mild or no abnormalities on pulmonary function tests (PFT) were studied. The results were compared against the clinical standards of PFT and low-dose computed tomography (CT). The results demonstrate the noninvasive ^{3}He lung morphometry detected alterations in acinar structure in smokers with clinically normal PFTs (Fig. 17.7). Compared to smokers with the largest FEV$_1$/FVC values, those with COPD had statistically significantly reduced alveolar depth (0.07 mm vs. 0.13 mm) and enlarged acinar ducts (0.36 mm vs. 0.30 mm). The mean alveolar geometry measurements in the healthiest subjects were in excellent quantitative agreement with literature values obtained using invasive techniques ($R = 0.30$ mm, $h = 0.14$ mm, at 1 T above FRC [81]). Importantly, ^{3}He lung morphometry detected greater abnormalities than either PFT or CT, and one feature of all of these maps was the relative homogeneity in normal lungs compared to significant disease-related heterogeneity in even early emphysema. In the latter case, a clear contrast is seen between the central portion of the lung and the lung periphery.

Hajari et al. [114] used in vivo lung morphometry to study the mechanisms of lung inflation and deflation in humans. In spite of decades of research, there is little consensus about whether lung inflation occurs due to the recruitment of new alveoli or by changes in the size and/or shape of alveoli and alveolar ducts. In this study, the average alveolar depth and alveolar duct radius was measured at three levels of inspiration in five healthy human subjects to calculate the average alveolar volume, surface area, and total number of alveoli at each level of inflation. The results indicated that during a 143 ± 18 % increase in lung-gas volume, the average alveolar depth decreases 21 ± 5 %, the average alveolar duct radius increases 7 ± 3 %, and the total number of alveoli increases by 96 ± 9 % (results are means $\pm$ SD between subjects), and that in healthy human subjects the lung inflates primarily by alveolar recruitment and, to a lesser extent, by anisotropic expansion of alveolar ducts.

17.5 Long-Range Diffusion

All of the methods discussed have used diffusion times of approximately 2 ms, corresponding to free displacements below 1 mm. Thus, most gas atoms start and end the diffusion interval (determined by the gradient pulse) in the same acinar airway. Additional information about lung airways is available from long-range ADC (LRADC) measurements.

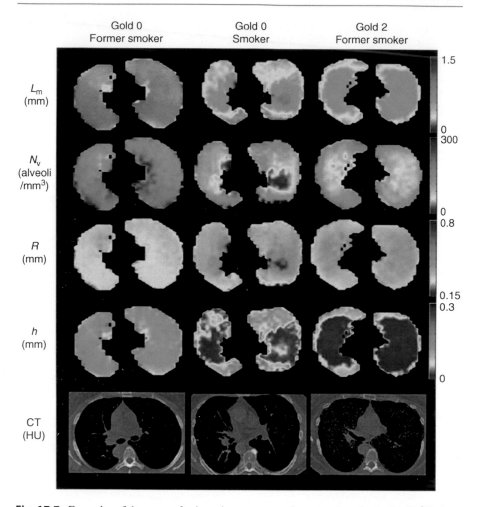

Fig. 17.7 Examples of the maps of acinar airways geometric parameters obtained with ³He lung morphometry and CT images (*bottom row*) for a GOLD 0 former smoker (*left*, $FEV_1 = 93$ % predicted, $FEV_1/FVC = 80$ %), a GOLD 0 smoker (*middle*, $FEV_1 = 94$ % predicted, $FEV_1/FVC = 71$ %), and a GOLD 2 former smoker (*right*, $FEV_1 = 62$ % predicted, $FEV_1/FVC = 56$ %). These images illustrate the heterogeneity of disease across the lungs and the significant increases in R and L_m and decreases in h and N_v with COPD. *Red pixels* on the CT images indicate regions of emphysema (attenuation less than −950 HU) (Adapted from Quirk et al. [99])

Diffusion over longer distances (e.g., 1–3 cm) requires much longer diffusion time intervals (several seconds) than the intravoxel T_2^* of approximately 20 ms at 1.5 T, which determines the lifetime of transverse magnetization in gradient-echo images. The solution is to let the *longitudinal* spin magnetization M_z carry the position information. To achieve this, a sequence of two $\pi/4$ rf pulses is used, separated by a gradient pulse in the x-direction [57]. The M_z is modulated from relative value 1 to 0 as a function of x,

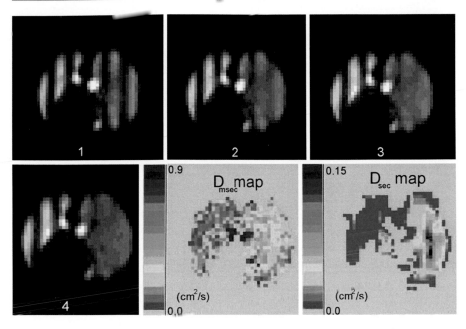

Fig. 17.0 Time sequence of tagged images in a canine with emphysema in the right lung only (*right side* of each image). The images have a tagging wavelength of 3 cm and were acquired 0–4.1 s after tagging, in equal increments of 1.36 s. The *LRADC* map at lower right is calculated from the decay rate of the fractional modulation on a pixel-by-pixel basis and shows a substantial difference in *LRADC* between the two lungs. The fast diffusion is evident from the rapid disappearance of the modulation in the right lung. An *ADC* map of short-range diffusion is also shown for comparison; note the different scales for *LRADC* and *ADC* (Adapted from Woods et al. [57])

$$M_z = \frac{1}{2}\left[1 - \cos\left(2\pi x / \lambda\right)\right] \tag{17.4}$$

where the wavelength of modulation λ is determined by the area of the gradient pulse, $\lambda = 2\pi/\gamma Gt$. A small-flip angle inspection image taken afterward in the *XY* plane reveals a stripe pattern superimposed on the lung image.

An example of stripe images with unilateral elastase-induced emphysema is shown in Fig. 17.8. Brownian motion (diffusion) of the gas will mix the bright (magnetized) and dark (unmagnetized) spins, leading to a decay of the spatial modulation [56]. That is, the stripes fade without losing average intensity, as in Fig. 17.8. To reveal *only* the effect of diffusion on the stripes, a normalizing scheme that corrects for overall T_1 decay of the signal as well as consumption of M_z by the rf imaging pulses usually is used [57, 58, 93].

Woods et al. [57] determined that in healthy canine lungs, the average *LRADC* was 0.015 ± 0.004 cm²/s, which is about ten times less than the average measured value for the traditional short-range *ADC* measured over milliseconds and hundreds of microns. In the emphysematous lung, the average *LRADC* varied from animal to animal, with significant increases from the normal lung in four of five animals. An average increase in *LRADC* by a factor of 2.7 in the emphysematous canine lungs implies that the technique may be used as a measure of tissue destruction, airway connectivity, and collateral ventilation over large distances.

The relevant length scale for diffusive motion is $\lambda/2$, approximately 1–1.5 cm [57]. In healthy lungs, the airways form a network of bifurcating paths over approximately 23 levels [115]. Thus, the airways are singly connected with a unique path between any two points. For example, a journey from one location at level 21 to level 22 at a point 1.5 cm away necessarily requires going from one acinus to another, since the acini have maximum linear dimensions of approximately 7 mm. Therefore, the atom must move from level 21 to at least level 16 (the level where the acini commence and interconnect) and back to level 22. At each of the many junctions, the atom must make the correct turn if it is to leave its starting acinus, and this tortuous path will make the long-range ADC quite small (0.02 cm^2/s has been measured in vivo in normal human lungs [58]) if gas motion is restricted along the airway tree. Further discussion of the diffusion physics behind LRADC measurements can be found in previous reports [59, 60, 91, 92, 94].

References

1. Yablonskiy DA et al (2009) Quantification of lung microstructure with hyperpolarized 3He diffusion MRI. J Appl Physiol 107(4):1258–1265
2. Leawoods JC et al (2001) Hyperpolarized 3He gas production and MR imaging of the lung. Concept Magn Reson 13(5):277–293
3. Cummings WJ et al (1995) Optical pumping of Rb vapor using high-power Ga1-xAlxAs diode laser arrays. Phys Rev A 51(6):4842–4851
4. Cates GD et al (1990) Laser production of large nuclear-spin polarization in frozen xenon. Phys Rev Lett 65(20):2591–2594
5. Driehuys B et al (1996) High-volume production of laser-polarized 129Xe. Appl Phys Lett 69(12):1668–1670
6. Rosen MS et al (1999) Polarized 129Xe optical pumping/spin exchange and delivery system for magnetic resonance spectroscopy and imaging studies. Rev Sci Instrum 70(2):1546–1552
7. Walker TG, Happer W (1997) Spin-exchange optical pumping of noble-gas nuclei. Rev Mod Phys 69(2):629–642
8. Nikolaou P et al (2009) Generation of laser-polarized xenon using fiber-coupled laser-diode arrays narrowed with integrated volume holographic gratings. J Magn Reson 197(2):249–254
9. Nelson IA, Chann B, Walker TG (2000) Spin-exchange optical pumping using a frequency-narrowed high power diode laser. Appl Phys Lett 76(11):1356–1358
10. Babcock E et al (2003) Hybrid spin-exchange optical pumping of 3He. Phys Rev Lett 91(12):123003
11. Jacob RE, Morgan SW, Saam B (2002) 3He spin exchange cells for magnetic resonance imaging. J Appl Phys 92(3):1588–1597
12. Jacob RE et al (2001) Wall relaxation of 3He in spin-exchange cells. Phys Rev Lett 87(14):143004
13. Schmiedeskamp J et al (2006) Relaxation of spin polarized 3He by magnetized ferromagnetic contaminants. Eur Phys J D 38(3):445–454
14. Becker J et al (1994) Study of mechanical compression of spin-polarized 3He gas. Nucl Instrum Methods Phys Res, Sect A 346(1–2):45–51

15. Gentile TR et al (2000) Demonstration of a compact compressor for application of metastability-exchange optical pumping of 3He to human lung imaging. Magn Reson Med 43(2):290–294
16. Gentile TR et al (2001) Compressing spin-polarized 3He with a modified diaphragm pump. J Res Natl Inst Stand Technol 106:709–729
17. van Beek EJ et al (2009) Hyperpolarised 3He MRI versus HRCT in COPD and normal volunteers: PHIL trial. Eur Respir J 34(6):1311–1321
18. Ruset IC, Ketel S, Hersman FW (2006) Optical pumping system design for large production of hyperpolarized. Phys Rev Lett 96(5):053002
19. Schrank G et al (2009) Characterization of a low-pressure high-capacity ^{129}Xe flow-through polarizer. Phys Rev A 80(6):063424
20. Nikolaou P et al (2013) Near-unity nuclear polarization with an open-source ^{129}Xe hyperpolarizer for NMR and MRI. Proc Natl Acad Sci U S A 110(35):14150–14155
21. Zheng J et al (2002) Combined MR proton lung perfusion/angiography and helium ventilation: potential for detecting pulmonary emboli and ventilation defects. Magn Reson Med 47(3):433–438
22. Dugas JP et al (2004) Hyperpolarized (3)He MRI of mouse lung. Magn Reson Med 52(6):1310–1317
23. Wang W et al (2011) Imaging lung microstructure in mice with hyperpolarized 3He diffusion MRI. Magn Reson Med 65(3):620–626
24. Caught by surprise: causes and consequences of the Helium 3 supply crisis. Comm Sci Technol (2010)
25. Salhi Z et al (2012) Recycling of 3He from lung magnetic resonance imaging. Magn Reson Med 67(6):1758–1763
26. Albert MS et al (1994) Biological magnetic resonance imaging using laser-polarized 129Xe. Nature 370(6486):199–201
27. O'Halloran RL et al (2010) Helium-3 MR q-space imaging with radial acquisition and iterative highly constrained back-projection. Magn Reson Med 63(1):41–50
28. Peterson ET et al (2011) Measurement of lung airways in three dimensions using hyperpolarized helium-3 MRI. Phys Med Biol 56(10):3107–3122
29. Deppe MH, Wild JM (2012) Variable flip angle schedules in bSSFP imaging of hyperpolarized noble gases. Magn Reson Med 67(6):1656–1664
30. Emami K et al (2013) Accelerated fractional ventilation imaging with hyperpolarized Gas MRI. Magn Reson Med 70(5):1353–1359
31. Johnson GA et al (2001) Registered (1)H and (3)He magnetic resonance microscopy of the lung. Magn Reson Med 45(3):365–370
32. Driehuys B et al (2007) 3He MRI in mouse models of asthma. Magn Reson Med 58(5):893–900
33. Deninger AJ et al (2002) Quantitative measurement of regional lung ventilation using 3He MRI. Magn Reson Med 48(2):223–232
34. Chen BT, Brau AC, Johnson GA (2003) Measurement of regional lung function in rats using hyperpolarized 3helium dynamic MRI. Magn Reson Med 49(1):78–88
35. Saam B et al (1999) Rapid imaging of hyperpolarized gas using EPI. Magn Reson Med 42(3):507–514
36. Gierada DS et al (2000) Dynamic echo planar MR imaging of lung ventilation with hyperpolarized (3)He in normal subjects and patients with severe emphysema. NMR Biomed 13(4):176–181
37. Wild JM et al (2003) Dynamic radial projection MRI of inhaled hyperpolarized 3He gas. Magn Reson Med 49(6):991–997
38. van Beek EJ et al (2004) Functional MRI of the lung using hyperpolarized 3-helium gas. J Magn Reson Imaging 20(4):540–554
39. Holmes JH et al (2009) Three-dimensional imaging of ventilation dynamics in asthmatics using multiecho projection acquisition with constrained reconstruction. Magn Reson Med 62(6):1543–1556

40. Holmes JH et al (2008) 3D hyperpolarized He-3 MRI of ventilation using a multi-echo projection acquisition. Magn Reson Med 59(5):1062–1071
41. Mistry NN et al (2010) Ventilation/perfusion imaging in a rat model of airway obstruction. Magn Reson Med 63(3):728–735
42. Salerno M et al (2001) Dynamic spiral MRI of pulmonary gas flow using hyperpolarized (3) He: preliminary studies in healthy and diseased lungs. Magn Reson Med 46(4):667–677
43. Stephen MJ et al (2010) Quantitative assessment of lung ventilation and microstructure in an animal model of idiopathic pulmonary fibrosis using hyperpolarized gas MRI. Acad Radiol 17(11):1433–1443
44. Altes TA et al (2001) Hyperpolarized 3He MR lung ventilation imaging in asthmatics: preliminary findings. J Magn Reson Imaging 13(3):378–384
45. de Lange EE et al (2009) Changes in regional airflow obstruction over time in the lungs of patients with asthma: evaluation with 3He MR imaging. Radiology 250(2):567–575
46. Costella S et al (2012) Regional pulmonary response to a methacholine challenge using hyperpolarized (3)He magnetic resonance imaging. Respirology 17(8):1237–1246
47. Kirby M et al (2011) Chronic obstructive pulmonary disease: quantification of bronchodilator effects by using hyperpolarized (3)He MR imaging. Radiology 261(1):283–292
48. Kirby M et al (2012) Evaluating bronchodilator effects in chronic obstructive pulmonary disease using diffusion-weighted hyperpolarized helium-3 magnetic resonance imaging. J Appl Physiol 112(4):651–657
49. McAdams HP et al (1999) Hyperpolarized 3He-enhanced MR imaging of lung transplant recipients: preliminary results. AJR Am J Roentgenol 173(4):955–959
50. Gast KK et al (2002) MRI in lung transplant recipients using hyperpolarized 3He: comparison with CT. J Magn Reson Imaging 15(3):268–274
51. Bannier E et al (2010) Hyperpolarized 3He MR for sensitive imaging of ventilation function and treatment efficiency in young cystic fibrosis patients with normal lung function. Radiology 255(1):225–232
52. Cadman RV et al (2013) Pulmonary 3He magnetic resonance imaging of childhood asthma. J Allergy Clin Immunol 131(2):369–76.e1–5
53. Fain S et al (2010) Imaging of lung function using hyperpolarized helium-3 magnetic resonance imaging: review of current and emerging translational methods and applications. J Magn Reson Imaging 32(6):1398–1408
54. Hong C et al (2005) Feasibility of combining MR perfusion, angiography, and 3He ventilation imaging for evaluation of lung function in a porcine model. Acad Radiol 12(2): 202–209
55. Stejskal EO (1965) Use of spin echoes in a pulsed magnetic-field gradient to study anisotropic, restricted diffusion and flow. J Chem Phys 43(10):3597–3603
56. Owers-Bradley JR et al (2003) MR tagging of human lungs using hyperpolarized 3He gas. J Magn Reson Imaging 17(1):142–146
57. Woods JC et al (2004) Magnetization tagging decay to measure long-range (3)He diffusion in healthy and emphysematous canine lungs. Magn Reson Med 51(5):1002–1008
58. Woods JC et al (2005) Long-range diffusion of hyperpolarized 3He in explanted normal and emphysematous human lungs via magnetization tagging. J Appl Physiol 99(5):1992–1997
59. Conradi MS et al (2008) The role of collateral paths in long-range diffusion of 3He in lungs. Acad Radiol 15(6):675–682
60. Bartel SE et al (2008) Role of collateral paths in long-range diffusion in lungs. J Appl Physiol 104(5):1495–1503
61. Wang C et al (2008) Assessment of the lung microstructure in patients with asthma using hyperpolarized 3He diffusion MRI at two time scales: comparison with healthy subjects and patients with COPD. J Magn Reson Imaging 28(1):80–88
62. Basser PJ, Mattiello J, LeBihan D (1994) MR diffusion tensor spectroscopy and imaging. Biophys J 66(1):259–267

63. Yablonskiy DA et al (2002) Quantitative in vivo assessment of lung microstructure at the alveolar level with hyperpolarized 3He diffusion MRI. Proc Natl Acad Sci U S A 99(5): 3111–3116

64. Chen XJ et al (2000) Detection of emphysema in rat lungs by using magnetic resonance measurements of 3He diffusion. Proc Natl Acad Sci U S A 97(21):11478–11481

65. Saam BT et al (2000) MR imaging of diffusion of (3)He gas in healthy and diseased lungs. Magn Reson Med 44(2):174–179

66. Salerno M et al (2002) Emphysema: hyperpolarized helium 3 diffusion MR imaging of the lungs compared with spirometric indexes–initial experience. Radiology 222(1): 252–260

67. West JB (1992) Pulmonary pathophysiology: the essentials, 4th edn. Williams and Wilkins, Baltimore

68. Peces-Barba G et al (2003) Helium-3 MRI diffusion coefficient: correlation to morphometry in a model of mild emphysema. Eur Respir J 22(1):14–19

69. Mata JF et al (2007) Evaluation of emphysema severity and progression in a rabbit model: comparison of hyperpolarized 3He and 129Xe diffusion MRI with lung morphometry. J Appl Physiol 102(3):1273–1280

70. Gierada DS et al (2009) Effects of diffusion time on short-range hyperpolarized (3)He dif-fusivity measurements in emphysema. J Magn Reson Imaging 30(4):801–808

71. Woods JC et al (2006) Hyperpolarized 3He diffusion MRI and histology in pulmonary emphysema. Magn Reson Med 56(6):1293–1300

72. Waters B, Owers-Bradley J, Silverman M (2006) Acinar structure in symptom-free adults by Helium-3 magnetic resonance. Am J Respir Crit Care Med 173(8):847–851

73. Fain SB et al (2005) Detection of age-dependent changes in healthy adult lungs with diffusion-weighted 3He MRI. Acad Radiol 12(11):1385–1393

74. Altes TA et al (2006) Assessment of lung development using hyperpolarized helium-3 diffu-sion MR imaging. J Magn Reson Imaging 24(6):1277–1283

75. Mugler JP et al (2004) The apparent diffusion coefficient of Xe-129 in the lung: preliminary human results. In: Proceedings of the ISMRM 12th annual scientific meeting & exhibition, Kyoto, 2004

76. Sindile A et al (2007) Human pulmonary diffusion weighted imaging at 0.2T with hyperpo-larized 129Xe. In: Proceedings of the 15th annual ISMRM meeting at the Joint Annual Meeting ISMRM-ESMRMB, Berlin, 2007

77. Kaushik SS et al (2011) Diffusion-weighted hyperpolarized 129Xe MRI in healthy volun-teers and subjects with chronic obstructive pulmonary disease. Magn Reson Med 65(4):1154–1165

78. Kirby M et al (2012) Hyperpolarized 3He and 129Xe MR imaging in healthy volunteers and patients with chronic obstructive pulmonary disease. Radiology 265(2):600–610

79. Driehuys B et al (2012) Chronic obstructive pulmonary disease: safety and tolerability of hyperpolarized 129Xe MR imaging in healthy volunteers and patients. Radiology 262(1):279–289

80. Boudreau M, Xu X, Santyr GE (2013) Measurement of 129Xe gas apparent diffusion coef-ficient anisotropy in an elastase-instilled rat model of emphysema. Magn Reson Med 69(1):211–220

81. Haefeli-Bleuer B, Weibel ER (1988) Morphometry of the human pulmonary acinus. Anat Rec 220(4):401–414

82. Mercer RR, Laco JM, Crapo JD (1987) Three-dimensional reconstruction of alveoli in the rat lung for pressure-volume relationships. J Appl Physiol 62(4):1480–1487

83. Sukstanskii AL, Yablonskiy DA (2008) In vivo lung morphometry with hyperpolarized 3He diffusion MRI: theoretical background. J Magn Reson 190(2):200–210

84. Sukstanskii AL, Conradi MS, Yablonskiy DA (2010) (3)He lung morphometry technique: accuracy analysis and pulse sequence optimization. J Magn Reson 207(2):234–241

85. Sukstanskii AL, Yablonskiy DA (2012) Lung morphometry with hyperpolarized 129Xe: theoretical background. Magn Reson Med 67(3):856–866
86. Mair RW et al (1998) Pulsed-field-gradient measurements of time-dependent gas diffusion. J Magn Reson 135(2):478–486
87. Mair RW et al (1999) Probing porous media with gas diffusion NMR. Phys Rev Lett 83(16):3324–3327
88. Fichele S et al (2004) Finite-difference simulations of 3He diffusion in 3D alveolar ducts: comparison with the "cylinder model". Magn Reson Med 52(4):917–920
89. Kitaoka H, Tamura S, Takaki R (2000) A three-dimensional model of the human pulmonary acinus. J Appl Physiol 88(6):2260–2268
90. Grebenkov DS (2007) Residence times and other functionals of reflected Brownian motion. Phys Rev E Stat Nonlin Soft Matter Phys 76(4 Pt 1):041139
91. Verbanck S, Paiva M (1990) Model simulations of gas mixing and ventilation distribution in the human lung. J Appl Physiol 69(6):2269–2279
92. Verbanck S, Paiva M (2007) Simulation of the apparent diffusion of helium-3 in the human acinus. J Appl Physiol 103(1):249–254
93. Perez-Sanchez JM, Rodriguez I, Ruiz-Cabello J (2009) Random walk simulation of the MRI apparent diffusion coefficient in a geometrical model of the acinar tree. Biophys J 97(2): 656–664
94. Conradi MS et al (2005) 3He diffusion MRI of the lung. Acad Radiol 12(11):1406–1413
95. Miller GW et al (2007) Simulations of short-time diffusivity in lung airspaces and implications for S/V measurements using hyperpolarized-gas MRI. IEEE Trans Med Imaging 26(11):1456–1463
96. Tsuda A et al (2008) Finite element 3D reconstruction of the pulmonary acinus imaged by synchrotron X-ray tomography. J Appl Physiol 105(3):964–976
97. Burrowes KS, Tawhai MH, Hunter PJ (2004) Modeling RBC and neutrophil distribution through an anatomically based pulmonary capillary network. Ann Biomed Eng 32(4): 585–595
98. Plotkowiak M et al (2009) Relationship between structural changes and hyperpolarized gas magnetic resonance imaging in chronic obstructive pulmonary disease using computational simulations with realistic alveolar geometry. Philos Transact A Math Phys Eng Sci 367(1896):2347–2369
99. Quirk JD et al (2011) In vivo detection of acinar microstructural changes in early emphysema with (3)He lung morphometry. Radiology 260(3):866–874
100. Ruppert K (2012) Lung morphometry using hyperpolarized Xenon-129: preliminary experience. In: Proceedings of the ISMRM 20th annual meeting & exhibition, Melbourne, 2012
101. Tanoli TS et al (2007) In vivo lung morphometry with hyperpolarized 3He diffusion MRI in canines with induced emphysema: disease progression and comparison with computed tomography. J Appl Physiol 102(1):477–484
102. Osmanagic E et al (2010) Quantitative assessment of lung microstructure in healthy mice using an MR-based 3He lung morphometry technique. J Appl Physiol 109(6):1592–1599
103. Jacob RE, Laicher G, Minard KR (2007) 3D MRI of non-Gaussian (3)He gas diffusion in the rat lung. J Magn Reson 188(2):357–366
104. Xu X et al (2012) Mapping of (3) He apparent diffusion coefficient anisotropy at sub-millisecond diffusion times in an elastase-instilled rat model of emphysema. Magn Reson Med 67(4):1146–1153
105. Voswinckel R et al (2004) Characterisation of post-pneumonectomy lung growth in adult mice. Eur Respir J 24(4):524–532
106. Soutiere SE, Mitzner W (2004) On defining total lung capacity in the mouse. J Appl Physiol 96(5):1658–1664
107. Fehrenbach H (2008) Commentaries on viewpoint: use of mean airspace chord length to assess emphysema. What does Lm tell us about lung pathology? J Appl Physiol 105(6):1984–1985; author reply 1986–7

108. Knudsen L et al (2007) Truncated recombinant human SP-D attenuates emphysema and type II cell changes in SP-D deficient mice. Respir Res 8:70
109. Mitzner W, Fallica J, Bishai J (2008) Anisotropic nature of mouse lung parenchyma. Ann Biomed Eng 36(12):2111–2120
110. Knudsen L et al (2010) Assessment of air space size characteristics by intercept (chord) measurement: an accurate and efficient stereological approach. J Appl Physiol 108(2):412–421
111. Lee J et al (2009) Lung alveolar integrity is compromised by telomere shortening in telomerase-null mice. Am J Physiol Lung Cell Mol Physiol 296(1):L57–L70
112. Knust J et al (2009) Stereological estimates of alveolar number and size and capillary length and surface area in mice lungs. Anat Rec (Hoboken) 292(1):113–122
113. Kang MJ et al (2008) Cigarette smoke selectively enhances viral PAMP- and virus-induced pulmonary innate immune and remodeling responses in mice. J Clin Invest 118(8):2771–2784
114. Hajari AJ et al (2012) Morphometric changes in the human pulmonary acinus during inflation. J Appl Physiol 112(6):937–943
115. Weibel ER (1963) Morphometry of the human lung. Springer, Berlin/Göttingen/Heidelberg

Dynamic MRI – Clinical Significance in Treatment for Patients with COPD

18

Koji Chihara and Akinari Hidaka

The chest wall consists of the rib cage and the diaphragm – abdomen. Actions of the inspiratory and expiratory respiratory muscles belonging to these compartments alternatively displace themselves resulting in pressure change of the pleural space, which yields respiration. As each compartment moves with a single degree of freedom in normal subject [1], the linear displacement or the cross-sectional area change of the rib cage and the abdomen obtained from the body surface has been measured with the magnetometer or the respiratory inductive plethysmograph in the analysis of chest wall mechanics[1, 2]. However, abnormal chest wall motions such as a biphasic motion of the abdomen during inspiration, the rib cage (abdomen paradox), or a phase difference between the rib cage and the abdomen were also observed in patients with COPD using these devices [3, 4].

There are limitations in interpretations for these curious phenomena, because the action of the diaphragm as the principal inspiratory muscle within the body is unable to estimate precisely with those tools. In fact, we found that the anterior part, the center (or dome), and the posterior of the diaphragm in patients with severe emphysema during breathing efforts analyzed by serial roentgenograms did not move as a simple piston as in normal, but did with a phase shift between the anterior and the other two parts. Some patients showed that the relationship between the

Electronic supplementary material
The online version of this chapter (doi:10.1007/978-88-470-5647-3_18) contains supplementary material, which is available to authorized users. Videos can also be accessed at http://www.springerimages.com/videos/978-88-470-5646-6

K. Chihara (✉)
Department of Thoracic Surgery, Shizuoka City Shizuoka Hospital,
10-93 Ohtemachi, Aoi-ku, Shizuoka 420-8630, Japan
e-mail: kojichihara420@hotmail.com

A. Hidaka
Department of Radiology, Kobe Teishin Hospital,
6-2-43 Kamitsutsui-dori, Kobe 651-8798, Japan
e-mail: a-hidaka@kobe-japanposthospital.jp

diaphragmatic length and peeling off the zone of apposition during inspiration was quite different between the right and left sides [5].

Magnetic resonance imaging (MRI) during rest has a potential advantage to provide a clearer shape of the diaphragm than other imaging modalities [6, 7].

As patients with emphysema feel dyspnea on exertion rather than during rest, MR images during breathing, namely, dynamic MRI, is a more preferable modality to study pathophysiology and mechanics of dyspnea in these patients. Dynamic MRI provides information regarding with not only chest wall motion but also movements of intrapleural structures such as the trachea, heart, great vessels, and pulmonary vascular trees. In terms of the latter aspect, opening during inspiration and folding during expiration of the pulmonary vascular trees suggest regional ventilation of the lung. In this chapter, we present some results obtained from the patients with severe emphysema who underwent lung volume reduction surgery (LVRS) [8] or giant bullectomy and show that dynamic MRI is a powerful modality in diagnosis and treatment for patients with emphysema.

18.1   MRI Instrument and Method

Dynamic MRI of the chest and the upper abdomen in the mid-coronal slice and the midsagittal slice were obtained with an MR instrument (1.5 T Signa-Advantage, G E) using fast spoiled GRASS method. The operating conditions were as follows: repetition time of 9.9 ms, echo time of 2.5 Fr, flip angle of $45°$, scan thickness of 10 mm, and field of view of the image in the sagittal and coronal directions of 450 or 480 mm.   One image was made every 1.4 s while a subject was asked to repeat a slow and deep breathing starting from the resting expiratory lung volume through the residual volume (RV) and the total lung capacity (TLC) lasting for approximately 30 s for one cycle [9].

18.2   PartI Chest Wall Motion and Configuration
of Patients with Emphysema

18.2.1 Subjects and Measurements

We studied six patients with emphysema who underwent bilateral LVRS and two patients undergoing unilateral LVRS via median sternotomy and 5 normal subjects who were recruited from our hospital personnel. The average age, height, and forced expiratory volume in one second (FEV1) of the patients were 69 ± 2 (SE) year, 162 ± 2 cm, 0.52 ± 0.06 L, respectively. The average of age and height of the normal subjects were 34 ± 4 year and 169 ± 2 cm. Dynamic MRI were obtained before and 1–6 months after LVRS in the patients group. In the mid-coronal slices, the zone of apposition (Di,zone) facing the lower rib cage, the part of the diaphragm dome facing the lung (Di,dome), and the transverse diameter of the lower rib cage at the upper point of the zone of apposition were measured at RV and TLC according to the method of Braun et al. In the midsagittal slices, the part of the diaphragm facing

Fig. 18.1 Relationship between Di,dome and Di,zone at the mid-coronal slice during slow and deep breathings in normal subjects (○) and in patients with emphysema before (□), and after (■) LVRS. Values are means ± SE. Each mean value at end-inspiration is plotted on a line of zero of Di,zone

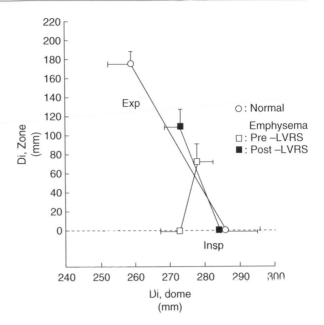

the lung(Di,dome), the anterior and posterior zones of apposition (Zone,app), and the anteroposterior diameter of the lower rib cage at the xiphoid process were measured at RV and TLC [10].

18.2.2   Results and Discussion

18.2.2.1 Coronal Slice

The relationship between the average of the sum of the right and left Di,dome and the average of the sum of the right and left Di,zone of the patients and the normal subjects at RV and TLC were shown in Fig. 18.1. Although the zone of apposition at TLC is not always zero [6], we plotted Di,zone at TLC on the line of zero in order to show its change from RV to TLC. The sum of the Di,dome of the both sides in the normal subjects increased while the sum of Di,zone decreased substantially from RV to TLC as shown in normal subjects [5, 9]. In contrast, Di,dome in the patients before LVRS started from a significantly longer point at RV than normal and reached a shorter point at TLC in the opposite way of normal. The average change from RV to TLC of Di,zone in the patients was approximately 40 % of normal. After LVRS, the change in Di,dome and that in Di,zone from RV to TLC returned to normal pattern, and the amounts of these changes were more than half of those in normal subjects.

This paradoxical pattern of change in Di,dome seen in the patients before LVRS could be explained as follows. In normal subjects the rib cage is conical so that the Di,dome increases from RV to TLC [11].

Although we did not measure Di,dome continuously through RV to TLC, we would expect that the lower rib cage of the patient with severe hyperinflation

Fig. 18.2 Relationship between Di,dome and anteroposterior diameter of the lower rib cage at the xiphoid process at the midsagittal slice during slow and deep breathings in normal subjects (○), patients with emphysema before (□), and after (■) LVRS. Values are means ± SE

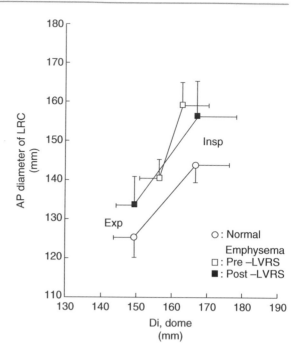

expands laterally so that the flattened diaphragm descends from a lower position at RV than normal and reaches a near point of an anatomical insertion to the rib cage of the diaphragm at TLC via a level of a maximum transverse diameter of the lower rib cage with excessive peeling off of the zone of apposition as shown in the stable patients with emphysema in the other study [5]. Decrease of lung volume after LVRS allowed the diaphragm to start a longer position at RV and to be a better shape of its dome, in other words, a longer zone of apposition. An increase of maximum lateral expansion of the lower rib cage from 4 ± 3 to 10 ± 3 mm (mean ± SE) ($p < 0.05$) before and after LVRS supported this explanation. Two patients showed decreasing lateral diameter during inspiration before LVRS, so-called Hoover's sign, and this abnormal motion disappeared after LVRS.

18.2.2.2 Sagittal Slice

Figure 18.2 shows the relationship between the average of the sum of the right Di,dome and the average of the sum of the anteroposterior diameter of the right lower rib cage at the xiphoid process in the normal subjects and the patients before and after LVRS. The xiphoid process of the patients at RV before LVRS shifted already to a similar position of the normal subjects at TLC due to hyperinflation resulting in shorter Di,dome of the patients. It was a striking finding that the anteroposterior diameter of the lower rib cage in the patients before LVRS could increase from that point to a higher point by 2 cm at TLC though the anterior zone at RV was almost zero. Actually, the anterior and posterior zones of apposition of the

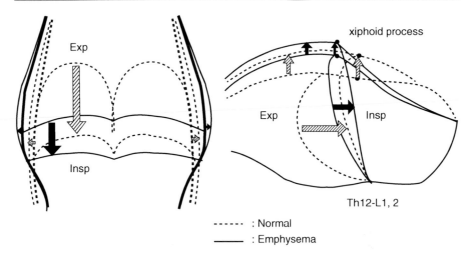

Fig. 18.3 Configuration of the rib cage, diaphragm, and abdomen in normal (*dotted line*) and patient with emphysema (*straight line*)

preoperative patients were 3 ± 2 and 36 ± 6 mm (mean $\pm$ SE), while those of the normal subjects were 52 ± 6 and 89 ± 5 mm, respectively. These results suggest that the rib cage expansion of the patients before LVRS is almost provided by strong recruitment of the rib cage muscles and the muscles in the neck whose recruitments tightly relate dyspnea sensation during respiratory loading [12, 13]. The point of the xiphoid process at RV, at which the diaphragm connected, descended after LVRS and gained more reserves for excursion that the anterior zone of apposition increased from 3 ± 2 to 14 ± 10 mm by LVRS ($p<0.05$).

We found geometrical changes not only in the diaphragm and but also in the rib cage in the patients before LVRS from both slices. In addition, the abdominal wall was flattened rather than round as in normal, which suggested a passive tension would work on the abdominal muscles. Taking these findings into account, the upward shift of the xiphoid process, which is the junction of these three compartments, and the flatted abdomen would restrict the motion of the anterior part of the diaphragm and induce a phase shift between the anterior, center, and posterior parts of the diaphragm (Fig. 18.3). We reported previously dis-coordination among the anterior, center, and posterior parts of the diaphragm and the upper and lower rib cages in a similar group with emphysema that were studied during effort breathing with serial roentgenograms [14]. In this study dynamic MRI was obtained during a slow and deep breathing, but similar discoordination among the chest wall components was seen before LVRS and was improved after LVRS (Fig. 18.4).

In summary, lung volume reduction surgery (LVRS) for patients with advanced emphysema improved the chest wall pump function by returning the position of the respiratory muscles of the chest wall compartments to near original positions, which results in improvement of their mechanical property and the relationships among the compartments as well.

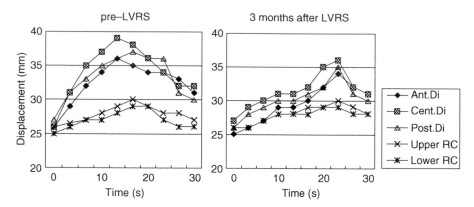

Fig. 18.4 Chest wall motion in an 80-year-old patient with emphysema before (*left*) and 3 months after LVRS (*right*). Note asynchrony among the compartments of the chest wall before LVRS and their synchronization after LVRS

18.3   Part 2: Patient Selection for LVRS

It is essential for successful outcome to select proper patients who might benefit from LVRS. Imaging modalities and physiological examinations show important roles in this process. Hyperinflation estimated by imaging and functional examination is mandatory. Heterogeneity of emphysematous lesions in CT scan and perfusion scan is necessary [8, 15–17], and the so-called worst or target area to be reduced in the upper lobe [8] has been a good predictor. Following these findings obtained from case studies, LVRS has been proved as a safe, effective, and durable treatment which improves life-span, exercise tolerance, QOL, and dyspnea in patients with severe COPD selected appropriately by distribution of emphysema (upper lobe vs. non-upper lobe) and exercise capacity (low vs. high) through National Emphysema Treatment Trial, NETT [18].

In addition to static imaging modalities noted above, we have been utilizing dynamic MRI to identify the target area which could be expressed as "airoma" characterized by trapped excessive air and poor perfusion since we started this treatment in 1995. Airoma holds intrinsic PEEP due to a longer time constant in ventilation and reduces pulmonary circulation as a resistance. This concept came from our clinical experience in the treatment of patients with emphysematous giant bullae as follows. In order to predict the outcome of bullectomy, we analyzed not only the diaphragm-rib cage motion but also regional ventilation with serial roentgenograms during breathing efforts in the supine posture before operation (Fig. 18.5) [19].

From the latter analysis, we found that the patients with giant bullae were subdivided into three groups according to relationship between the diaphragmatic motion as a representative of ventilation of adjacent normal lung and the change of the size of the giant bulla as follows:

1. Synchronized type: patients whose bullae changed the size in phase with the diaphragmatic excursion complained breathlessness after bullectomy rather than

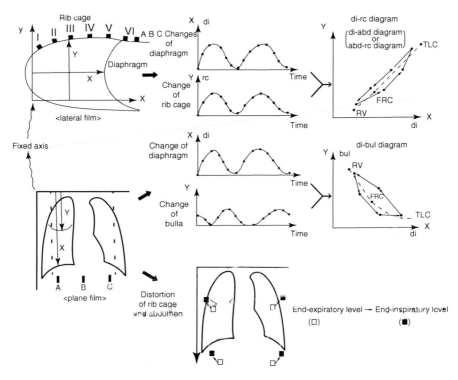

Fig. 18.5 Radiographic method for analysis of the chest wall motion. Lead markers are attached on body surface. Craniocaudal displacement of the diaphragm and posteroanterior displacement of the rib cage during breathing efforts are measured with serial lateral roentgenograms. Craniocaudal displacements of the diaphragm and the bulla are measured in the serial posteroanterior roentgenograms. There is a complete paradox between the diaphragm and the bulla in this illustration. Rib cage distortion can be detected with tracing of leads during breathing (From Chihara and Hitomi [19])

improvement while FEV1 dropped postoperatively, and returned to the preoperative values approximate 1 year after bullectomy.

2. Paradoxical type: patients whose bullae reached a maximum size at the end-expiration, in other words, showing a 180° phase shift with the diaphragmatic motion. It is suggested that no changes in the size of bulla mean little ventilation through the bulla. Those benefited from bullectomy from early postoperative period because of improvement of breathlessness and spirometry.

3. Intermediate type: patients whose bullae reached maximum size at early expiration showed an intermediate pattern between the two groups.

These results suggest that a patient who has a less ventilated, more air-trapped emphysematous part in the lung might get improvement soon after the resection of the part. Although we could not define a clear line like a bulla to estimate local area ventilation in patients with diffuse emphysema, we were able to utilize opening and closing motions of vascular trees during breathing with dynamic MRI which would reflect regional ventilation because the pulmonary arteries run along the bronchiole. We defined little changes of vascular trees of a region of the lung as little ventilation to the region.

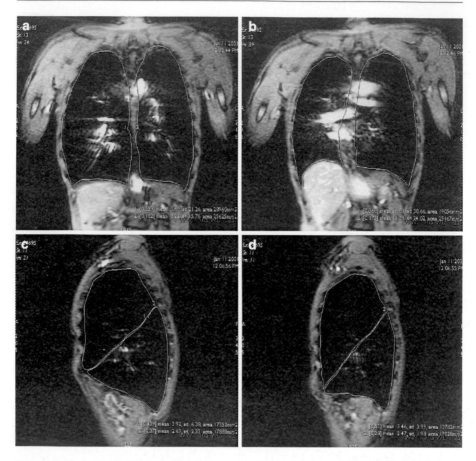

Fig. 18.6 Dynamic MRI in the coronal slices at TLC (**a**) and RV (**b**), and the left sagittal slices at TLC (**c**) and at RV (**d**) before LVRS of a 60-year-old male patient whose FEV1 was 0.28 L. The left lung pushes the heart to the right during expiration before LVRS (**b**). Ventilation fraction of the right and left lung before LVRS were 25 and −3 %, respectively. The vascular trees of the left upper lobe in the sagittal slices changed few during breathing (**c**, **d**), and VF of the left upper lobe was only 5 %. It was 21 % for the lower lobe

18.3.1 Coronal Slice

The amplitude of the right and left diaphragmatic motion was simple and useful information about ventilation of each lung. We found a phase shift between the two hemi-diaphragms in some patients. The most impressive sign of more air trapping of either lung was that the heart was pushed to the opposite side during expiration by the lung (Fig. 18.6a, b). Similar shifts of the trachea or the superior vena cava were seen in these patients. It was easy to detect the worse side with these findings. For qualitative estimation of the air trapping in the interested lung, we measured the ratio of lung area at RV to that at TLC as a ventilation fraction (VF).

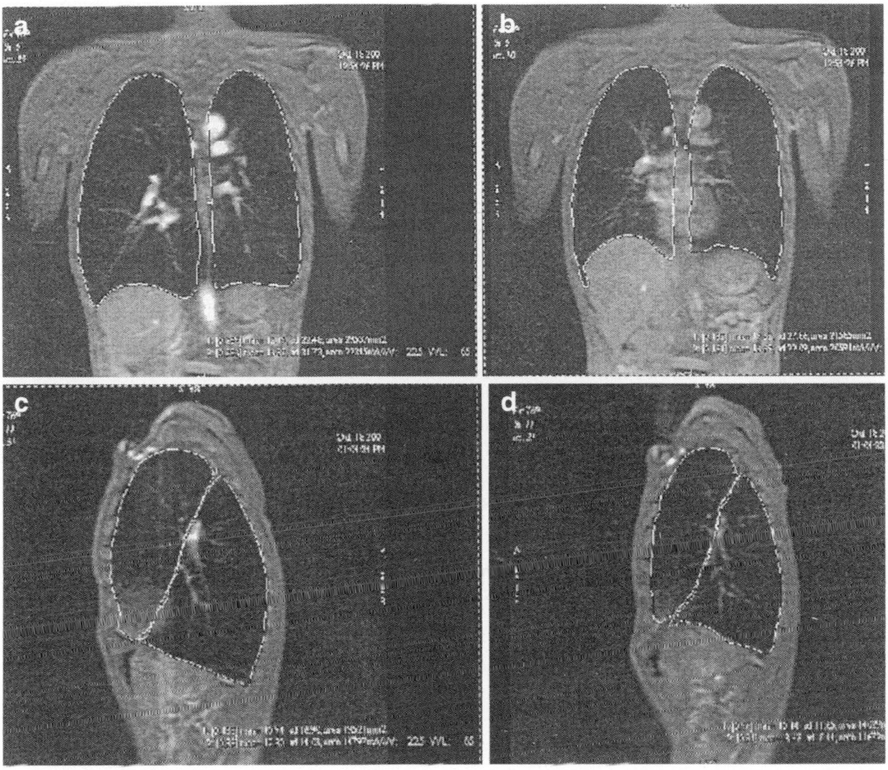

Fig. 18.7 Dynamic MRI in the coronal slices at TLC (**a**) and RV (**b**), and the left sagittal slices at TLC (**c**) and at RV (**d**) 7 months after LVRS. VF of the right and the left lung were 30 and 8 %, respectively, in the coronal slices. VF of the upper lobe and the lower lobe were 21 and 28 %, respectively. VF of the whole lung increased from 12 to 19 % in the coronal slices, and that of the left lung increased from 13 to 25 % by LVRS. Configuration of the chest wall was remarkably improved after LVRS. Vital capacity, FEV1, and 6-min walk increased from 1.9 to 2.9 L, from 0.28 to 0.34 L, and from 220 to 338 m, respectively, and RV decreased from 5.66 (385 %) to 3.52 L (243 %) after LVRS

In the coronal slices it was easy to evaluate the respiratory changes of the vascular trees during breathing for the upper lobe, but not always for the middle or lower lobes.

18.3.2 Sagittal Slice

Dynamic MRI in the sagittal slices gave us more information than that in the coronal slices. By identifying each lobe by interlober fissure with the absence of vascular structures, we could measure VF for each lobe and define the severity of air trapping. A representative case who had the worst part in the left upper lobe and the second worst part in the right upper lobe is showed in Figs. 18.6 and 18.7.

18.3.3 Clinical Results

Thirty-one patients were selected for LVRS between October 1995 and June 2003. Their characteristics and mean values in function testing were as follows: a mean age of 68 year (range 52–80), BMI of 18 Kg/m^2 (15–23), %FEV$_1$ of 27 % (11–46), %RV of 263 % (178–385), and 6 MWD of 287 m (75–450). We defined airoma in the upper lobes of 12 patients, in the lower lobes of 12 patients, in both lobes of 6 patients, and in the middle lobe of 1 patient. Bilateral LVRS through median sternotomy were performed in 17 patients, while unilateral procedure by video-assisted thoracoscopic surgery or thoracotomy was done in others. All patients were followed ranging from 1.8 to 9.5 years (median 6.5 years). There was no in-hospital mortality. Two patients underwent reexploration for air leak. Two patients needed mechanical ventilation for a few months after LVRS and recovered. All patients except one reported decrease in dyspnea and were satisfied with surgery. Patient selection based on functional imaging gave us promising early results.

Eleven patients out of 22 patients who underwent LVRS by Dec 1999 survived more than 5 years. Survival ratio at 1,2,3,4,and 5 years with Kaplan-Meier method were 97, 94, 90, 72 and 49 %, respectively. Respiratory failure and newly founded cancer were two major reasons of mortality. There was no difference between survival ratios in patients with upper lobe airoma and those with lower lobe airoma. Lung volume reduction surgery for patients with emphysema selected by functional imaging modalities produces symptomatic improvement in early term, and better survival for at least 3 years. Lung volume reduction surgery is a good and promising palliative treatment for patients with advanced emphysema wherever the airoma is located [20].

18.4 In Conclusion

Dynamic MRI with two dimensions has limitation unable to infer something about the whole respiratory system. However, it provides not only insights about the interaction between the chest wall motion and regional ventilation of the lung but also reliable information to select the patients who might benefit from LVRS.

Case Presentations by Dynamic MRI and Brief Summary of Clinical Results

Normal: 49-Year-Old Male

Coronal slice: Both diaphragms move in coordinated fashion. The motion of the lower rib cage and the diaphragm expressed as a widening piston is well understood (Video 18.1).

Sagittal slice: The diaphragm and the rib cage move in phase (Videos 18.2 and 18.3).

Patient with Severe COPD: 60-Year-Old Male

1. Before left LVRS
   Coronal slice (Video 18.4)
   Sagittal slice (Video 18.5)
2. After left LVRS
   Coronal slice (Video 18.6)
   Sagittal slice (Video 18.7)
   Details about this patient were described in the text. See Figs. 18.6 and 18.7.

Patient with Bilateral Giant Bullae: 41-Year-Old Male

He underwent bilateral bullectomy 15 years ago. He felt dyspnea during walking and was referred to our hospital.
1. Before left bullectomy
   Coronal slice: It is suggested that the left giant bulla was more air trapped than the right giant bulla because it pushes the heart and the trachea to the right side during end-expiration phase.
   Left sagittal slice: The left giant bulla compressed the hilum structures significantly. The areas of the bulla at end-inspiration and at end-expiration were 183 and 187 cm^2, respectively. No changes in area of the bulla meaning little connection to the main airway was concise with the operative findings that the bulla remained in its shape by intrinsic PEEP of 3 cmH_2O within the bulla when the left bronchus opens to atmospheric pressure.
2. 6 months after left bullectomy
   Coronal slice: The right lung remained giant bulla and in turn compressed the left lung significantly.
   Left sagittal slice: The left vascular trees were restored well.
   As significant improvement both in exertional dyspnea and functional examinations were obtained after left bullectomy, he returned to his job.
   Vital capacity (% predicted), forced vital capacity, forced expiratory volume in one second, and residual volume before left bullectomy were 2.7 L(68), 2.49 L(62), 0.77 L(21), and 4.47 L(292), respectively. Those 6 months after operation were 3.5 L(88), 3.22 L(81), 1.72 L(48), and 2.69 L(177), respectively. Exercise capability improvements were as follows: 6-min walk distance and exercise tolerance in Bruce protocol ECG were 380 m and 4 min before bullectomy, and those increased to 440 m and 10 min after left bullectomy. He subsequently underwent right giant bullectomy 8 months after the left bullectomy.

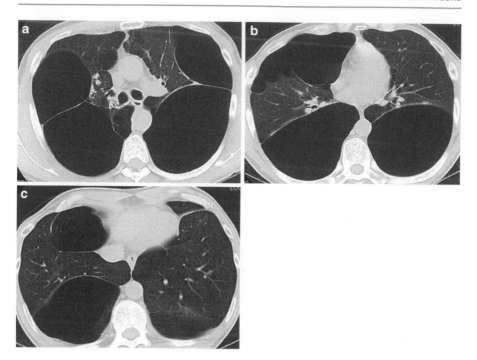

Fig. 18.8 Chest CT before left bullectomy. (**a-c**) The giant bullae of the both sides presented through the apex to the bottom of the pleural space, and compressed the lungs. The left lung parenchyme was more preserved than the right

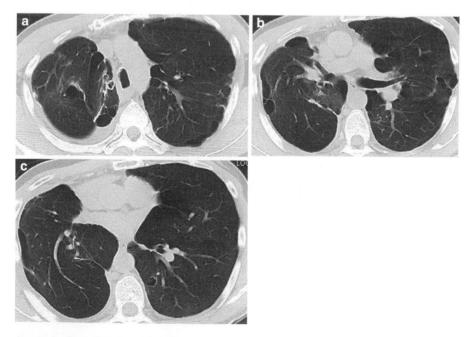

Fig. 18.9 Chest CT after right bullectomy. (**a-c**) The pulmonary vascular beds were well recovered by sequential giant bullectomies

References

1. Konno K, Mead J (1967) Measurement of the separate volume changes of rib cage and abdomen during breathing. J Appl Pysiol 24:544–548
2. Sackner JD, Nixon AJ, Davis B et al (1980) Non-invasive measurement of ventilation during exercise using a respiratory inductive plethysmograph. Am Rev Respir Dis 122:867–871
3. Ashutosh K, Gilbert R, Auchincloss JH et al (1975) Asynchronous breathing movements in patients with chronic obstructive pulmonary disease. Chest 67:553–557
4. Gillemartin JJ, Gibson GJ (1986) Mechanisms of paradoxical rib cage motion in patients with chronic obstructive pulmonary disease. Am Rev Respir Dis 134:683–687
5. Chihara K, Yoshimura T, Itoi S et al (1995) Excessive peel-off of the zone of apposition in emphysema during inspiration. Am J Respir Crit Care Med 151:A117
6. Gauthier AP, Verbanck S, Estenne M et al (1994) Three-dimensional reconstruction of the in vivo human diaphragm shape at different lung volumes. J Appl Physiol 76:495–506
7. Paiva M, Verbanck S, Estenne M et al (1992) Mechanical implications of in vivo human diaphragm shape. J Appl Physiol 72:1407–1412
8. Cooper JD, Trulock EP, Triantafillou AN et al (1995) Bilateral pneumonectomy (volume reduction) for chronic obstructive pulmonary disease. J Thorac Cardiovasc Surg 116:109–119
9. Hidaka A, Chihara K, Nakai M et al (1997) Chest wall motion in patients with emphysema analyzed by dynamic MRI before and after volume reduction surgery (VRS) Am J Respir Crit Care Med 155:A520
10. Braun NMT, Arora NS, Rochester DF (1982) Force-length relationship of the normal human diaphragm. J Appl Physiol 53:405–412
11. Petrolll WM, Knight H, Rochester DF (1990) Effect of lower rib cage expansion and diaphragm shortening of the zone of apposition. J Appl Physiol 68:484–488
12. Sharp JT, Druz WS, Moisan T et al (1980) Postural relief of dyspnea in severe COPD. Am Rev Respir Dis 122:201–211
13. Ward ME, Eidelman D, Stubbing DG et al (1988) Respiratory sensation and pattern of respiratory muscle activation during diaphragm fatigue. J Appl Physiol 65:2181–2189
14. Sahara H, Nakai S, Tsuda T et al (1998) Diaphragm – rib cage motion before and after lung volume reduction surgery. Chest 114:351S
15. Stirling GR, Babidge WJ, Peacock MJ et al (2001) Lung volume reduction surgery in emphysema: a systematic review. Ann Thorac Surg 72:641–648
16. Weder W, Thurnheer R, Stammberger UZ et al (1997) Radiologic emphysema morphology is associated with outcome after surgical lung volume reduction. Ann Thorac Surg 64:313–320
17. Rogers RM, Coxson HO, Scuiba FC et al (2000) Preoperative severity of emphysema predictive of improvement after lung volume reduction surgery. Use of CT morphometry. Chest 118:1240–1247
18. Naunheim KS, Wood DE, Mohsenifar Z et al (2006) Long-term follow-up of patients receiving lung-volume-reduction surgery versus medical therapy for severe emphysema by the National Emphysema Treatment Trial Research Group. Ann Thorac Surg 82:431–443
19. Chihara K, Hitomi S (1990) Classification for bullous emphysema based on analysis of chest wall motion and pulmonary function before and after bullectomy. Nihon Kyobu Shikkan Gakkai Zasshi 28:239–245
20. Chihara K, Nakajima D, Yamashina A et al (2005) Early and long-term results of lung volume reduction surgery for patients with emphysema. Chest 128:311S

Pulmonary Functional Imaging with Positron Emission Tomography

19

Jose G. Venegas, Dominic Layfield, Scott Harris, Elliot Greenblatt, and Tilo Winkler

19.1 Introduction

In most diseases of the lung, both function and structure are spatially heterogeneous. As a result, global measures of lung function obtained from measurements at the mouth may be insensitive to localized pathological changes in the lungs and usually fail to detect the true extent of the functional impairment. With the development of imaging methods capable of providing detailed information in three dimensions, the field of functional imaging has emerged to fill these gaps.

Pulmonary functional imaging can be broadly defined as the quantitative topographical assessment of functional, mechanical, and structural characteristics of the lung and its local responses to environmental stress, injury, and infection (Table 19.1). Topographically, each of these parameters can be affected differently by disease and may be assessed by imaging modalities such as X-ray computerized tomography (CT), positron or single-photon emission tomography (PET and SPECT), and magnetic resonance imaging (MRI). Functional parameters include, but are not limited to, regional ventilation $\left(s\dot{V}_A\right)$, perfusion $\left(\dot{Q}\right)$, $\dot{V}_A / \dot{Q}$ ratio, and shunt fraction $\left(\dot{Q}_{shunt} / \dot{Q}_r\right)$, among others. Mechanical characteristics include parameters such as airway pathway resistance, regional tissue elastance and viscoelasticity, airway wall distensibility that can be estimated by a combination of imaging, and measured mechanical variables at the airway opening such as pressure. Structural parameters characterize the airway wall by its luminal area (A_i) or radius (r_i) and its wall thickness aspect ratio (wall thickness to total diameter, ω) and the parenchyma by its degree of fractional air content (F_{gas}) and tissue content. Finally, the regional response to infection or injury can be characterized by parameters such as vascular permeability, extravascular lung water, and cellular inflammatory responses measured mostly with PET.

J.G. Venegas (✉) • D. Layfield • S. Harris • E. Greenblatt • T. Winkler
Department of Anesthesia, Pain Medicine and Critical Care,
Massachusetts General Hospital, Boston, MA 01907, USA
e-mail: jvenegas@alum.mit.edu

A. Aliverti, A. Pedotti (eds.), *Mechanics of Breathing*,
DOI 10.1007/978-88-470-5647-3_19, © Springer-Verlag Italia 2014

Table 19.1 Imaging Parameters used to characterize lung function, mechanics, structure and response to injury

	Parameter	Symbol	Imaging method
Functional	Regional ventilation or ventilation per unit volume	$\dot{V}_A$ or $s\dot{V}_A$	PET [1]
			CT [2]
			MRI [3]
	Regional perfusion	$\dot{Q}$	PET [4]
			CT [5]
			MRI [6]
	Ventilation-perfusion ratio	$\dot{V}_A / \dot{Q}$	PET [7]
			MRI [8]
	Regional shunt fraction	$\dot{Q}_{shunt} / \dot{Q}_r$	PET [7, 9]
Mechanical	Airway pathway resistance	R_p	PET [10]
	Tissue elastance	E_{tiss}	CT [2]
	Airway wall distensibility		CT [11]
Structural	Airway luminal area or radius	A_i or r_i	CT [12]
			MRI [13]
	Wall thickness or aspect ratio	tor $w = t/r_i$	CT [14]
	Fractional air content	F_{gas}	PET [15]
			CT [2]
			MRI [16]
Response to injury	Vascular permeability		PET [17]
	Extravascular lung water		PET [18]
	Inflammation		PET [19]

Because of the short half-life of many of the isotopes used in PET, and its exquisitely high sensitivity to detect isotopes in trace concentrations, this imaging modality is suitable for imaging most of the physiological parameters mentioned above, all within a short period of time and without physically affecting the process being measured.

This chapter is an expansion of a recent article but is not a comprehensive review of the functional imaging field. Instead, it is limited to presenting examples of PET and PET-CT applications in pulmonary functional imaging, developed and validated in our lab over the past two decades. For more detailed and broader descriptions on these topics, the reader is referred to recent reviews in the imaging and physiologic literature [20].

19.2 PET and PET-CT (the Basics)

19.2.1 Physical Principles

PET imaging is based on the characteristic of certain isotopes that, upon radioactive decay, emit a positron (the antimatter counterpart of an electron), thus their name: positron-emitting isotopes. Where it can interact with surrounding atoms for a short distance (typically less than 1 mm in solid tissue, but could be ~3 mm or more in the lung), it looses kinetic energy to the point where it interacts with an electron. This encounter annihilates both electron and positron, producing a pair of gamma photons, moving in almost exactly opposite directions (due to conservation of momentum), that, when detected in opposing photon counters simultaneously, are counted as a true "coincidence event" by the PET scanning device, and the source of radiation is known to have occurred in the path between the detectors [21]. After correction for photon energy attenuation by surrounding tissues and other factors [22], the local concentration of an isotope-labeled substance within the body can be recovered in 3D by reconstruction of the local decay coincident events collected over a period of time. In PET-CT attenuation correction is based on the density data from CT scan of the imaged area.

19.2.2 Temporal and Spatial Characteristics of PET-CT

Modern PET-CT scanners provide spatial resolutions as small as 1 mm^3 for small animal micro-PET [23] and <0.25 cm^3 in clinical scanners that is complemented by the much higher resolution of CT <1 mm^3. More importantly, PET-CT can provide spatial and temporal co-registered 3D images of structure and function. PET-CT scanners consist of the two imaging devices mounted next to each other. First a CT scan is used to collect a short (~15 s for a full high-resolution chest scan) scan, and then the imaged part of the body is moved to the PET gantry to collect a series of dynamic scans that can be as short as a few seconds each but typically take several minutes. To exploit the high spatial resolution of CT and avoid blurring by motion, the CT scan is acquired during a breath-hold. In contrast, most PET scans, due to their longer imaging time, have to be acquired during breathing, thus degrading their spatial resolution to ~1 cm^3 for images of the lung. Although newer PET and CT scanners allow imaging to be gated by breathing to reduce motion blurring of the data, in clinical studies this is rarely done because of increased radiation dose and/or prolonging scanning time. Instead, spatial misregistration errors, resulting from combining the static CT scan with breathing PET scans, can be minimized by acquiring the CT at a lung volume equivalent to that of the average volume during breathing. In our studies we use impedance plethysmography [1] to estimate a mean lung volume during a period of breathing prior to imaging. We present this value, and an instantaneous lung volume signal, to the subject via video display goggles for visual feedback during imaging (Fig. 19.1). Using this system, the subject is coached to stop breathing at a mean lung volume during the CT image acquisition. For positron emitters of short half-life, PET-CT allows acquisition of serial 3D data sets of multiple parameters of lung physiology and aerosol deposition during relatively short periods of time including airway tree structure at high resolution (Fig. 19.2).

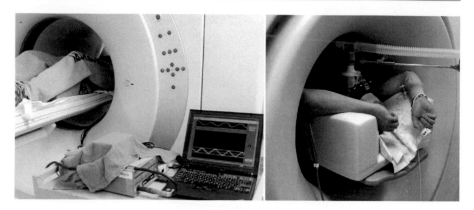

Fig. 19.1 Lung volume display during PET-CT imaging. A signal of dynamic lung volume is obtained with an impedance plethysmograph (SomnostarPT, Sensormedics Corp, Yorba Linda, CA) and displayed in real time on the screen of a laptop and presented to the subject on video display goggles. The computer calculates the average lung volume during breathing and displays a line on the screen to guide the subject to stop breathing at that volume during the CT scan. In this manner, the high-resolution CT data is collected at a volume equivalent to the average lung volume during breathing, and thus similar to that during the acquisition of the PET imaging scan

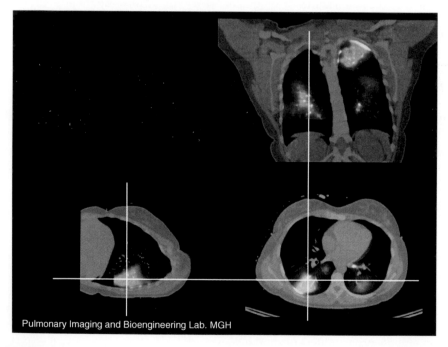

Fig. 19.2 Three-dimensional imaging data merging the residual Nitrogen-13 gas after a washout period of 2 minutes collected with PET, and the high-resolution structure obtained with CT. Because the PET imaging field is limited to a length of 20 cm, the PET data does not include the most caudal part of the lung. Color code for the PET scan is yellow for the highest tracer concentration and black for the lowest concentration. Note the patchy distribution of tracer residual demonstrating large regions of the lung with very low ventilation surrounded by well ventilating lung (Pulmonary Imaging and Bioengineering Lab. MGH)

19.3 PET Imaging of Lung Function and Aerosol Deposition

19.3.1 N^{13}-Saline Imaging of Ventilation and Perfusion

19.3.1.1 The Basics

Nitrogen-13 is a positron-emitting isotope of nitrogen that can be produced in gas form (^{13}N-N$_2$) or as part of other compounds such as ammonia (^{13}N-NH$_3$). In this application ^{13}N is used in gas form and, as N$_2$, is highly insoluble in water, blood, and lung tissues (partition coefficient of N$_2$ in water at body temperature ~0.98). The nitrogen-13-labeled gas is dissolved into degassed saline and injected into a peripheral vein. Once carried to the pulmonary circulation, upon reaching gas-containing alveoli, the isotope will diffuse into the airspaces of the lung with minimal absorption by other tissues. Because of its low solubility, we had to develop methods such that ^{13}N-N$_2$ could be forced into saline solution at concentrations that yield adequate activity for imaging. For this purpose we built an automatic device [24] including quality control and injection safety features (Fig. 19.3). Once in saline solution, the tracer is injected intravenously during a breath-hold. The isotope is carried by venous blood, and, when it reaches the capillary bed, it diffuses across the thin alveolar membrane into the airspace at first pass. Then, in the gas phase the tracer remains at a plateau concentration until ventilation is restarted. Since the isotope is transported by blood flow, the local plateau concentration of ^{13}N-N$_2$ during the breath-hold is proportional to the fraction of blood flow (perfusion, $\dot{Q}$) feeding that region (Fig. 19.4).

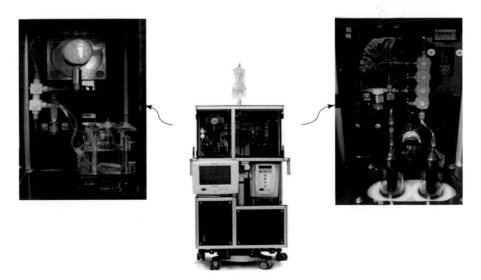

Fig. 19.3 Front view and details of a three generation apparatus for labeling processing and injecting Nitrogen-13 in saline solution SALSA-3G. The system is based on a modern Stelant MEDRad injector and, under computer control, purifies the gas sent by a cyclotron, mixes it with degassed saline and injects it to the patient [24]

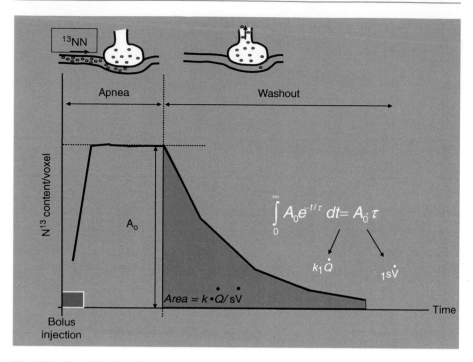

Fig. 19.4 Quantification of regional ventilation and perfusion with PET from the tracer kinetics of Nitrogen-13. The plot represents the local concentration of the tracer gas versus time following a bolus intravenous injection during apnea. Due to the low solubility of nitrogen in blood and tissues, upon arrival to the pulmonary capillary bed it diffuses to the alveolar air space and remains at a plateau level during the apnea. The tracer concentration at the plateau level, A_0, is proportional to the regional perfusion ($\dot{Q}$) reaching that region. After a short apnea, the subject begins to breathe and the tracer is washed out with a concentration following a single exponential function, if the ventilation is uniform within the region. The time constant ($t?$) is inversely proportional to the regional ventilation per unit of gas volume ($s\dot{V}$). It can thus be shown that the area under the washout curve is proportional to the ratio of $\dot{Q}/s\dot{V}$ Thus, from the injection of a single isotope, one can obtain co-registered images of $\dot{Q}$, $s\dot{V}$ and $\dot{Q}/V$

As breathing is restarted, the tracer is ventilated out of the lung, and its regional washout rate is proportional to regional alveolar ventilation per unit of gas volume $\left(s\dot{V}_A\right)$. For a single-compartment model (uniform $s\dot{V}_A$ and $\dot{Q}$ within the resolution element), the area under the concentration-time plot, normalized by the plateau value, is proportional to the ratio of perfusion to specific ventilation $\left(\dot{Q}/s\dot{V}_A\right)$, an index of gas transport efficiency. Although this model applies well to the healthy lung, it does not work well in disease. Analysis of local washout kinetics in a bronchoconstricted lung shows the existence of multi-compartment behavior suggesting important ventilation-perfusion mismatch within the resolution of imaging (sub-resolution heterogeneity) [25, 26]. This type of behavior can be modeled assuming that the local blood flow is distributed between a slow and a fast sub-resolution compartments that substantially improved gas exchange predictions [7] (Fig. 19.5).

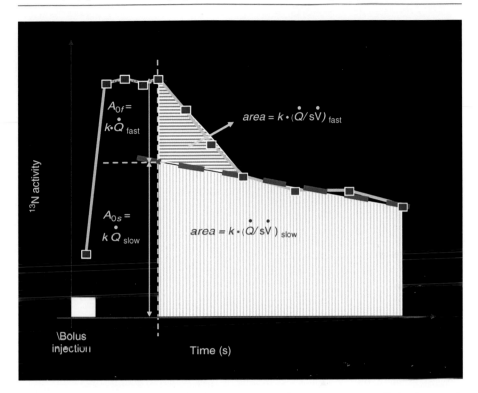

Fig. 19.5 Two-compartment analysis of VQ: In regions of the lung where ventilation is not uniform, the kinetics during the tracer washout do not follow a single exponential function. Instead, the data can be approximated by a double compartment with a fast compartment that washes out early; and a slow compartment that washes out at a lower rate. With this analysis the fraction of the blood flow from each compartment can be estimated

19.3.1.2 Pulmonary Shunt

In diseased or injured lung, areas of edematous tissue, alveolar flooding, or atelectasis involve blood flow that does not contact aerated spaces. This blood, therefore, does not participate in gas exchange and is said to *shunt*.

Within any region of the lung, shunting can be visualized with the ^{13}N-saline infusion/washout technique (Fig. 19.6). The total tracer content has two components: (1) tracer that is carried by blood that reaches aerated alveoli, redistributes into the airspace, and is retained during apnea and (2) tracer that is carried by blood reaching collapsed or flooded regions, in which the tracer passes rapidly through the lung, arriving and leaving without the retention of the tracer caused by a preferential partition coefficient.

During apnea, local tracer content rapidly reaches a peak whose magnitude is proportional to the total perfusion to the region (Q_R). Thereafter, its concentration falls as tracer carried in shunting blood is removed from the lung. The level to which the content falls at the end of apnea[1] is proportional to the blood flow to aerated lung (Q_A).

---

[1] If the duration of the apnea is very short, the kinetics may not exhibit a plateau. In this case, Q_A can be estimated by extrapolating an exponential function fitted to the apnea curve.

Fig. 19.6 Tracer kinetics of partially shunting lung. Tracer that is delivered to the collapsed compartment passes rapidly through the lung without significant redistribution, while tracer that reaches inflated lung diffuses almost completely into the airspace. The kinetics during the apnea phase represents the sum of these two components

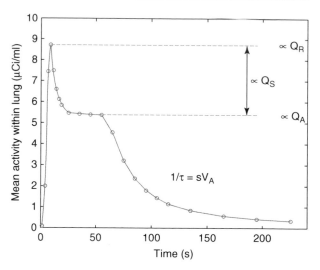

The local shunt fraction can thus be deduced as $1-(Q_A/Q_R)$. As with normal lung, the ventilation of aerated lung is given by the tracer washout rate.

The description given above is based on an idealized model of the lung and tracer kinetics, which has several deficiencies: for example, the infusion of tracer is implicitly assumed to be instantaneous; mixing in the heart is not modeled; the time-averaging effect of the PET scanner is not accounted for.

Improved parameter estimates can be made by matching the PET data to the output of a more complete model of the cardiopulmonary system [24]. In the model shown in Fig. 19.7, the heart is considered to be a single, well-mixed chamber; the effective heart volume (V_H) implicitly includes mixing effects in the vena cava and pulmonary artery. The tracer is convected through the pulmonary artery, modeled with a time delay (Δt_{TD}), and reaches the lungs, which are divided into a number of regions of interest (ROIs). The blood flow to each ROI is considered to enter one of two parallel compartments: the first compartment is aerated and retains tracer during apnea; in the second compartment, tracer shunts through the lung. The contribution of both compartments is added to describe the kinetics of the tracer through the region. Finally, since the PET scanner essentially measures mean tracer concentration over an imaging period, this effect is incorporated into the model.

Using nonlinear optimization techniques, the model parameters are adjusted to provide an optimal fit to the experimental data. For each region of the lung, the following parameters are estimated: perfusion to aerated compartment (Q_A), perfusion to shunt compartment (Q_S), and specific ventilation of the aerated compartment $\left(s\dot{V}_A\right)$.

Regional $s\dot{V}_A$ and $\dot{Q}$ of normal lungs and animal models with heterogeneous disease were analyzed using these methods [25] (Fig. 19.8). The analysis gave excellent correlations between measured blood gases and those predicted from calculations using the imaged values of regional ventilation, perfusion, and shunt

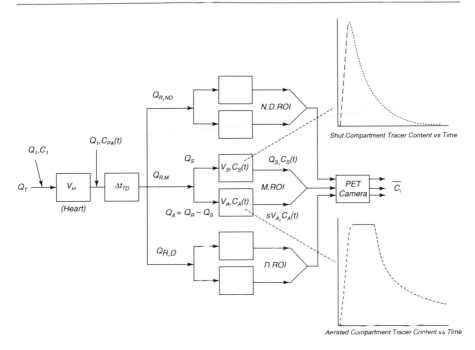

Fig. 19.7 Enhanced model of the lung including regional shunt. The injected tracer is mixed in the heart of volume V_H and convected to the lung with a time delay (Δt_{TD}). Each region of interest is composed of two compartments, one aerated and the other pure shunt. Finally, the effect of PET imaging is included. An equivalent model can be formulated to evaluate regions with heterogeneous ventilation

(Fig. 19.9). The study also demonstrated that if the sub-resolution heterogeneity was ignored, the correlations were poor [25], indicating that in diseased lungs $s\dot{V}_A$ to $\dot{Q}$ mismatching, at length scales smaller than the spatial resolution of PET, is substantial but can be recovered by analysis of the temporal information of the data.

19.3.1.3 Patchy Ventilation in Asthma

Using a similar analysis it was shown that methacholine-induced bronchoconstriction resulted in patchy and bimodal distributions of regional ventilation (Fig. 19.10) in animals [26], in asthmatic subjects [27, 28], and in normal lungs [29]. Of interest was the substantial, although incomplete, attempt of the lung to maintain VQ matching in the presence of severe bronchoconstriction [27].

Such a patchy distribution is also observed with MR hyperpolarized gases [30] and is consistent with a mathematical model of the lung that includes its bronchial structure and short and long distance interactions between the airway wall and its surrounding parenchyma [31]. Predictions from that model have been consistent and unified several apparently paradoxical observations such as dilation of some airways following MCh inhalation [32] or worsening of airway constriction with deep inhalations or after albuterol administrations (described below).

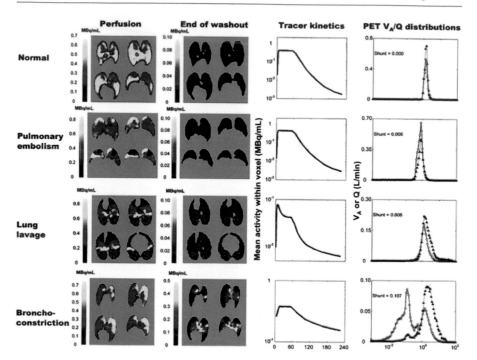

Fig. 19.8 Examples of data from sheep showing the regional distributions of Perfusion (*first column from the left*), tracer retention at end washout (*second column*), the tracer kinetics in a semi-log plot (*third column*), and the distribution of V/Q in terms of fraction of ventilation or fraction of perfusion. Data from a normal lung in the prone position (*first row from the top*) shows relatively linear tracer kinetics and narrow uni-modal distribution of VQ. The data from a model of pulmonary embolism, also in the prone position (*second row*), shows regions with perfusion defects and some broadening of the V/Q distributions but no shunt and minimal tracer retention. For the model of Acute Lung Injury caused by saline lavage (*third row*) imaged in the supine position, the image of perfusion is collected at the end of the breath hold, and shows dependent regions with reduced tracer due to an elevated shunt. Note some tracer is also retained in regions of the lung and there is a broadening of the V/Q distribution. Finally, for a bronchoconstricted prone animal following inhalation of methacholine (*fourth row*), the data exhibits regions of elevated tracer retention showing ventilation defective patches and a multi-exponential washout curve. The V/Q plot shows clear bimodal distributions (Vidal Melo et al. [7])

Fig. 19.10 The regional distribution of ventilation in bronchoconstricted lungs is patchy and bimodal. The top figure is 3D rendering of the chest wall (*gray*), airways (*brown*), and ventilation defects (*magenta*). The bottom plots are distributions of mean-normalized ventilation of a subject with asthma at baseline (*left*) and after Mch Challenge (*right*). Note that both at baseline and Post challenge the distributions are bimodal. At baseline there is a small fraction of voxels ventilated with less than one tenth of the ventilation in the rest of the lung. Post Mch, the fraction of hypoventilated voxels is substantially increased (greater area under the low ventilation mode)

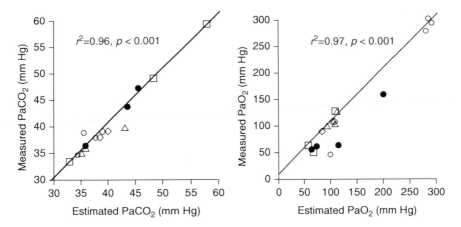

Fig. 19.9 Values of blood gases estimated from PET imaging data (*x*-axis) plotted against measured blood gases in animals with severe gas exchange impairment shown in Fig. 19.8, show excellent correlation. Excellent correlations where obtained when the imaging data was analyzed with the multi-compartment model of Figs. 19.5 and 19.7. The correlation was lost when the data was analyzed with the single compartment model, suggesting that a large fraction of the gas exchange impairment is caused by sub-resolution heterogeneity in V/Q (Taken from Melo Ref [7])

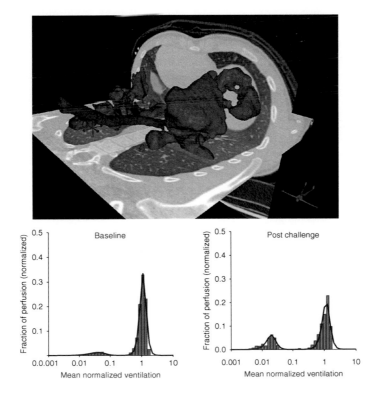

Although not well characterized, the impact of a patchy distribution of ventilation on peripheral distribution and airway deposition of an inhaled medication was intuitively understandable. Indeed, given that the primary transport mechanism for aerosol particles is convection along the inhaled gas stream, one can expect that (1) the transport of aerosol particles into severely hypoventilated regions of the lung periphery should be reduced and (2) to compensate for the reduced airflow through airways leading to patches of ventilation defective alveoli, there should be an elevation of airflow through airway leading to the well-ventilated regions; thus from mathematical modeling it can be inferred that deposition of the aerosol in those airways will be increased by inertial effects [33]. One could therefore theorize that delivery of an aerosol to a patchy lung may cause exaggerated bronchoreactivity if the aerosol contains an agonist or has reduced effectiveness if the aerosol contains a bronchodilator [34]. The following examples illustrate how a preexisting patchy $\dot{V}$ distribution can affect the regional response to inhaled bronchoactive aerosols.

19.3.1.4 Sequential Methacholine (MCh) Challenges

We reasoned that if a first bronchial challenge by MCh aerosol produced a patchy distribution of ventilation, a second challenge, by depositing the agonist on preferentially ventilated regions, should dramatically alter the pattern of ventilation heterogeneity. In this example, we imaged with PET ventilation distribution in one asthmatic after each of two consecutive MCh challenges, both at the same PC20 concentration determined days before the scanner. The first challenge was used to create an initial patchy ventilation distribution, and the second challenge was given 30 min later to evaluate the effects on ventilation heterogeneity.

In this case, ventilation defects formed in the dependent part of each lung after the first challenge (Fig. 19.11, top left panel). Note that although the left lung ventilation defect retained a lower fraction of activity than that of the right lung at the end of the washout (0.30 vs. 0.40), the rest of the lung had a residual activity of only 3 % of the initial one. In contrast, after the second challenge the previously poorly ventilated dependent region of the right left lung showed not only an increase in perfusion but also a substantial reduction in tracer retention fraction compared with that following the first challenge (from 0.3 to 0.02). The ventilation defect of the right lung also reduced its tracer retention (from 0.4 to 0.16), although not as much as the left lung. This illustrates how the reduced ventilation in those regions, after the first challenge, partially protected them from receiving the second dose of the agonist compared with the rest of the lung that tripled its fraction of tracer retained (from 0.03 to 0.09). Since the sequential challenges were given separated by 30 min of each other, it is possible that the regional degree of constriction of the lungs, including its dependent parts, may have spontaneously decreased. However, this would not explain why the less-ventilated regions increased ventilation while the rest of the lung decreased it. Instead, the result is consistent with previous observations in bronchoconstricted sheep [26] and supine human subjects [28] where regions that became ventilation defects with methacholine were being preferentially ventilating prior to the aerosol challenge. This result also supports the hypothesis that bronchoprovocation in the presence of heterogeneous $\dot{V}$ distribution, by concentrating the agonist in well-ventilated areas, can exaggerate a regional hyperreactive response [35].

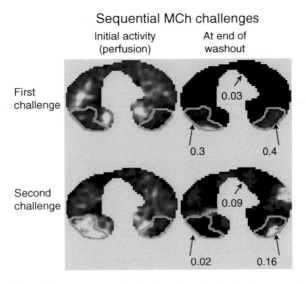

Fig. 19.11 The effect of heterogeneous distribution of ventilation during aerosol injalation can be seen from the changes in regional perfusion and ventilation following sequential methacholine challenges. The figure shows the distribution of tracer concentration, in a transverse slice of the thorax following IV injection during the apnea (perfusion, *left column*) and after a 3 min period of ventilation (tracer retention, *right column*). The *upper images* were obtained following an initial methacholine challenge, and the *lower images* after a second agonist challenge. The regions with low ventilation (high tracer retention) after the first challenge are *circled by a green line* and numbers show the average fraction of tracer remaining in them and in the rest of the lung at end washout. Note that the regions with low ventilation following the first challenge increased their ventilation after the second challenge at the expense of the rest of the lung. This clearly demonstrates how the initial heterogeneity of ventilation can modify the local effects of an inhaled bronchoconstrictive agent

19.3.1.5 Methacholine (MCh) Challenge of an Initially Patchy Lung

A similar effect can be seen following an MCh challenge to a subject originally showing with mild but visible ventilation defects (Fig. 19.12). In this case, the MCh inhalation results in increase of ventilation and blood flow in regions that were poorly ventilated at baseline and a reduction of regional ventilation and blood flow in well-ventilated regions at baseline (Fig. 19.13).

19.3.1.6 Paradoxical Effects of Albuterol

Opposite effects can be expected if a bronchodilator is delivered to a heterogeneously constricted lung. The following example illustrates such a case, where regional changes in ventilation and increased global measures of obstruction were observed in a spontaneously bronchoconstricted asthmatic after inhalation of albuterol aerosol. In this case, mild obstructive symptoms were noted prior to the baseline study, and the ^{13}N-saline scans showing substantial ventilation defects scatter within the lung (Fig. 19.14 left). For this reason, instead of methacholine, the subject was then given inhalation of albuterol in a ^{13}N-NH_3-labeled saline solution (2.5 mg in 0.5 ml) with a standard jet nebulizer during normal tidal breathing. Local deposition of the isotope-labeled aerosol was imaged with PET (Fig. 19.14 right).

Baseline

Perfusion   Tracer retention

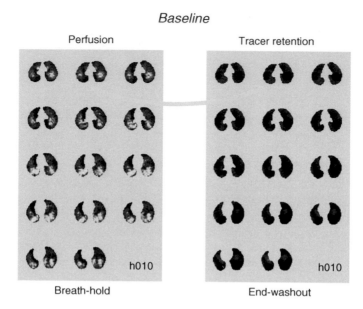

Breath-hold   End-washout

Fig. 19.12 Cross-sectional images of regional perfusion (*left*) and tracer retention after 2 minutes of washout (*right*) of an asthmatic subject at baseline. Starting from *top* to *bottom*, and *left* to *right*, are tomograms from the cranial to the caudal direction. The *yellow arrow* points at regions of lower perfusion on the left lung that coincide with areas of mild tracer retention

Twenty minutes after albuterol inhalation, a second set of ^{13}N-saline PET scans were conducted (Fig. 19.14, middle).

From the ^{13}N-saline PET scan (Fig. 19.14), it can be seen that the anatomical location, and extent, of tracer-retaining regions at baseline, of this spontaneously constricted patient, was not noticeably different from those observed in asthmatics with MCh-induced bronchoconstriction after the second challenge of MCh (Fig. 19.11). Furthermore, after albuterol inhalation, this subject had a paradoxical reduction in FEV1 of 14 %, an increase of 12 % in the heterogeneity in $\dot{V}$ assessed as the mean-normalized standard deviation of regional $\dot{V}$, and an increase of 22 % in low-frequency airway resistance (R_{low}) and of 91 % in low-frequency tissue elastance (E_{low}), both measured with the forced oscillatory flow technique. In addition, from the 3D rendering of the ventilation defective regions (Fig. 19.14), it is clearly visible a striking peripheral shift of regions of low $\dot{V}$ at the expense of central regions. This shift correlated with the mostly central deposition of the albuterol inhaled from a jet nebulizer during shallow tidal breathing. Simultaneous to the paradoxical deterioration in FEV1, the fraction of volume occupied by ventilation defects (VDef's Vol) increased by 44 % and their ventilation relative to that of the rest of the lung $\dot{V}_{\text{Def/out}}$ was reduced by 18 %. This example illustrates how a patchy $\dot{V}$ distribution during bronchoconstriction can result in unexpected results due to a heterogeneous deposition of the bronchodilator, a mechanism that could provide an explanation for paradoxical clinical observations [36]. The study also underlines the usefulness of combining imaging of aerosol deposition with imaging of lung function for interpreting global measures of airway function such as FEV1 or airway resistance.

After inhalation of agonist (Mch)

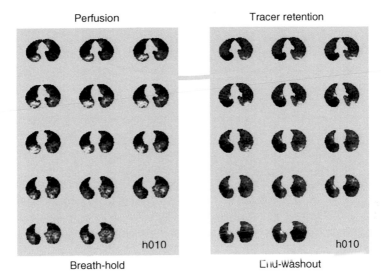

Perfusion

Tracer retention

h010

h010

Breath-hold

End-washout

Fig. 19.13 Cross-sectional images of regional perfusion (*left*) and tracer retention (*right*) of the same asthmatic subject of Fig. 19.12 after a metacholine (*Mch*) challenge. The *yellow arrow* points at the same regions of Fig. 19.12, but this time shows high blood flow and no tracer retention on the left lung. This illustrates how the regions of high ventilation at baseline, became hypo ventilated, while the regions of ventilation defects at baseline were protected from the agonist and became well ventilated

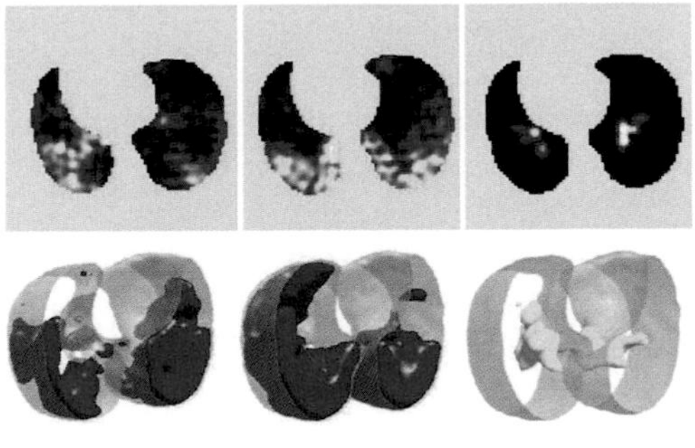

Paradoxical effects of aluterol

	Contol	Post albuterol	Distrib. albuterol		% change
FEV1/TLC					−12
R_{low}					22
E_{low}					91
cov $\dot{V}$					12
$\dot{V}$Def/Out					−18
VDef's Vol.					44

Fig. 19.14 Paradoxical response to a broncho-dilator. Representative tomographic slices of tracer retention and the corresponding 3D rendering of ventilation defects at control condictions (*Left*) and after inhalation of albuterol (*Center*), and the distribution of the bronchodilator (*right*). The table shows the percent change caused by the albuterol on: Forced exhaled volume during the first second devided by functional residual capacity (FEV1/TLC), Lung resistance (R_{low}) and elastance (E_{low}) measured with forced oscillations at 0.2 Hz, the heterogeneity of ventilation covV, the ratio of specific ventilation between the ventilation defective regions and the rest of the lung, and the relative volume covered by the ventilation defects. For explanation see text

Direct clinical implications of these examples may not be critical for inhalation of short-acting bronchodilators, given that elevated doses of these drugs may be effective in most cases to relieve obstructive symptoms with minor side effects. However, the mechanism of heterogeneously distributed aerosol medication may explain why inhaled therapies tend to fail in severe asthma attacks and intravenous bronchodilators may be required. More relevant could be the potential implications of these results for inhalation of long-acting bronchodilator medications. It is not difficult to envision how, if these medications are repeatedly given into a heterogeneous lung with ventilation defects, systematically constricted regions that are deprived of the drug could over time undergo airway remodeling or become chronically constricted [37]. Although the well-ventilated lung would be kept dilated under treatment, a sudden exacerbation could result in severe bronchoconstriction of the ventilating lung with a reduced capacity to dilate the remodeled regions. This could explain the observed increase in mortality in subjects receiving inhaled long-acting bronchodilators without corticosteroids [38] and the persistence of ventilation defects over time regardless of disease severity or treatment [30, 39].

19.4 PET-CT Imaging of Aerosol Deposition

Previous PET imaging studies had evaluated [^{18}F] fluorodeoxyglucose (^{18}F-FDG)-inhaled aerosol to provide detailed 3D quantification of the intrapulmonary distribution of aerosol deposition [40]. Similar information, although at reduced spatial resolution, can be obtained from SPECT-CT imaging [41]. The short half-life of ^{13}NNH$_3$ (10 min) as a tracer, compared with that of ^{18}F-FDG (110 min) or SPECT agents (6 h), opens the possibility of sequential imaging of aerosol deposition in the same subject at short intervals and substantially reduced (approximately one-tenth) radiation dose compared with ^{18}F-FDG. ^{13}NNH$_3$, as a tracer, is currently limited to imaging saline-based aerosols (Fig. 19.15). Longer half-life isotopes may be needed to assess aerosol deposition from other therapeutic inhalers such as MDIs or DPIs that require special loading of the agent. PET can also be used for imaging the deposition and bio-distribution of directly labeled drugs and examine the resulting clinical correlates [42].

19.5 PET-CT Provides the Link Between Global Mechanical Obstruction and Airway Constriction

Global airflow obstruction and heterogeneities in airway constriction and ventilation distribution are prominent features of asthma. However, the mechanistic link between these global and regional features had not been defined. Based on simultaneous studies of oscillatory mechanics and regional ventilation distribution, it was theorized that heterogeneous peripheral airway resistance was responsible for mechanical obstruction in asthma [43, 44]. That hypothesis was recently tested using a combination of PET, to image the distribution of regional ventilation, and

Fig. 19.15 3D renderings of the central airways tree and aerosol depostion. The peripheral deposition of the aerosol is seen as a cloud following the direction of the airways. Note the substantial amount of tracer in the esophagus and the spot of high deposition on the right upper lobar bronchus

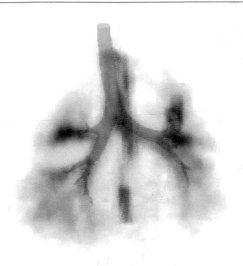

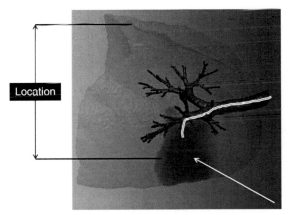

Central airways

Gas velocity and flow rate
Pathway Resistance
Airway deposition dose
Wall thickness
Airway distensibility

Lung periphery

Ventilation and Perfusion
Volumes (Gas, tissue, blood)
Peripheral Resistance
Tissue Elastance
Aerosol Deposition
Inflammation

Location

Fig. 19.16 (Pulmonary Imaging and Bioengineering Lab. MGH)

CT, to obtain detailed parenchyma and airway morphology [45]. Subjects with and without asthma were imaged before and after MCh challenges, and global obstruction was assessed with spirometry. Image-derived structure, analyzed using Apollo software (VIDA, Iowa City, IA, USA), and ventilation data measured with PET (Fig. 19.16) were used as inputs to a subject-specific computational model of lung mechanics. The model estimated the anatomical distribution of peripheral resistance that was consistent with the measured distribution of ventilation and the global degree of airway obstruction measured by spirometry. Results from this study (Fig. 19.17) show that peripheral specific conductance ($sG = G/V_{gas}$) in both groups was substantially lower than that from central airways (diameter >2 mm), and the

MCh effect on central and peripheral airways conductance

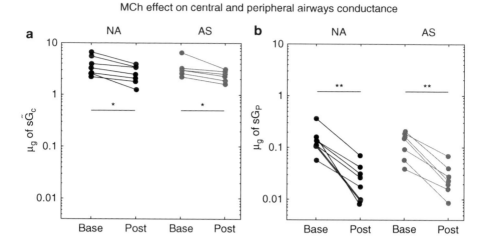

Fig. 19.17 Changes in the mean value of specific pathway conductance for central (*left*) and peripheral (*right*) airways resulting from a methacholine challenge (Base vs Post), measured from a group of eight nonasthmatic (*NA*) and one of seven asthmatic (*AS*) subjects. For explanations see text * $p<0.05$, ** $p<0.005$

reduction in conductance due to MCh was much greater in peripheral airways than in central ones. It was thus concluded that peripheral airways are mostly responsible for the elevation in airway resistance during bronchoconstriction confirming previous theoretical predictions [46].

19.5.1 Imaging of Pulmonary Inflammation with ¹⁸F-FDG

Florine-18-labeled fluorodeoxyglucose (¹⁸F-FDG) is an analog of glucose mostly used as a PET radiotracer to detect elevated metabolism of cancerous tumors. When injected intravenously, the uptake of the ¹⁸F-FDG radiotracer by normal lung tissues is low, but it is elevated within inflamed tissues by ventilator-induced lung injury [47, 48, 49] (Fig. 19.18), smoke inhalation [50], infection [51], or allergic reaction [52]. This elevated uptake rate (K_i, min⁻¹) is mostly localized on high metabolically active leukocytes, but other cells may also be involved [49]. In a model of unilateral cigarette smoke inhalation [50], we imaged regional K_i in addition to regional gas content (F_{gas}), ventilation ($\dot{V}_r$), and perfusion (Q_r) (Fig. 19.19) and derived K_i and $\dot{V}_r / Q_r$ distributions for each lung for one of the animals (Fig. 19.20). These distributions showed lower $\dot{V}_r / Q_r$ and higher K_i for the smoke-exposed lung, with consistent higher spread in both distributions for that lung. However, although all animals were given the same cigarette dose to the left lung, there was a substantial variability in both the K_i and $\dot{V}_r / Q_r$ distributions between animals (Fig. 19.21). The variability in response to smoke inhalation between animals unveiled important correlations between the shunt fraction for each lung and the maximal values of K_i ($K_{i, max}$), defined as the mean plus the standard deviation of the distribution.

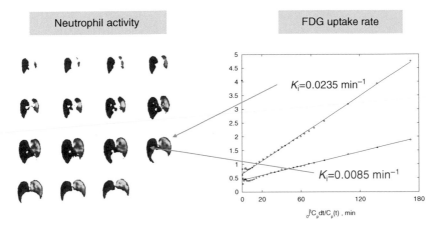

Fig. 19.18 Neutrophilic inflamation imaged in a sheep with unilateral (left lung) ventilation induced lung injury (VILI). The tomography images seen from head to tail (left lung on the right side of the prone sheep) show elevated 18F-FDG uptake. The graph on the right shows the elevated uptake rate (K_i) of the 18F-FDG on the left (injured) lung, measured from the slop of the plot

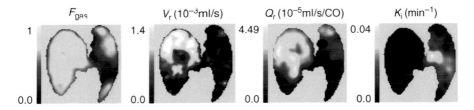

Fig. 19.19 Regional lung function and inflammation following unilateral (left lung) tobacco smoke inhalation. The images show a representative slices of a gas fraction (F_{gas}), regional ventilation (V_r), regional Perfusion Q_r, and FDG uptake rate K_i seen from tail to head (*left lung* on the *right side*) of this prone sheep. Color code is defined for each image (Schroeder et al. [50])

Fig. 19.20 Distributions of k_i and ventilation–perfusion ratio V/Q following unilateral exposure to cigarette smoke. Control (*thin line*) refers to the right lung that was not exposed to cigarette smoke. *Thick line* represents the distributions on the left lung that was exposed to smoke from ten cigarettes (Schroeder et al. [50])

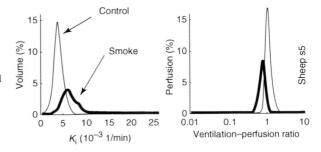

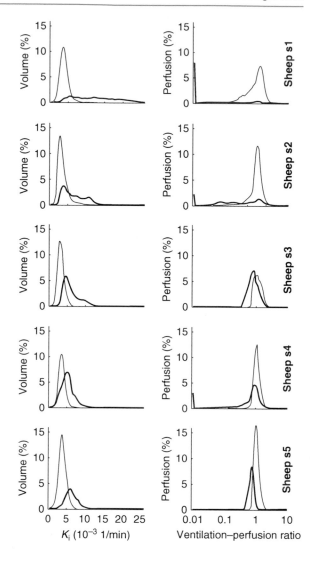

Fig. 19.21 (*Left*) Graphs of K_i in control lung (*thin line*) and smoke-exposed lung (*heavy line*) in sheep s1–s5. (*Right*) Corresponding mean normalized distributions of V/Q. Animals are ordered by heterogeneity of K_i distribution (SD(K_i)) in the smoke-exposed lung. Note the substantial inter-animal variability in the functional and inflammatory responses to smoke

In other words, this correlation demonstrated the connection between the degree of functional gas exchange impairment and the degree of inflammation (Fig. 19.22). The data also showed a strong correlation between the mean-normalized variance of $\log\left(\dot{V}_r / Q_r\right)$ of the control lung and of the smoke-exposed lung (Fig. 19.23). It is reasonable to assume that the heterogeneity in $\dot{V}_r / Q_r$ measured from the control lung represents the degree of heterogeneity preexisting before the exposure to smoke. Based on this assumption, the correlation between $\mathrm{cov}^2\left(\dot{V}_r / Q_r\right)$ of control and exposed lung would be consistent with the hypothesis that the degree of preexisting heterogeneity in the lung may be responsible for the variability in its response to cigarette smoke inhalation.

Fig. 19.22 Regional shunt fraction plotted against $K_{i,max}$ in control lung (*cirles*) and smoke-exposed lung (*black dots*), showing the correlation of highest level of local inflammation ($K_{i,max}$) with lung functional parameters within each lung field

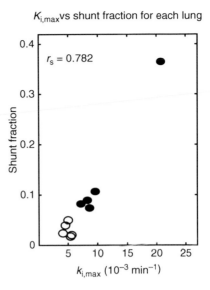

$K_{i,max}$vs shunt fraction for each lung

$r_s = 0.782$

Fig. 19.23 Heterogeneity of ventilation/perfusion (cov^2(V/Q) for the control lung is highly correlated with that of the smoke-exposed lung. Note the one order of magnitude difference of the scales

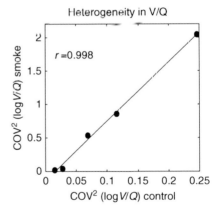

Heterogeneity in V/Q

$r = 0.998$

19.6 Relationship Between Airway Inflammation, Airway Hyperresponsiveness, and Lung Function in Asthma

These following paragraphs illustrate a method for assessment of these relationships noninvasively in human subjects and demonstrates that ^{18}F-FDG K_i can serve as a biomarker of eosinophilic inflammation and local lung function [52]. In subjects with demonstrated atopic asthma, we used PET-CT to assess regional $\dot{Q}$, $s\dot{V}_A$, fractional gas content (F_{gas}), airway wall thickness aspect ratio (ω), and regional K_i, after 10 h of segmental allergen challenge to the right middle bronchus. These parameters, measured on the allergen-challenged lobe, were compared to those on

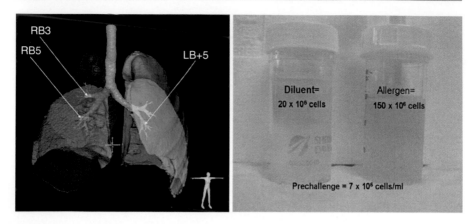

Fig. 19.24 *Left*: Bronchial Allergen Challenge in Atopic Asthma. Airway tree and lung lobes from one subject's HRCT scan showing the segmental allergen challenged segment (Lower airway segment, *RB5*) and the dilluent segment RB3. *Right*: Samples of BAL fluid from one of the subject studied. Bal from the diluent-challenged segment is moderately cellular; but clear while the BAL from the allergen challenged segment is cloudy and highly cellular

the right upper lobe, where diluent only was applied as a control. Wall thickness aspect ratio, ω, of the allergen-challenged airway was compared to those of similarly sized airways from unaffected areas of the lung. The ratio in local K_i between allergen and diluent segments was compared to the ratio in cell counts obtained, 24 h after the allergen challenge, by bronchoalveolar lavage of the respective segments (Fig. 19.24).

The data showed systematic regional reductions in $\dot{Q}$, $s\dot{V}_A$, and F_{gas} and increased ω and K_i in challenged versus controlled regions in all subjects (Fig. 19.25). Figure 19.26 shows that the ratio of eosinophil count (allergen/diluent) was linearly related with the ratio in ^{18}F-FDG K_i ($R^2 = 0.9917$, $p < 0.001$). What is remarkable about this strong correlation is that the variables were measured 14 h apart, suggesting that the K_i ratio predicts the degree of eosinophilic cellular infiltrate into the alveoli many hours later. This may be because the K_i signal comes from marginating eosinophils (that are activated and avidly taking up plasma ^{18}F-FDG), and these cells then migrate into the alveolar compartment over the ensuing hours. Also evident from this data was that the absolute K_i in a region was not correlated to the absolute eosinophil count. Instead K_i and eosinophil counts were correlated when normalized by the values from the diluent lobe. This suggests that there might be a generalized inflammatory response that is variable among individuals, which is amplified by the allergen-specific response. The data suggests that regional K_i, may be a noninvasive and highly predictive biomarker of eosinophilic airway inflammation and its functional effects in asthma. The method may serve to help understand the mechanisms of allergic inflammation and to test the therapeutic effectiveness of novel drugs or treatments.

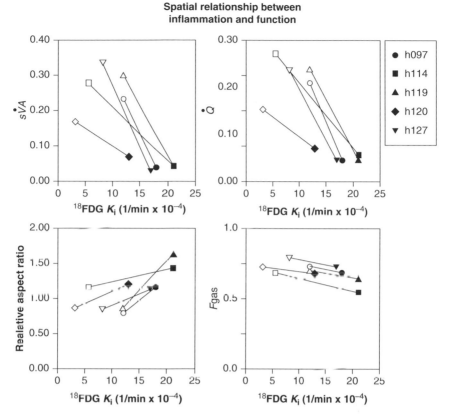

Fig. 19.25 Functional variables versus K_i. Clockwise from upper *left*: sV_A, Q, relative aspect ratio, and F_{gas}. Each symbol represents individual subject, with open symbols representing diluent and closed symbols allergen. Allergen systematically increased K_i, with reductions in ventilation, perfusion gas content, and an increase in airway wall thickness

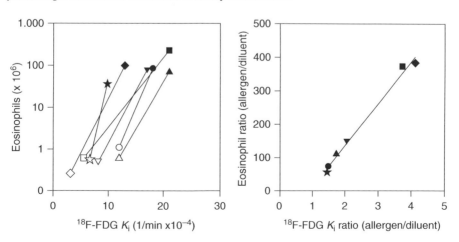

Fig. 19.26 Eosinophil count versus K_i and eosinophil count ratio (allergen to diluent) versus K_i ratio. Each subject is represented by different symbols. All subjects had increase in K_i and eosinophil count in allergen-challenged region (*dark symbols*), compared with diluent region (*open symbols*). Eosinophil count ratio was highly correlated ($R^2=0.9917$, $P<0.001$) with K_i ratio

34. Venegas J, Winkler T, Harris RS (2013) Lung physiology and aerosol deposition imaged with positron emission tomography. J Aerosol Med Pulm Drug Deliv 26(1):1–8
35. Venegas J (2007) Linking ventilation heterogeneity and airway hyperresponsiveness in asthma. Thorax 62(8):653–654
36. Eckert B, Armstrong JG, Mitchell CA (1993) Paradoxical bronchoconstriction in patients with stable asthma. Med J Aust 159(8):566
37. Grainge CL, Lau LC, Ward JA, Dulay V, Lahiff G, Wilson S, Holgate S, Davies DE, Howarth PH (2011) Effect of bronchoconstriction on airway remodeling in asthma. N Engl J Med 364(21):2006–2015
38. Salpeter SR, Buckley NS, Ormiston TM, Salpeter EE (2006) Meta-analysis: effect of long-acting beta-agonists on severe asthma exacerbations and asthma-related deaths. Ann Intern Med 144(12):904–912
39. de Lange EE, Altes TA, Patrie JT, Parmar J, Brookeman JR, Mugler JP 3rd, Platts-Mills TA (2007) The variability of regional airflow obstruction within the lungs of patients with asthma: assessment with hyperpolarized helium-3 magnetic resonance imaging. J Allergy Clin Immunol 119(5):1072–1078
40. Dolovich MB (2009) 18F-fluorodeoxyglucose positron emission tomographic imaging of pulmonary functions, pathology, and drug delivery. Proc Am Thorac Soc 6(5):477–485
41. Fleming JS, Conway JH, Bolt L, Holgate ST (2003) A comparison of planar scintigraphy and SPECT measurement of total lung deposition of inhaled aerosol. J Aerosol Med 16(1):9–19
42. Dolovich MB (2001) Measuring total and regional lung deposition using inhaled radiotracers. J Aerosol Med 14(Suppl 1):S35–S44
43. Tgavalekos NT, Venegas JG, Suki B, Lutchen KR (2003) Relation between structure, function, and imaging in a three-dimensional model of the lung. Ann Biomed Eng 31(4):363–373
44. Wongviriyawong C, Harris RS, Greenblatt E, Winkler T, Venegas JG (2013) Peripheral resistance: a link between global airflow obstruction and regional ventilation distribution. J Appl Physiol 114(4):504–514
45. Wongviriyawong C, Harris RS, Zheng H, Kone M, Winkler T, Venegas JG (2012) Functional effect of longitudinal heterogeneity in constricted airways before and after lung expansion. J Appl Physiol 112(1):237–245
46. Tgavalekos NT, Musch G, Harris RS, Vidal Melo MF, Winkler T, Schroeder T, Callahan R, Lutchen KR, Venegas JG (2007) Relationship between airway narrowing, patchy ventilation and lung mechanics in asthmatics. Eur Respir J 29(6):1174–1181
47. Costa EL, Musch G, Winkler T, Schroeder T, Harris RS, Jones HA, Venegas JG, Vidal Melo MF (2010) Mild endotoxemia during mechanical ventilation produces spatially heterogeneous pulmonary neutrophilic inflammation in sheep. Anesthesiology 112(3):658–669
48. de Prost N, Costa EL, Wellman T, Musch G, Winkler T, Tucci MR, Harris RS, Venegas JG, Vidal Melo MF (2011) Effects of surfactant depletion on regional pulmonary metabolic activity during mechanical ventilation. J Appl Physiol 39(3):179–182
49. de Prost N, Tucci MR, Vidal Melo MF (2010) Assessment of lung inflammation with 18F-FDG PET during acute lung injury. Am J Roentgenol 195(2):292–300
50. Schroeder T, Vidal Melo MF, Musch G, Harris RS, Winkler T, Venegas JG (2007) PET imaging of regional 18F-FDG uptake and lung function after cigarette smoke inhalation. J Nucl Med 48(3):413–419
51. Servaes S (2011) Imaging infection and inflammation in children with (18)F-FDG PET and (18)F-FDG PET/CT. J Nucl Med Technol 39(3):179–182
52. Harris RS, Venegas JG, Wongviriyawong C, Winkler T, Kone M, Musch G, Vidal Melo MF, de Prost N, Hamilos DL, Afshar R, Cho J, Luster AD, Medoff BD (2011) 18F-FDG uptake rate is a biomarker of eosinophilic inflammation and airway response in asthma. J Nucl Med 52(11):1713–1720

Part IV

Different Treatment and Mechanics of Breathing

Pharmacological Treatment: an Update

20

Peter Calverley

Pharmacological treatment is a key component of integrated COPD management. Over the last decade, many overviews and treatment guidelines have been published, including those by the ATS/ERS, UK National Institute for Health and Care Excellence (NIHCE) and the Global initiative for chronic Obstructive Lung Disease (GOLD) [1, 2, 3]. Updated advice relative to these last two documents is now available [4, 5]. This chapter considers aspects of COPD treatment in relationship to their impact on lung mechanics and examines whether other treatments, without a direct mechanical effect on the lungs, can also benefit patients suffering from COPD.

20.1 Lung Mechanics and COPD Treatment

Although the definition of COPD has been modified over time, all recent versions emphasise the role of persistent and usually progressive airflow obstruction, as a defining feature. Hence, abnormalities in lung mechanics lie at the heart of COPD and explain many, but not, of the problems experienced by these patients.

Although defined in terms of airflow limitation, COPD diagnosis relies not only on the presence of a reduced FEV_1/FVC ratio but also on the absolute reduction in FEV_1 which is normally reported in terms of the post-bronchodilator value. This approach has been widely adopted in clinical trials of COPD treatment, but to be accepted as clinically useful, treatments must also modify outcomes other than objectively measured lung function, as measured in Table 20.1. Many studies reflect the excellent reproducibility and effort independence of this measurement. Unfortunately, the relationship of the FEV_1 to the degree of reported symptoms is

P. Calverley, DSc, FMedSci
Clinical Sciences Department, Institute of Ageing and Chronic Diseases,
University Hospital Aintree, Lower Lane, Liverpool L9 7AL, UK
e-mail: pmacal@liverpool.ac.uk

A. Aliverti, A. Pedotti (eds.), *Mechanics of Breathing*,
DOI 10.1007/978-88-470-5647-3_20, © Springer-Verlag Italia 2014

Table 20.1 Pharmacological management of COPD exacerbations

Drug	Setting	Route	Dose	Comment
Bronchodilator (SABA/SAMA)	O.P.	Inhaled	2 puffs every 3–4 hours	Frequency of use should decrease over 48 h or seek help
Bronchodilator (SABA/SAMA)	I.P.	Inhaled	Salbutamol 2.5 or 5 mg and ipratropium 500 mcg every 6 hours	Nebulised till symptoms resolve
Corticosteroids	O.P. and I.P.	Oral	Prednisolone 30 mg	Give for 7–10 days and stop
Antibiotics	O.P.	Oral	Drug with appropriate sensitivity	Give for 5–7 days in patient with worse cough and sputum and dyspnoea
Antibiotics	I.P.	Oral	Drug with appropriate sensitivity	Give for 5–7 days in patient with worse cough and sputum and dyspnoea. Parenteral route seldom needed

O.P. outpatient, *I.P.* hospitalised inpatient or ER attendee
For other abbreviations, see text.

relatively weak. This is because symptoms relate not primarily to the presence of airflow obstruction but to changes in other physiological variables.

The earliest mechanical change in COPD is a rise in residual volume, which reflects the onset of expiratory flow limitation and/or airway closure in the peripheral airways [6]. Reductions in mid-expiratory flow and an increased gradient between the total and peripheral respiratory system resistance may detect these abnormalities when spirometry is still relatively normal, but problems with between-subject reproducibility have made these difficult techniques to apply in clinical trial populations. As residual volume rises, so does end-expiratory lung volume (EELV) and this reflects the impact of both static and dynamic changes in lung mechanics [7]. Certainly, dynamic hyperinflation during exercise is an important determinant of symptoms, as illustrated elsewhere in this volume. Studies with anticholinergic bronchodilator drugs, at the early stages of COPD, have shown that the absolute degree of dynamic hyperinflation at any point during exercise can be modified, although this does not necessarily translate into important changes in exercise capacity [8].

In practice, bronchodilator treatment is not used regularly until the patient begins to report more persistent symptoms, by which time more significant deteriorations in lung mechanics have occurred.

As EELV increases, the inspiratory capacity falls, and in consequence, the end-inspiratory volume during tidal breathing more readily approaches the inspiratory reserve volume, particularly during exercise. As a result, inspiratory muscle function is compromised and more effort is required to generate a smaller volume change, which translate into a rapid rise in the patient's breathlessness. This has been well documented during exercise [9, 10], but similar factors are likely to apply during exacerbations when both static and dynamic increases in lung volume occur [11, 12].

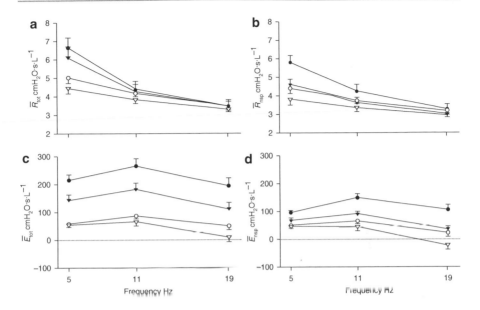

Fig. 20.1 Multifrequency impedance spectra for (**a**) mean whole breath resistance ($\bar{R}_{tot}$), (**b**) mean inspiration resistance ($\bar{R}_{insp}$), (**c**) mean whole breath respiratory elastance at 5 Hz ($\bar{E}_{tot}$) and (**d**) mean inspiratory elastance at 5 Hz ($\bar{E}_{insp}$) in flow-limited (*closed symbols*) and nonflow-limited (*open symbols*) patients at baseline before (*circles*) and after (*triangles*) bronchodilatation (Reproduced from Ref. [17] with permission)

Bronchodilator drugs both decrease residual volume and increase inspiratory capacity at rest, which means that a larger tidal volume is possible and/or exercise can continue for longer, before critical levels of breathlessness develop [13].

There are now good studies that have shown these effects with all classes of bronchodilators, irrespective of their duration of action [14, 15]. It is likely that the reduction in symptoms seen after bronchodilator treatment during an exacerbation is due to this effect. This has been noted even under resting conditions in severe COPD patients with marked hyperinflation, who were given both beta-agonists and anticholinergic [16]. In this setting, where tidal expiratory flow limitation is present, there is little evidence that is modified by the bronchodilator drugs, although lung volume decreases [17]. Studies using the forced oscillation technique have shown that in flow-limited COPD patients, bronchodilators have much more impressive effects on inspiratory rather than expiratory respiratory system resistance [18] (Fig. 20.1). In practice, the respiratory system prefers to reduce dynamically regulated EELV rather than expiratory flow limitation presumably because the volume changes are directly sensed symptomatically and influence the breathing pattern. From the above, it is clear that bronchodilators can have important effects on both breathlessness and exercise tolerance by shifting the critical choke points of flow limitation more proximally and aiding lung emptying, before the onset of flow limitation.

The effects of bronchodilator drugs in the prevention of exacerbation are more subtle but again are more likely to be related to their actions on lung mechanics. At present, exacerbations are considered to be sustained, symptomatically defined events, which may (or may not) require the use of additional medical treatment [19]. By increasing inspiratory capacity, a larger lung volume change is possible before symptoms (the defining feature of the exacerbation event) develop. Hence, regular long-acting inhaled bronchodilator treatment is associated with episodes which are reported as exacerbations, and hence, exacerbation frequency is lower in studies where effective bronchodilatation is given [20, 21]. As health status is influenced both by the number of exacerbations [22] and the degree of exercise limitation, sustained-acting bronchodilators will also improve this outcome.

Effects on gas exchange are more complex. In some studies, particularly those using short-acting beta-agonists have shown that there is deterioration in ventilation-perfusion matching, possibly by local relief of hypoxic vasoconstriction [23]. The result in changes in arterial oxygen percentage is small and not likely to be clinically significant, and at present, this effect of these drugs is not one that seems to restrict their use or be associated with safety hazards. The close interactions between lung volumes and pulmonary artery pressure mean that bronchodilators can produce apparent reductions in the degree of pulmonary hypertension seen in COPD [24]. Whether this is a real effect on intravascular pressure or simply a consequence of the way in which pulmonary artery is measured and the effects of lung volume on trans-pulmonary arterial wall pressure gradient is less clear.

While bronchodilators have predictable effects on lung mechanics, this is much less true for anti-inflammatory treatment. Trials with both inhaled corticosteroids (ICS) and PDE4 inhibitor roflumilast have shown small but consistent increases of FEV1 over 12 months of treatment [25, 26]. This is reflected in treatments of quality of life, at least with ICS, especially when they are combined with long-acting beta-antagonists (LABA) [27]. Exercise tolerance can be increased by adding an anti-inflammatory to a beta-antagonist [28]. These changes reflect the small but important reductions in lung volumes secondary to control of airway inflammation. Whether the same change explains the decrease in exacerbation frequency seen with anti-inflammatory drugs is less clear. Recent data about a combination of a once-daily inhaled corticosteroid and LABA showed that exacerbation rates can be reduced even in the absence of changes in FEV1 [29], suggesting that anti-inflammatories may not simply work by modifying lung mechanics.

20.2　Current Treatment Approaches in COPD

The pharmacological management of acute exacerbations has not changed over the last decade. Patients received increased doses of both short-acting beta-antagonists and antimuscarinic often given from a wet nebuliser when they attend a hospital. Oral corticosteroids accelerate the rate of recovery from the exacerbation and reduce the chances of early relapse [30, 31] with doses of 30 mg prednisolone or equivalent being given for 7–10 days. Antibiotics in patients reporting cough and increased

Fig. 20.2 A multicomponent COPD assessment. When assessing risk, choose the highest risk according to GOLD spirometric grade or exacerbation history (Reproduced from Ref. [5] with permission)

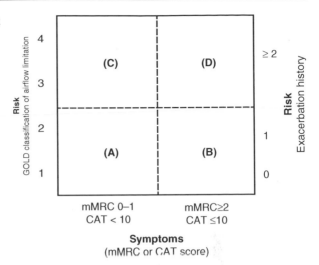

sputum volume and breathlessness reduce the duration of the events, irrespective of the background treatment [32]. However, adding parenteral theophylline has no beneficial effects and may be harmful.

Approaches to chronic management have changed and are no longer driven exclusively by relating treatment to the FEV₁, although lung function remains an important consideration in treatment choices. Two rather different management algorithms have been proposed. The GOLD group now suggests that patients should be classified by combining information about the intensity of their symptoms (normally evaluated by the MRC breathlessness score and/or the COPD assessment test [CAT]), together with information about the risk of future events (assessed by the post-bronchodilator FEV1 and the prior exacerbation history). This scheme is described in Fig. 20.2.

By contrast, NICE (like the ATS/ERS guidelines [1] and using formal evidence-based review) proposes that patients should be stratified by whether their initial FEV₁ is above or below 50 % of predicted and therapy assigned accordingly.

In practice, the first-line choices of the different approaches are very similar and can be summarised as:

GOLD group A – Short-acting inhaled bronchodilators to relieve symptoms. This is equivalent to the first step in the NICE guidelines.

GOLD group B – Long-acting inhaled bronchodilators as monotherapy. This corresponds to the second step in NICE for patients with an FEV₁ above 50 % predicted. There are now good data to suggest that once-daily tiotropium is better than twice-daily salmeterol [21], but whether this is a pharmacological effect or simply the result of the longer duration of action of tiotropium is unclear. This issue is likely to be resolved when more data about truly once-daily LABAs such as indacaterol, which has already been shown to produce equivocal changes to tiotropium in lung function [33], becomes available.

GOLD group C – These patients with relatively few symptoms but worse lung function and/or exacerbation history appear to be infrequent in hospital practice [34] but form a significant component of the COPD population in the community. Here, either type of inhaled long-acting bronchodilator would be appropriate, with a marginal preference for LAMA.

GOLD group D – This forms the commonest group in hospital practice, and here either LAMA or a combination of LABA and ICS would be first-line treatment. There is somewhat more evidence in favour of combination treatment based on secondary outcomes and the one clinical trial which conducted a head-to-head comparison in this group of patients [35].

20.3　Practical Issues

Although there are good data to support all of the above approaches, no therapy for COPD abolishes symptoms and/or exacerbations in every subject. In general, treatment decreases the magnitude of these problems, as is shown by data with roflumilast, which illustrates the conversion of frequent exacerbators to individuals who are less frequent exacerbators [36]. Realistic alternative treatments in patients, who continue to have troublesome symptoms, have been recommended by NICE. For patients with an FEV_1 of above 50 % predicted, they advise adding a second inhaled bronchodilator. The evidence for this was initially rather weak but recently has been strengthened by data with a new once-daily combination of indacaterol and glycopyrronium, which improves lung function better than either of the components of 12 weeks [37] and which is better than either of its component drugs at preventing exacerbations in more severe disease [38]. In patients with an FEV_1 up to 60 % predicted, reanalysis of the TORCH data has shown benefits of an LABA/ICS combination on both lung function and the rate of exacerbations [39]. For those patients whose FEV_1 is below 50 % predicted, but still have problems, triple treatment with an LAMA/LABA and ICS is associated with few exacerbations and morning symptoms [40]. Whether roflumilast helps this group of patients is less clear and a clinical trial to resolve this issue is under way [41]. However, for patients who do not wish to use inhaled corticosteroids and have a history of bronchitis, this PDE4 inhibitor is a useful alternative treatment [42].

Why treatment is unexpectedly ineffective has been little studied. The interaction between the behaviour of the chest wall and lungs is likely to be significant, at least in terms of bronchodilator actions. In general, patients with COPD increase the EELV during exercise as a result of the increased breathing frequency and the presence of tidal flow limitation. In most patients, the chest wall also hyperinflates to accommodate the increased lung volume [43]. This is not the response of the chest wall during exercise in healthy subjects where volume tends to decrease [44]. We have shown that some subjects who decrease their lung volumes after bronchodilators seem to adopt a more normal chest wall response, which is disadvantageous, because they still show lung hyperinflation [45] (Fig. 20.3). Whether this pattern of behaviour persists, or the patient adapts to it with repeated dosing, has not been established, but it does explain why some patients report that they are not helped by the bronchodilator treatment, even though the lung function appears to improve.

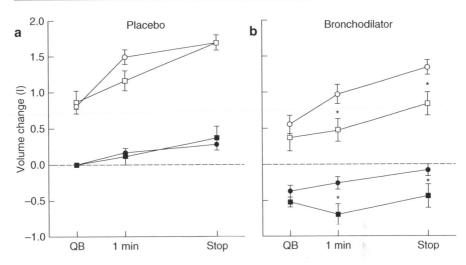

Fig. 20.3 Changes in end-expiratory chest wall volumes (*closed symbols*) and end-inspiratory volumes (*open symbols*) after (**a**) placebo and (**b**) bronchodilator during quiet breathing (*QB*), after 1 min of exercise and in the 30 s before stopping exercise (Stop). The data are divided into those who improved exercise time after bronchodilator (improvers: denoted by circles, $n = 12$) and those who did not (non-improvers: denoted by squares, $n = 6$). All values are referred to end-expiratory volumes during QB after placebo treatment. Data are expressed as mean (SE). *$p < 0.05$ (improvers vs. non-improvers) (Reproduced from Ref. [45] with permission)

Other patients unresponsive to bronchodilators include those whose exercise perfor-mance is limited by leg fatigue [46] reflecting the importance of interaction of hyperinflation and intrinsic cardiac disease and cardiac function. Other treatment approaches directed at these exercise-limiting problems are more likely to be effec-tive than simply relying on improving lung function.

All drug classes have adverse effects, which are well appreciated. The inhaled route is preferred for bronchodilators, as it significantly decreases the incidence of side effects, but beta-antagonists are still associated with tremor, if used excessively, particularly in elderly subjects where they can produce palpitations. Dry mouth and even urinary retention have been reported with regular tiotropium treatment [47]. The inhaled route mitigates many of the anticipated side effects of corticosteroids, particularly osteoporosis and cataracts [48], but pneumonia is more common in patients who take inhaled corticosteroids, particularly those corticosteroids belong-ing to the fluticasone group [49, 50]. This risk does not seem to be associated with an increase in mortality rate [27] but may reflect the poor resolution of previous COPD exacerbations [50]. This area merits further research if pneumonia is to be effectively prevented.

Despite concerns about the cardiovascular safety of beta-antagonists, the most recent data is reassuring and suggests that use of this class of agents may be benefi-cial, even in those with a history of myocardial infarction [51]. Similar concerns are being raised around antimuscarinic drugs, but the data reported by the large 4-year UPLIFT study is reassuring [52]. Recent further anxieties about cardiovascular mortality have been discussed in connection with the soft mist inhalation device used to deliver tiotropium [53]. A large clinical trial to assess the safety of this treatment is due to report in 2003 [54].

20.4   Future Developments

Despite hopes for more dramatic disease-modifying treatments in COPD, none of the candidate drugs have so far progressed to large-scale clinical trials. At present, most attention has been focused on once-daily inhaled treatments, with members of the existing bronchodilator classes, alone or in combination or together with corticosteroids. Additionally, the twice-daily drug aclidinium bromide also shows promise [55] and is now being tested in combination with formoterol. Small improvements in overall outcomes appear possible with these treatments, although the gains compared with earlier treatments are likely to be modest. Exacerbation prevention without modifying lung mechanics is possible by giving long-term antibiotics such as azithromycin [56], but whether this drug should be used widely is uncertain, given the potential impact on antimicrobial resistance.

New agents such as MAP kinase antagonists and biological treatments are under tests at present and may yet change our approaches to COPD management. However, for the time being, we are likely to get most gains by effectively using the treatments which have already been developed, rather than seeing new agents, with which to manage this disease.

References

1. Celli BR, MacNee W (2004) Standards for the diagnosis and treatment of patients with COPD: a summary of the ATS/ERS position paper. Eur Respir J 23(6):932–946
2. National Collaborating Centre for Chronic Conditions (2004) Chronic obstructive pulmonary disease. National clinical guideline on management of chronic obstructive pulmonary disease in adults in primary and secondary care. Thorax 59(Suppl 1):1–232
3. Pauwels RA, Buist AS, Calverley PMA, Jenkins CR, Hurd SS (2001) Global strategy for the diagnosis, management and prevention of chronic obstructive pulmonary disease. Am J Respir Crit Care Med 163:1256–1276
4. O'Reilly J, Jones MM, Parnham J, Lovibond K, Rudolf M (2010) Management of stable chronic obstructive pulmonary disease in primary and secondary care: summary of updated NICE guidance. BMJ 340:c3134. doi:10.1136/bmj.c3134.:c3134
5. Vestbo J, Hurd SS, Agusti AG, Jones PW, Vogelmeier C, Anzueto A et al (2012) Global strategy for the diagnosis, management and prevention of chronic obstructive pulmonary disease, GOLD executive summary. Am J Respir Crit Care Med 187(4):347–365
6. Macklem PT (2010) Therapeutic implications of the pathophysiology of COPD. Eur Respir J 35(3):676–680
7. Calverley PM, Koulouris NG (2005) Flow limitation and dynamic hyperinflation: key concepts in modern respiratory physiology. Eur Respir J 25(1):186–199
8. O'Donnell DE, Laveneziana P, Ora J, Webb KA, Lam YM, Ofir D (2009) Evaluation of acute bronchodilator reversibility in patients with symptoms of GOLD stage I COPD. Thorax 64(3): 216–223

9. Laveneziana P, Webb KA, Ora J, Wadell K, O'Donnell DE (2011) Evolution of dyspnea during exercise in chronic obstructive pulmonary disease: impact of critical volume constraints. Am J Respir Crit Care Med 184(12):1367–1373

10. Parshall MB, Schwartzstein RM, Adams L, Banzett RB, Manning HL, Bourbeau J et al (2012) An official American Thoracic Society statement: update on the mechanisms, assessment, and management of dyspnea. Am J Respir Crit Care Med 185(4):435–452

11. Parker CM, Voduc N, Aaron SD, Webb KA, O'Donnell DE (2005) Physiological changes during symptom recovery from moderate exacerbations of COPD. Eur Respir J 26(3):420–428

12. Stevenson NJ, Walker PP, Costello RW, Calverley PM (2005) Lung mechanics and dyspnea during exacerbations of chronic obstructive pulmonary disease. Am J Respir Crit Care Med 172(12):1510–1516

13. Newton MF, O'Donnell DE, Forkert L (2002) Response of lung volumes to inhaled salbutamol in a large population of patients with severe hyperinflation. Chest 121(4):1042–1050. JID – 0231335

14. O'Donnell DE, Voduc N, Fitzpatrick M, Webb KA (2004) Effect of salmeterol on the ventilatory response to exercise in chronic obstructive pulmonary disease. Eur Respir J 24(1): 86–94

15. O'Donnell DE, Fluge T, Gerken F, Hamilton A, Webb K, Aguilaniu B et al (2004) Effects of tiotropium on lung hyperinflation, dyspnoea and exercise tolerance in COPD. Eur Respir J 23(6):832–840

16. Hadcroft J, Calverley PM (2001) Alternative methods for assessing bronchodilator reversibility in chronic obstructive pulmonary disease. Thorax 56(9):713–720

17. Dellaca RL, Pompilio PP, Walker PR, Duffy N, Pedotti A, Calverley PM (2009) Effect of bronchodilatation on expiratory flow limitation and resting lung mechanics in COPD. Eur Respir J 33(6):1329–1337

18. Aliverti A, Dellaca R, Pelosi P, Chiumello D, Pedotti A, Gattinoni L (2000) Optoelectronic plethysmography in intensive care patients. Am J Respir Crit Care Med 161(5):1546–1552

19. Wedzicha JA, Seemungal TA (2007) COPD exacerbations: defining their cause and prevention. Lancet 370(9589):786–796

20. Niewoehner DE, Rice K, Cote C, Paulson D, Cooper JA Jr, Korducki L et al (2005) Prevention of exacerbations of chronic obstructive pulmonary disease with tiotropium, a once-daily inhaled anticholinergic bronchodilator: a randomized trial. Ann Intern Med 143(5):317–326

21. Vogelmeier C, Hederer B, Glaab T, Schmidt H, Rutten-van Molken MP, Beeh KM et al (2011) Tiotropium versus salmeterol for the prevention of exacerbations of COPD. N Engl J Med 364(12): 1093–1103

22. Spencer S, Calverley PM, Burge PS, Jones PW (2004) Impact of preventing exacerbations on deterioration of health status in COPD. Eur Respir J 23(5):698–702

23. Khoukaz G, Gross NJ (1999) Effects of salmeterol on arterial blood gases in patients with stable chronic obstructive pulmonary disease. Comparison with albuterol and ipratropium. Am J Respir Crit Care Med 160(3):1028–1030

24. MacNee W, Wathen CG, Hannan WJ, Flenley DC, Muir AL (1983) Effects of pirbuterol and sodium nitroprusside on pulmonary haemodynamics in hypoxic cor pulmonale. Br Med J (Clin Res Ed) 287(6400):1169–1172

25. Calverley P, Pauwels R, Vestbo J, Jones P, Pride N, Gulsvik A et al (2003) Combined salmeterol and fluticasone in the treatment of chronic obstructive pulmonary disease: a randomised controlled trial. Lancet 361(9356):449–456

26. Calverley PM, Rabe KF, Goehring UM, Kristiansen S, Fabbri LM, Martinez FJ (2009) Roflumilast in symptomatic chronic obstructive pulmonary disease: two randomised clinical trials. Lancet 374(9691):685–694

27. Calverley PM, Anderson JA, Celli B, Ferguson GT, Jenkins C, Jones PW et al (2007) Salmeterol and fluticasone propionate and survival in chronic obstructive pulmonary disease. N Engl J Med 356(8):775–789

28. O'Donnell DE, Sciurba F, Celli B, Mahler DA, Webb KA, Kalberg CJ et al (2006) Effect of fluticasone propionate/salmeterol on lung hyperinflation and exercise endurance in COPD. Chest 130(3):647–656

29. Dransfield MT, Bourbeau J, Jones PW, Hanania NA, Mahler DA, Vestbo J et al (2013) Once-daily inhaled fluticasone furoate and vilanterol versus vilanterol only for prevention of exacerbations of COPD: two replicate double-blind, parallel-group, randomised controlled trials. Lancet Respir Med 1(3):210–223

30. Davies L, Angus RM, Calverley PMA (1999) Oral corticosteroids in patients admitted to hospital with exacerbations of chronic obstructive pulmonary disease: a prospective randomised controlled trial. Lancet 354(9177):456–460

31. Niewoehner DE, Erbland ML, Deupree RH, Collins D, Gross NJ et al (1999) Effect of systemic glucocorticoids on exacerbations of chronic obstructive pulmonary disease. N Engl J Med 340(25):1941–1947

32. Daniels JM, Snijders D, de Graaff CS, Vlaspolder F, Jansen HM, Boersma WG (2010) Antibiotics in addition to systemic corticosteroids for acute exacerbations of chronic obstructive pulmonary disease. Am J Respir Crit Care Med 181(2):150–157

33. Donohue JF, Fogarty C, Lotvall J, Mahler DA, Worth H, Yorgancioglu A et al (2010) Once-daily bronchodilators for chronic obstructive pulmonary disease: indacaterol versus tiotropium. Am J Respir Crit Care Med 182(2):155–162

34. Han MK, Muellerova H, Curran-Everett D, Dransfield MT, Washko G, Regan EA et al (2013) GOLD 2011 disease severity classification in COPDGene:a prospective cohort study. c Respir Med 1:43–49

35. Wedzicha JA, Calverley PM, Seemungal TA, Hagan G, Ansari Z, Stockley RA (2008) The prevention of chronic obstructive pulmonary disease exacerbations by salmeterol/fluticasone propionate or tiotropium bromide. Am J Respir Crit Care Med 177(1):19–26

36. Wedzicha JA, Decramer M, Seemungal TA (2012) The role of bronchodilator treatment in the prevention of exacerbations of COPD. Eur Respir J 40(6):1545–1554

37. Vogelmeier C, Bateman ED, Pallante J, Allagappan VKT, Andrea P, Chen H et al (2013) Efficacy and safety of once-daily QVA149 compared with twice-daily salmeterol–fluticasone in patients with chronic obstructive pulmonary disease (ILLUMINATE): a randomised, double-blind, parallel group study. Lancet Respir Med 1:51–60

38. Wedzicha JA, Decramer M, Ficker JH, Niewoehner DE, Sandstrom T, Taylor AF et al (2013) Analysis of chronic obstructive pulmonary disease exacerbations with the dual bronchodilator QVA149 compared with glycopyrronium and tiotropium (SPARK): a randomised, double-blind, parallel-group study. Lancet Respir Med 1(3):199–209

39. Jenkins CR, Jones PW, Calverley PM, Celli B, Anderson JA, Ferguson GT et al (2009) Efficacy of salmeterol/fluticasone propionate by GOLD stage of chronic obstructive pulmonary disease: analysis from the randomised, placebo-controlled TORCH study. Respir Res 10:59

40. Welte T, Miravitlles M, Hernandez P, Eriksson G, Peterson S, Polanowski T et al (2009) Efficacy and tolerability of budesonide/formoterol added to tiotropium in patients with chronic obstructive pulmonary disease. Am J Respir Crit Care Med 180(8):741–750

41. Calverley PM, Martinez FJ, Fabbri LM, Goehring UM, Rabe KF (2012) Does roflumilast decrease exacerbations in severe COPD patients not controlled by inhaled combination therapy? The REACT study protocol. Int J Chron Obstruct Pulmon Dis 7:375–382. doi:10.2147/COPD.S31100. Epub;%2012 Jun;%20

42. Bateman ED, Rabe KF, Calverley PM, Goehring UM, Brose M, Bredenbroker D et al (2011) Roflumilast with long-acting beta2-agonists for COPD: influence of exacerbation history. Eur Respir J 38(3):553–560

43. Calverley PM (2006) Dynamic hyperinflation: is it worth measuring? Proc Am Thorac Soc 3(3):239–244

44. Aliverti A, Cala SJ, Duranti R, Ferrigno G, Kenyon CM, Pedotti A et al (1997) Human respiratory muscle actions and control during exercise. J Appl Physiol 83(4):1256–1269

45. Aliverti A, Rodger K, Dellaca RL, Stevenson N, Lo MA, Pedotti A et al (2005) Effect of salbutamol on lung function and chest wall volumes at rest and during exercise in COPD. Thorax 60(11):916–924

46. Pepin V, Saey D, Whittom F, LeBlanc P, Maltais F (2005) Walking versus cycling: sensitivity to bronchodilation in chronic obstructive pulmonary disease. Am J Respir Crit Care Med 172(12):1517–1522

47. Stephenson A, Seitz D, Bell CM, Gruneir A, Gershon AS, Austin PC et al (2011) Inhaled anticholinergic drug therapy and the risk of acute urinary retention in chronic obstructive pulmonary disease: a population-based study. Arch Intern Med 171(10):914–920

48. Ferguson GT, Calverley PM, Anderson JA, Jenkins CR, Jones PW, Willits LR et al (2009) Prevalence and progression of osteoporosis in patients with COPD: results from the TOwards a Revolution in COPD Health study. Chest 136(6):1456–1465

49. Crim C, Calverley PM, Anderson JA, Celli B, Ferguson GT, Jenkins C et al (2009) Pneumonia risk in COPD patients receiving inhaled corticosteroids alone or in combination: TORCH study results. Eur Respir J 34(3):641–647

50. Calverley PM, Stockley RA, Seemungal TA, Hagan G, Willits LR, Riley JH et al (2011) Reported pneumonia in patients with COPD: findings from the INSPIRE study. Chest 139(3):505–512

51. Calverley PM, Anderson JA, Celli B, Ferguson GT, Jenkins C, Jones PW et al (2010) Cardiovascular events in patients with COPD: TORCH study results. Thorax 65(8):719–725

52. Celli B, Decramer M, Kesten S, Liu D, Mehra S, Tashkin DP (2010) Mortality in the 4 year trial of tiotropium (UPLIFT) in patients with COPD. Am J Respir Crit Care Med 182:948–955

53. Singh S, Loke YK, Enright PL, Furberg CD (2011) Mortality associated with tiotropium mist inhaler in patients with chronic obstructive pulmonary disease: systematic review and meta-analysis of randomised controlled trials. BMJ 342:d3215. doi:10.1136/bmj.d3215.:d3215

54. Wise RA, Anzueto A, Calverley P, Dahl R, Dusser D, Pledger G et al (2013) The Tiotropium Safety and Performance in Respimat(R) Trial (TIOSPIR(R)), a large scale, randomized, controlled, parallel-group trial-design and rationale. Respir Res 14:40. doi:10.1186/1465-9921-14-40

55. Jones PW, Singh D, Bateman ED, Agusti A, Lamarca R, de Miquel G et al (2012) Efficacy and safety of twice-daily aclidinium bromide in COPD patients: the ATTAIN study. Eur Respir J 40(4):830–836

56. Albert RK, Connett J, Bailey WC, Casaburi R, Cooper JA Jr, Criner GJ et al (2011) Azithromycin for prevention of exacerbations of COPD. N Engl J Med 365(8):689–698

Respiratory and Non-respiratory Muscle Dysfunction in COPD

21

Didier Saey, Marc-André Caron, Richard Debigaré, and François Maltais

21.1 Introduction

Chronic obstructive pulmonary disease (COPD) is a multisystemic disease where exercise intolerance is a common feature and has a profound impact on the quality of life. Exercise intolerance in patients with COPD results from a complex interplay of central and peripheral factors in which both respiratory [1] and limb [2, 3] muscle dysfunction could significantly contribute. Dysfunction of respiratory and limb muscles is recognized as a major systemic manifestation of COPD [4]. Interestingly, adaptation of limb muscles in response to COPD differs from adaptation of respiratory muscles [5]. The aim of this chapter is to summarize the current knowledge on the structural and functional adaptations of both muscle groups in response to COPD.

21.2 Structural and Functional Alterations in Respiratory and Limb Muscles

Several structural and functional alterations affect both respiratory and limb muscles. It should be noted that most of the data published on the skeletal muscle adaptations in COPD have been obtained by studying the diaphragm and the *vastus lateralis*. This section will therefore focus on the adaptations reported in these two muscles and, when data are available, will provide insights on the situation observed in other muscles.

D. Saey • M.-A. Caron • R. Debigaré • F. Maltais (✉)
Department of Respiratory, Institut Universitaire de Cardiologie et de Pneumologie de Québec, 2725, chemin Sainte-Foy, Quebec City, QC G1V 4G5, Canada
e-mail: didier.saey@criucpq.ulaval.ca; marc-andre.caron@criucpq.ulaval.ca; richard.debigare@rea.ulaval.ca; francois.maltais@fmed.ulaval.ca

A. Aliverti, A. Pedotti (eds.), *Mechanics of Breathing*,
DOI 10.1007/978-88-470-5647-3_21, © Springer-Verlag Italia 2014

21.2.1 Structural Alterations

21.2.1.1 Muscle Mass

Approximately 15 % of COPD patients present a reduced whole body muscle mass, as defined by a fat-free mass index (FFMI) <14.62 m^2 in women and <17.05 kg/m^2 in men [6]. The reduction in muscle mass is more frequent in the severe stage of the disease but can be observed as early as in GOLD I stage [6]. Muscle mass decline may occur independently of body mass index (BMI), since a proportion of COPD patients exhibit lowered FFMI despite a normal BMI [6, 7].

Respiratory Muscles

Diaphragm muscle mass is difficult to quantify directly in living human subjects. Diaphragm fiber cross-sectional area (CSA) is reduced by 40–60 % in patients with severe COPD [8]. Patients with mild-to-moderate COPD present a 30 % reduction in myosin heavy chain content isolated from diaphragm samples [9], suggesting that an atrophic process or at least a change in the morphology of this muscle is occurring early in the development of COPD. The CSA of type I diaphragm fibers is decreased in patients with COPD compared to subjects with normal lung function [10]. This finding is not universal to all respiratory muscles since parasternal intercostal muscle does not present a decreased fiber size in COPD [11]. However, patients with COPD and frequent exacerbations (4 or more in the past 12 months) exhibit a decline in the intercostal and abdominal muscles' CSA, as measured by computed tomography, when compared to patients with COPD without frequent exacerbations (first hospital admission) [12]. Finally, sternocleidomastoid muscle CSA is equivalent when patients with severe COPD are compared to age-matched subjects with normal lung function [13].

Limb Muscles

It is reported that 15–20 % of moderate COPD patients present a reduced mid-thigh CSA when compared to age-matched controls [14, 15]. Similarly, about 20–25 % of *vastus lateralis* muscle fibers present a reduced CSA in COPD patients [16]. Quadriceps *rectus femoris* CSA is also reduced in all the severity stages of COPD when compared to age-matched healthy controls [17]. This decreased fiber CSA can be observed in all muscle fiber types [18], although type IIa and IIx fibers appear to be preferably impaired [16, 19].

21.2.1.2 Shift in Fiber-Type Distribution

Respiratory Muscles

A muscle fiber-type shift, in favor of type I fibers, is observed in the diaphragm of severe COPD patients [8]. The increased proportion of type I fibers is correlated with disease severity [10] and can be observed even in mild-to-moderate COPD patients [20]. A fiber-type shift is also observed in accessory respiratory muscles. In fact, parasternal intercostal muscles exhibit increased proportion of type I fibers in COPD patients [11] while external intercostal muscles present increased proportion of type II fibers. However, this latter finding is not universal, since others have reported a similar myosin heavy chain isoforms proportion in external intercostal muscle when comparing severe COPD patients and control subjects [21].

Limb Muscles

A shift in fiber-type proportion is consistently observed in the quadriceps of patients with COPD. Whereas healthy subjects present a decreased proportion of type II fibers with aging [22], patients with COPD exhibit a decreased proportion of oxidative type I fibers in favor of type IIx glycolytic fibers [18, 23]. The magnitude in this fiber shift reported in quadriceps correlates with disease severity [24]. Interestingly, this fiber shift is not observed in the deltoid, an upper body muscle [25].

21.2.1.3 Capillarization

Capillarization is an essential component of the body's oxygen delivery system. Adequate capillary network ensures proper blood distribution throughout muscle tissue and, ultimately, adequate oxygen delivery to individual myofibers. Sufficient oxygen delivery is essential to ensure an optimal muscle function.

Respiratory Muscles

The capillary network is expanded in the diaphragm of patients with COPD as supported by the observation of an enhanced number of capillaries per fiber on all fiber types in these individuals [20].

Limb Muscles

In absolute number, the amount of capillaries is decreased in the *vastus lateralis* of patients with COPD [18]. However, when considering the number of capillaries per fiber, the ratio is typically comparable between healthy subjects and patients with COPD [18]. Interestingly, patients with COPD who develop quadriceps muscle fatigue after a submaximal exercise exhibit fewer capillaries per fiber in the *vastus lateralis* compared to patients with COPD that do not experience fatigue in the same conditions [26].

21.2.1.4 Contractility

Respiratory Muscles

It is unclear if a defect in the contractile apparatus is present in the diaphragm of patients with COPD. The average and maximal tensions produced by isolated diaphragm fibers are similar when patients with COPD of all GOLD stages and healthy subjects are compared [10]. On the contrary, a reduced passive tension is reported in diaphragm muscle fibers isolated from patients with mild COPD [27]. In the same line, these fibers display a reduced sensitivity to calcium, a parameter that likely results in a reduced force generation [9].

Limb Muscles

Muscle bundles isolated from the *vastus lateralis* of patients with COPD and healthy subjects exhibit similar maximum tetanic tensions, indicating that its contractile properties are preserved in COPD [28]. In support of this finding, the ratio of quadriceps strength over muscle CSA is preserved in COPD when compared to healthy subjects [14]. This may not be the case in patients chronically exposed to systemic corticosteroids [29].

21.2.1.5 Metabolic and Mitochondrial Alterations

Respiratory Muscles

In accordance with the predominance of type I fiber proportion in the diaphragm of patients with COPD, an increase in oxidative enzyme activity along with a decrease in glycolytic enzyme activity are reported [20, 30]. In patients with moderate [31] and severe [21] COPD, increased mitochondrial respiratory chain capacity has been observed in the diaphragm when compared to healthy subjects. This finding is also reported in external intercostal muscle of patients with severe COPD [21].

Limb Muscles

The activity of a number of oxidative enzymes is decreased in the *vastus lateralis* of patients with COPD. Although conflictual data exist concerning cytochrome c oxidase activity [32, 33], hydroxyacyl-coenzyme A dehydrogenase (HADH) and citrate synthase enzymatic activities are all lower in COPD when compared to healthy population [34–36]. Interestingly, oxidative enzyme activities are reduced in type IIa fibers isolated from the *vastus lateralis* of patients with COPD compared to healthy subjects [37]. Glycolytic enzyme activity is not clearly modulated in the *vastus lateralis* in COPD, but when oxidative-to-glycolytic enzymatic ratios are considered, a glycolytic-dominant metabolism is observed in COPD [34, 36].

A reduction in the number of mitochondria per μm^2 of fiber is found in the *vastus lateralis* and the *tibialis anterior* of patients with COPD when compared to age-matched controls [24]. Furthermore, a decreased expression of mitochondrial transcription factor A (TFAM) and proliferator-activated receptor-γ coactivator (PGC-1α), two important contributors in mitochondria biogenesis, is found in the *vastus lateralis* of patients with COPD [38]. Interestingly, the respiratory properties of individual mitochondria isolated from the *vastus lateralis* are similar between patients with COPD and healthy individuals [39], indicating that the impaired oxidative capacity of the *vastus lateralis* is the result of a decrease in the density of the mitochondria rather than a functional defect in these organelles.

21.2.2 Functional Alterations

Strength, endurance, and resistance to fatigue, the main muscle function components [40], are commonly decreased in patients with COPD [4], but there are substantial differences between respiratory and non-respiratory muscles.

21.2.2.1 Respiratory Muscles

Respiratory muscle dysfunction is a cardinal feature of acute and chronic respiratory failure and is frequently observed in patients with COPD [41–43]. Hypercapnic respiratory failure due to respiratory muscle weakness [2, 44] is associated with morbidity in patients with COPD [45], and maximum inspiratory pressure is an independent determinant of survival in these patients [46]. Moreover, respiratory muscle dysfunction has been associated with an increased risk for repeated hospital admissions [47].

Due to increased lung resistance and elastance, as well as an amplified ventilatory demand in COPD, the diaphragm and the accessory inspiratory muscles face chronic increased load. Given its role as the primary inspiratory muscle, the majority of studies have focused on the diaphragm. However, when the ventilatory demand increases as a result of aging, respiratory diseases, and/or exercise, the accessory respiratory muscles, such as the intercostal and scalene muscles, contribute in a progressive manner to the breathing effort [48–50]. Despite their relevance, limited data on accessory respiratory muscle function are available.

Patients with COPD generate lower maximal inspiratory and transdiaphragmatic pressures through voluntary maneuvers but also when induced by phrenic nerve electrical or magnetic stimulation when compared to healthy subjects [42, 43, 51–53]. The decrease in diaphragmatic force has been attributed to two main factors. First, hyperinflation-induced diaphragm shortening places the diaphragm at a mechanical disadvantage [1]. Second, a shorter length of the diaphragmatic fibers [54] makes the diaphragm contracting on the ascending branch of its length-tension relationship. However, when corrected for reduced muscle length, diaphragm strength production is preserved or even increased in patients with severe COPD [42].

Whether the respiratory muscle endurance is altered in COPD is still unclear and, because of technical difficulties, limited data are available. Given the mechanical impairment of inspiratory muscles in COPD, decreased endurance has been suggested to take place in this disease [55]. However, inspiratory muscle endurance during repeated maximal voluntary contractions was found to be slightly superior in patients with severe chronic airflow limitation when compared to healthy subjects [51]. Adaptive response to the chronic respiratory load and the shorter duty cycle was evocated to explain the relative preservation of inspiratory muscle endurance [56]. This is in line with greater oxidative capacity [8, 57, 58] and higher resistance to fatigue of the diaphragm [59, 60]. A qualitative systematic review [61] has shown that overloading of the inspiratory muscles by diverse methods (such as inspiratory resistive loading, whole body exercise, and hyperpnoea under normocapnic, hypoxic, or hypercapnic conditions) can induce muscle fatigue in patients with COPD. However, the extent of muscle fatigue varies widely between studies, ranging from 5 to 67 %, and the functional significance of inspiratory muscle fatigue is still unclear [61].

Although expiration is normally a passive process, air exhalation can be facilitated by the contraction of other muscle groups, including those of the abdominal wall and the internal intercostal muscles. Patients with COPD exhibit a relatively preserved [62] or decreased [41, 63] expiratory muscle strength, as well as reduced expiratory muscle endurance [64]. The latter is decreased proportionally with disease severity in patients with COPD [64].

21.2.2.2 Limb Muscles

A decrease in muscle strength and/or endurance is common in patients with COPD [2, 14, 65–67]. A 15–25 % decline in upper and lower limb muscle strength is usually observed when compared to age-matched healthy subjects [2, 14, 68, 69]. The degree of weakness and reduced endurance vary among muscle groups: Strength and endurance of the upper limb muscles is better preserved than that of the lower

Table 21.1 Evidence of limb and respiratory muscle dysfunction in COPD

Limb	Diaphragm
Structural adaptations	
Muscle atrophy	
↓ Muscle mass	↓ Muscle mass
Morphological changes	
↓ Proportion of type I fibers	↑ Proportion of type I fibers
↑ Proportion of type IIx fibers atrophy of type I and IIa fibers	↓ Proportion of type IIx fibers
↓ Capillarization	↑ Capillarization
Altered metabolic capacity	
↓ Intramuscular pH	↑ Oxidative enzyme activities
↓ ATP concentration	↓ Glycolytic enzyme activities
↑ Muscle lactate concentration	↑ Mitochondrial enzyme activities
↑ Ionosine monophosphate	
↓ Mitochondrial enzyme activities	
Functional adaptations	
↓ Strength	↓ Inspiratory and transdiaphragmatic pressures
↓ Endurance	Preserved or ↓ endurance
↑ Fatigability	Fatigability unclear

limb muscles [14, 51, 68, 70–72]. This heterogeneity in muscle dysfunction between various limb muscles suggests a role for disuse in the development of limb muscle dysfunction in COPD. The similar muscle strength/CSA ratio between patients with COPD and healthy subjects [14] supports the notion that muscle atrophy is the main mechanism of weakness in this disease. However, under certain circumstances such as chronic or repeated exposure to systemic corticosteroids, a reduction in strength that is out of proportion with the degree of atrophy may occur [14, 29].

Quadriceps fatigue is observed in up to 50 % of patients with COPD after a localized exercise [73] or cycling exercise [3, 74, 75]. Although susceptibility to muscle fatigue has been mostly reported in the quadriceps after cycling exercise [75], it has also been observed in plantiflexors and dorsiflexors of the ankle after walking tasks [69]. Muscle fatigue after exercise is not abnormal in itself; the concern in COPD is that fatigue occurs at a much lower intensity than in age-matched healthy subjects [69, 74].

Interestingly, quadriceps strength and muscle CSA are positively correlated with FEV_1 [14]. In addition, quadriceps strength also correlates with exercise capacity and 6 min walking distance [2, 14]. Consequently, along with impaired lung function, patients with COPD have to deal with weaker and fatigue-prone muscles to perform their daily tasks. This situation has direct implications for exercise tolerance. Premature leg fatigue [3, 69, 76], early muscle acidosis [77, 78], and heightened perception of leg fatigue [14, 79] are all mechanisms through which lower limb muscle dysfunction may lead to exercise intolerance in COPD. Moreover, muscle weakness is also associated with other relevant clinical consequences of the disease such as decreased quality of life [80], impaired functional status [14], rate of hospitalization, and utilization of healthcare resources (Table 21.1) [81].

21.3   Etiology of Muscle Dysfunction in COPD

21.3.1 Muscle Disuse

Patients with COPD are less active than age-matched healthy controls [82, 83], and the sedentary lifestyle is already present early in the course of the disease [84]. Inactivity initiates structural and functional modifications that are similar to what is seen in COPD limb muscles, including a decrease in type I muscle fibers, a reduction in oxidative enzymatic capacity, and muscle atrophy [85]. In contrast, the increased activity observed in respiratory muscles is in agreement with the increased type I muscle fiber proportion observed in the diaphragm of patients with COPD. In addition to disuse, multiple evidences support the existence of a myopathy in COPD that could act in synergy with inactivity to further worsen muscle function. For example, training does not improve muscle fiber typing in COPD patients [18], and muscle function is weakly correlated to physical activity level and physical fitness in these patients [86], suggesting that mechanisms other than inactivity are involved in the development of limb muscle dysfunction.

This section proposes a quick overview of the possible implication of the inflammatory response, oxidative stress, medication, hypoxia, low anabolism, and cigarette smoking in the development of muscle dysfunction in COPD.

21.3.2   Inflammatory Response

COPD pathogenesis is associated with a severe inflammatory response in the airways and lungs [87]. Review articles have concluded that the reduction in lung function in COPD is associated with increased levels of circulating inflammatory markers (circulating leukocytes, serum tumor necrosis factor alpha, fibrinogen, and c-reactive protein) [88]. Inflammation by itself can induce skeletal muscle modifications such as atrophy and impaired contractility [89, 90]. Furthermore, systemic inflammation is a risk factor for limb muscle weakness and exercise intolerance in COPD [91, 92]. Interestingly, exacerbation events in COPD are associated with a worsening in systemic inflammatory response [93]. These periods of exacerbation could therefore represent critical events in the progressive development of muscle dysfunction in COPD. At the muscle level, it is not clear whether inflammation is present [94, 95]. Perhaps exacerbation episodes could be key moments where local inflammation is increased.

21.3.3   Oxidative Stress

Oxidative stress results from an imbalance between reactive oxygen species production and the level of antioxidant defenses. Evidence of oxidative stress is found in the *vastus lateralis* and the diaphragm of patients with COPD [96–98]. Oxidative stress can be deleterious for muscle tissue. For instance, it is known to promote protein catabolism [99], a key cell event in skeletal muscle atrophy development, and is also directly associated to muscle endurance in patients with severe COPD [96].

21.3.4 Medication

Prolonged usage of systemic corticosteroid is known to induce myopathy [100]. In COPD, the steroid-induced myopathy is associated with peripheral and respiratory muscle weaknesses, as well as a reduction in quadriceps fiber CSA when compared to healthy subjects and patients with COPD not chronically using corticosteroids [101].

21.3.5 Hypoxia

Chronic exposure to a hypoxic atmosphere induces a significant reduction of the mid-thigh CSA and the *vastus lateralis* muscle CSA in human subjects [102]. Impaired tissue oxygenation or decreased PaO_2 in COPD is associated with lower body weight [103, 104]. Moreover, patients with hypoxemic COPD exhibit evidences of increased oxidative stress in the *vastus lateralis* when compared to non-hypoxemic COPD after a knee extension exercise protocol [105]. In addition, hypoxia can induce an inflammatory response [106, 107] and may promote protein degradation while reducing protein synthesis [5].

21.3.6 Low Anabolism

Low levels of testosterone have been reported in patients with COPD [108, 109]. However, the impact of low testosterone on muscle dysfunction development is unclear since hypogonadism does not further alter limb muscle strength and endurance in patients with COPD [110]. Testosterone can promote muscle hypertrophy by stimulating protein synthesis [111]. When combined to a training program, testosterone therapy appears to increase lean body mass in COPD patients [112].

21.3.7 Cigarette Smoking

Cigarette smoking is the main causal agent of COPD [113]. Interestingly, vastus lateralis muscle specimens sampled from non-COPD smokers exhibit decreased type I fiber proportion along with an increase in glycolytic enzymatic activity [114]. These data show that skeletal muscle from smokers could be already impaired prior to development of COPD.

Figure 21.1 summarizes the main factors involved in muscle adaptations in COPD.

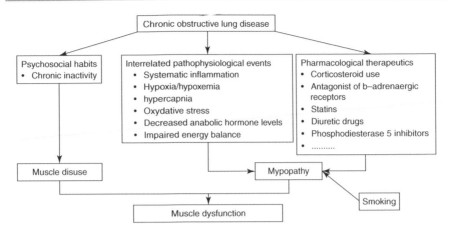

Fig. 21.1 Main factors involved in muscle adaptations in COPD

21.4   Muscle Dysfunction Reversibility

Exercise training does not improve lung function. As a result, other physiological adaptations have to be invoked to explain improvements in exercise capacity and health status occurring after exercise training in COPD. Limb and respiratory muscle adaptations are among these positive modifications.

Exercise training is a powerful intervention to improve limb muscle strength and fatigue susceptibility [115, 116]. This therapy may also prevent further worsening in limb muscle function during an acute exacerbation of the disease [117]. Although most of the studies have focused on lower limbs, emerging literature demonstrates that upper limb muscle training is also efficient in COPD [118, 119]. The response to exercise training is nevertheless heterogeneous in patients with COPD and is commonly smaller compared to what is observed in healthy subjects [120]. Response to exercise at the cellular level is a complex and highly regulated process. Recent literature elegantly demonstrates that metabolic responses [121] and regulation of the cellular stresses after exercise [122, 123] are distinct in lower limb muscle of patients with COPD when compared to healthy subjects. In addition, regenerative capacity could be altered in patients with severe disease and muscle atrophy [124]. Knowledge about the molecular response to exercise training in COPD is at its infancy, but further development on this topic will be instrumental to better understand the impact of COPD on muscle tissue adaptation to training and in designing better training programs.

Various others interventions such as nutritional support, growth hormone and its analogs, antioxidants, and vitamin D supplementation have been investigated for their potential ability to improve muscle mass and function [4]. The actual clinical efficacy and application of these interventions are still uncertain.

Conclusion

Muscle dysfunction is a common manifestation in patients with COPD. Mechanical imbalance due to increased preloads and hyperinflation constitute the main factors contributing to respiratory muscle dysfunction, whereas deconditioning due to reduced physical activity appears to be a significant driver of limb muscle dysfunction. Although disuse plays an important role in muscle dysfunction, it cannot fully explain the muscle adaptations observed in this disease. Many mechanisms including local and systemic factors are likely to be involved in this process. Interestingly, muscle dysfunction is, at least, partially reversible with exercise training. Because of its relevance in chronic respiratory diseases, it is crucial to be able to recognize, characterize, and promote interventions aimed to maintain adequate function in respiratory and limb muscles in these patients.

References

1. Laghi F, Tobin MJ (2003) Disorders of the respiratory muscles. Am J Respir Crit Care Med 168:10–48
2. Gosselink R, Troosters T, Decramer M (1996) Peripheral muscle weakness contributes to exercise limitation in COPD. Am J Respir Crit Care Med 153:976–980
3. Saey D, Debigare R, LeBlanc P, Mador MJ, Cote CH, Jobin J, Maltais F (2003) Contractile leg fatigue after cycle exercise: a factor limiting exercise in patients with chronic obstructive pulmonary disease. Am J Respir Crit Care Med 168:425–430
4. American Thoracic Society/European Respiratory S (1999) Skeletal muscle dysfunction in chronic obstructive pulmonary disease. Am J Respir Crit Care Med 159:S1–S40
5. Caron MA, Debigare R, Dekhuijzen PN, Maltais F (2009) Comparative assessment of the quadriceps and the diaphragm in patients with COPD. J Appl Physiol 107:952–961
6. Vestbo J, Prescott E, Almdal T, Dahl M, Nordestgaard BG, Andersen T, Sorensen TI, Lange P (2006) Body mass, fat-free body mass, and prognosis in patients with chronic obstructive pulmonary disease from a random population sample: findings from the Copenhagen City Heart study. Am J Respir Crit Care Med 173:79–83
7. Vermeeren MA, Creutzberg EC, Schols AM, Postma DS, Pieters WR, Roldaan AC, Wouters EF (2006) Prevalence of nutritional depletion in a large out-patient population of patients with COPD. Respir Med 100:1349–1355
8. Levine S, Kaiser L, Leferovich J, Tikunov B (1997) Cellular adaptation in the diaphragm in chronic obstructive pulmonary disease. N Engl J Med 337:1799–1806
9. Ottenheijm CA, Heunks LM, Sieck GC, Zhan WZ, Jansen SM, Degens H, de Boo T, Dekhuijzen PN (2005) Diaphragm dysfunction in chronic obstructive pulmonary disease. Am J Respir Crit Care Med 172:200–205
10. Stubbings AK, Moore AJ, Dusmet M, Goldstraw P, West TG, Polkey MI, Ferenczi MA (2008) Physiological properties of human diaphragm muscle fibres and the effect of chronic obstructive pulmonary disease. J Physiol 586:2637–2650
11. Levine S, Nguyen T, Friscia M, Zhu J, Szeto W, Kucharczuk JC, Tikunov BA, Rubinstein NA, Kaiser LR, Shrager JB (2006) Parasternal intercostal muscle remodeling in severe chronic obstructive pulmonary disease. J Appl Physiol 101:1297–1302
12. Guerri R, Gayete A, Balcells E, Ramirez-Sarmiento A, Vollmer I, Garcia-Aymerich J, Gea J, Orozco-Levi M (2010) Mass of intercostal muscles associates with risk of multiple exacerbations in COPD. Respir Med 104:378–388
13. Peche R, Estenne M, Gevenois PA, Brassinne E, Yernault JC, De Troyer A (1996) Sternomastoid muscle size and strength in patients with severe chronic obstructive pulmonary disease. Am J Respir Crit Care Med 153:422–425
14. Bernard S, Leblanc P, Whittom F, Carrier G, Jobin J, Belleau R, Maltais F (1998) Peripheral muscle weakness in patients with chronic obstructive pulmonary disease. Am J Respir Crit Care Med 158:629–634

15. Mathur S, Takai KP, Macintyre DL, Reid D (2008) Estimation of thigh muscle mass with magnetic resonance imaging in older adults and people with chronic obstructive pulmonary disease. Phys Ther 88:219–230

16. Natanek SA, Gosker HR, Slot IG, Marsh GS, Hopkinson NS, Man WD, Tal-Singer R, Moxham J, Kemp PR, Schols NM, Polkey MI (2013) Heterogeneity of quadriceps muscle phenotype in chronic obstructive pulmonary disease (COPD): implications for stratified medicine? Muscle Nerve 48(4):488–497

17. Shrikrishna D, Patel M, Tanner RJ, Seymour JM, Connolly BA, Puthucheary ZA, Walsh SL, Bloch SA, Sidhu PS, Hart N, Kemp PR, Moxham J, Polkey MI, Hopkinson NS (2012) Quadriceps wasting and physical inactivity in patients with COPD. Eur Respir J 40:1115–1122

18. Whittom F, Jobin J, Simard PM, Leblanc P, Simard C, Bernard S, Belleau R, Maltais F (1998) Histochemical and morphological characteristics of the vastus lateralis muscle in COPD patients. Comparison with normal subjects and effects of exercise training. Med Sci Sports Exerc 30:1467–1474

19. Gosker HR, Engelen MP, van Mameren H, van Dijk PJ, van der Vusse GJ, Wouters EF, Schols AM (2002) Muscle fiber type IIx atrophy is involved in the loss of fat-free mass in chronic obstructive pulmonary disease. Am J Clin Nutr 76:113–119

20. Doucet M, Debigare R, Joanisse DR, Cote C, Leblanc P, Gregoire J, Deslauriers J, Vaillancourt R, Maltais F (2004) Adaptation of the diaphragm and the vastus lateralis in mild-to-moderate COPD. Eur Respir J 24:971 979

21. Ribera F, N'Guessan B, Zoll J, Fortin D, Serrurier B, Mettauer B, Bigard X, Ventura-Clapier R, Lampert E (2003) Mitochondrial electron transport chain function is enhanced in inspiratory muscles of patients with chronic obstructive pulmonary disease. Am J Respir Crit Care Med 167: 873–879

22. Larsson L (1983) Histochemical characteristics of human skeletal muscle during aging. Acta Physiol Scand 117:469–471

23. Maltais F, Sullivan MJ, Leblanc P, Duscha BD, Schachat FH, Simard C, Blank JM, Jobin J (1999) Altered expression of myosin heavy chain in the vastus lateralis muscle in patients with COPD. Eur Respir J 13:850–854

24. Gosker HR, Hesselink MK, Duimel H, Ward KA, Schols AM (2007) Reduced mitochondrial density in the vastus lateralis muscle of patients with COPD. Eur Respir J 30:73–79

25. Gea J, Orozco-Levi M, Barreiro E, Ferrer A, Broquetas J (2001) Structural and functional changes in the skeletal muscles of COPD patients: the "compartments" theory. Monaldi Arch Chest Dis 56:214–224

26. Saey D, Michaud A, Couillard A, Cote CH, Mador MJ, LeBlanc P, Jobin J, Maltais F (2005) Contractile fatigue, muscle morphometry, and blood lactate in chronic obstructive pulmonary disease. Am J Respir Crit Care Med 171:1109–1115

27. Ottenheijm CA, Heunks LM, Hafmans T, van der Ven PF, Benoist C, Zhou H, Labeit S, Granzier HL, Dekhuijzen PN (2006) Titin and diaphragm dysfunction in chronic obstructive pulmonary disease. Am J Respir Crit Care Med 173:527–534

28. Debigaré R, Cote CH, Hould FS, Leblanc P, Maltais F (2003) In vitro and in vivo contractile properties of the vastus lateralis muscle in males with COPD. Eur Respir J 21:273–278

29. Decramer M, Lacquet LM, Fagard R, Rogiers P (1994) Corticosteroids contribute to muscle weakness in chronic airflow obstruction. Am Rev Respir Dis 150:11–16

30. Levine S, Gregory C, Nguyen T, Shrager J, Kaiser L, Rubinstein N, Dudley G (2002) Bioenergetic adaptation of individual human diaphragmatic myofibers to severe COPD. J Appl Physiol 92:1205–1213

31. Wijnhoven JH, Janssen AJ, van Kuppevelt TH, Rodenburg RJ, Dekhuijzen PN (2006) Metabolic capacity of the diaphragm in patients with COPD. Respir Med 100:1064–1071

32. Puente-Maestu L, Perez-Parra J, Godoy R, Moreno N, Tejedor A, Gonzalez-Aragoneses F, Bravo JL, Alvarez FV, Camano S, Agusti A (2009) Abnormal mitochondrial function in locomotor and respiratory muscles of COPD patients. Eur Respir J 33:1045–1052

33. Sauleda J, García-Palmer F, Wiesner RJ, Tarraga S, Harting I, Tomás P, Gómez C, Saus C, Palou A, Agusí AGN (1998) Cytochrome oxidase activity and mitochondrial gene expression

in skeletal muscle of patients with chronic obstructive pulmonary disease. Am J Respir Crit
Care Med 157:1413–1417

34. Green HJ, Burnett ME, D'Arsigny CL, O'Donnell DE, Ouyang J, Webb KA (2008) Altered
metabolic and transporter characteristics of vastus lateralis in chronic obstructive pulmonary
disease. J Appl Physiol 105:879–886

35. Maltais F, Leblanc P, Whittom F, Simard C, Marquis K, Belanger M, Breton MJ, Jobin
J (2000) Oxidative enzyme activities of the vastus lateralis muscle and the functional status
in patients with COPD. Thorax 55:848–853

36. Maltais F, Simard AA, Simard C, Jobin J, DesgagnÇs P, Leblanc P (1996) Oxidative capacity
of the skeletal muscle and lactic acid kinetics during exercise in normal subjects and in
patients with COPD. Am J Respir Crit Care Med 153:288–293

37. Gosker HR, van Mameren H, van Dijk PJ, Engelen MP, van der Vusse GJ, Wouters EF,
Schols AM (2002) Skeletal muscle fibre-type shifting and metabolic profile in patients with
chronic obstructive pulmonary disease. Eur Respir J 19:617–625

38. Remels AH, Schrauwen P, Broekhuizen R, Willems J, Kersten S, Gosker HR, Schols AM
(2007) Peroxisome proliferator-activated receptor expression is reduced in skeletal muscle in
COPD. Eur Respir J 30:245–252

39. Picard M, Godin R, Sinnreich M, Baril J, Bourbeau J, Perrault H, Taivassalo T, Burelle Y
(2008) The mitochondrial phenotype of peripheral muscle in chronic obstructive pulmonary
disease: disuse or dysfunction? Am J Respir Crit Care Med 178:1040–1047

40. Saey D, Troosters T (2008) Measuring skeletal muscle strength and endurance, from bench
to bedside. Clin Invest Med 31:E307–E311

41. Rochester DF, Braun NM, Arora NS (1979) Respiratory muscle strength in chronic obstructive pulmonary disease. Am Rev Respir Dis 119:151–154

42. Similowski T, Yan S, Gauthier AP, Macklem PT, Bellemare F (1991) Contractile properties
of the human diaphragm during chronic hyperinflation. N Engl J Med 325:917–923

43. Bellemare F, Cordeau MP, Couture J, Lafontaine E, Leblanc P, Passerini L (2002) Effects of
emphysema and lung volume reduction surgery on transdiaphragmatic pressure and diaphragm length. Chest 121:1898–1910

44. Begin P, Grassino A (1991) Inspiratory muscle dysfunction and chronic hypercapnia in
chronic obstructive pulmonary disease. Am Rev Respir Dis 143:905–912

45. Zielinski J, MacNee W, Wedzicha J, Ambrosino N, Braghiroli A, Dolensky J, Howard P,
Gorzelak K, Lahdensuo A, Strom K, Tobiasz M, Weitzenblum E (1997) Causes of death in
patients with COPD and chronic respiratory failure. Monaldi Arch Chest Dis 52:43–47

46. Gray-Donald K, Gibbons L, Shapiro SH, Macklem PT, Martin JG (1996) Nutritional status and
mortality in chronic obstructive pulmonary disease. Am J Respir Crit Care Med 153:961–966

47. Vilaro J, Ramirez-Sarmiento A, Martinez-Llorens JM, Mendoza T, Alvarez M, Sanchez-
Cayado N, Vega A, Gimeno E, Coronell C, Gea J, Roca J, Orozco-Levi M (2010) Global
muscle dysfunction as a risk factor of readmission to hospital due to COPD exacerbations.
Respir Med 104:1896–1902

48. Casadevall C, Coronell C, Ramirez-Sarmiento AL, Martinez-Llorens J, Barreiro E, Orozco-
Levi M, Gea J (2007) Upregulation of pro-inflammatory cytokines in the intercostal muscles
of COPD patients. Eur Respir J 30:701–707

49. DiMarco AF, Romaniuk JR, Supinski GS (1992) Parasternal and external intercostal
responses to various respiratory maneuvers. J Appl Physiol 73:979–986

50. Duiverman ML, de Boer EW, van Eykern LA, de Greef MH, Jansen DF, Wempe JB, Kerstjens
HA, Wijkstra PJ (2009) Respiratory muscle activity and dyspnea during exercise in chronic
obstructive pulmonary disease. Respir Physiol Neurobiol 167:195–200

51. Newell SZ, McKenzie DK, Gandevia SC (1989) Inspiratory and skeletal muscle strength and
endurance and diaphragmatic activation in patients with chronic airflow limitation. Thorax
44:903–912

52. Polkey MI, Kyroussis D, Hamnegard CH, Mills GH, Green M, Moxham J (1996) Diaphragm
strength in chronic obstructive pulmonary disease. Am J Respir Crit Care Med 154:
1310–1317

53. Criner G, Cordova FC, Leyenson V, Roy B, Travaline J, Sudarshan S, O'Brien G, Kuzma AM, Furukawa S (1998) Effect of lung volume reduction surgery on diaphragm strength. Am J Respir Crit Care Med 157:1578–1585

54. Cassart M, Pettiaux N, Gevenois PA, Paiva M, Estenne M (1997) Effect of chronic hyperinflation on diaphragm length and surface area. Am J Respir Crit Care Med 156:504–508

55. Klimathianaki M, Vaporidi K, Georgopoulos D (2011) Respiratory muscle dysfunction in COPD: from muscles to cell. Curr Drug Targets 12:478–488

56. Ottenheijm CA, Heunks LM, Dekhuijzen RP (2008) Diaphragm adaptations in patients with COPD. Respir Res 9:12

57. Orozco-Levi M (2003) Structure and function of the respiratory muscles in patients with COPD: impairment or adaptation? Eur Respir J Suppl 46:41s–51s

58. Orozco-Levi M, Gea J, Lloreta JL, Felez M, Minguella J, Serrano S, Broquetas JM (1999) Subcellular adaptation of the human diaphragm in chronic obstructive pulmonary disease. Eur Respir J 13:371–378

59. Polkey MI, Kyroussis D, Hamnegard CH, Mills GH, Hughes PD, Green M, Moxham J (1997) Diaphragm performance during maximal voluntary ventilation in chronic obstructive pulmonary disease. Am J Respir Crit Care Med 155:642–648

60. Mador MJ, Kufel TJ, Pineda LA, Sharma GK (2000) Diaphragmatic fatigue and high-intensity exercise in patients with chronic obstructive pulmonary disease. Am J Respir Crit Care Med 161:118–123

61. Janssens JP, Perrin E, Bennani I, de Muralt B, Titelion V, Picaud C (2001) Is continuous transcutaneous monitoring of pco₂ (tcpco₂) over 8 h reliable in adults? Respir Med 95:331–335

62. Morrison NJ, Richardson J, Dunn L, Pardy RL (1989) Respiratory muscle performance in normal elderly subjects and patients with COPD. Chest 95:90–94

63. Nishimura Y, Tsutsumi M, Nakata H, Tsunenari T, Maeda H, Yokoyama M (1995) Relationship between respiratory muscle strength and lean body mass in men with COPD. Chest 107:1232–1236

64. Ramirez-Sarmiento A, Orozco-Levi M, Barreiro E, Mendez R, Ferrer A, Broquetas J, Gea J (2002) Expiratory muscle endurance in chronic obstructive pulmonary disease. Thorax 57:132–136

65. Serres I, Gautier V, Varray AL, PrÇfaut CG (1998) Impaired skeletal muscle endurance related to physical inactivity and altered lung function in COPD patients. Chest 113:900–905

66. Coronell C, Orozco-Levi M, Mendez R, Ramirez-Sarmiento A, Galdiz JB, Gea J (2004) Relevance of assessing quadriceps endurance in patients with COPD. Eur Respir J 24:129–136

67. Koechlin C, Couillard A, Simar D, Cristol JP, Bellet H, Hayot M, Prefaut C (2004) Does oxidative stress alter quadriceps endurance in chronic obstructive pulmonary disease? Am J Respir Crit Care Med 169:1022–1027

68. Gosselink R, Troosters T, Decramer M (2000) Distribution of muscle weakness in patients with stable chronic obstructive pulmonary disease. J Cardiopulm Rehabil 20:353–360

69. Gagnon P, Maltais F, Bouyer L, Ribeiro F, Coats V, Brouillard C, Noel M, Rousseau-Gagnon M, Saey D (2013) Distal leg muscle function in patients with COPD. COPD 10:235–242

70. Man WDC, Soliman MGG, Nikoletou D, Harris ML, Rafferty GF, Mustfa N, Polkey MI, Moxham J (2003) Non-volitional assessment of skeletal muscle strength in patients with chronic obstructive pulmonary disease. Thorax 58:665–669

71. Gea JG, Pasto M, Carmona MA, Orozco-Levi M, Palomeque J, Broquetas J (2001) Metabolic characteristics of the deltoid muscle in patients with chronic obstructive pulmonary disease. Eur Respir J 17:939–945

72. Heijdra YF, Pinto-Plata V, Frants R, Rassulo J, Kenney L, Celli BR (2003) Muscle strength and exercise kinetics in COPD patients with a normal fat-free mass index are comparable to control subjects. Chest 124:75–82

73. Mador MJ, Deniz O, Aggarwal A, Kufel TJ (2003) Quadriceps fatigability after single muscle exercise in patients with chronic obstructive pulmonary disease. Am J Respir Crit Care Med 168:102–108

74. Mador MJ, Bozkanat E, Kufel TJ (2003) Quadriceps fatigue after cycle exercise in patients with COPD compared with healthy control subjects. Chest 123:1104–1111

75. Man WDC, Soliman MGG, Gearing J, Radford SG, Rafferty GF, Gray BJ, Polkey MI, Moxham J (2003) Symptoms and quadriceps fatigability after walking and cycling in chronic obstructive pulmonary disease. Am J Respir Crit Care Med 168:562–567

76. Amann M, Regan MS, Kobitary M, Eldridge MW, Boutellier U, Pegelow DF, Dempsey JA (2010) Impact of pulmonary system limitations on locomotor muscle fatigue in patients with COPD. Am J Physiol Regul Integr Comp Physiol 299:R314–R324

77. Casaburi R, Patessio A, Ioli F, Zanaboni S, Donner CF, Wasserman K (1991) Reductions in exercise lactic acidosis and ventilation as a result of exercise training in patients with obstructive lung disease. Am Rev Respir Dis 143:9–18

78. Maltais F, Jobin J, Sullivan MJ, Bernard S, Whittom F, Killian KJ, Desmeules M, BÇlanger M, Leblanc P (1998) Metabolic and hemodynamic responses of the lower limb during exercise in patients with COPD. J Appl Physiol 84:1573–1580

79. Hamilton AL, Killian KJ, Summers E, Jones NL (1995) Muscle strength, symptom intensity and exercise capacity in patients with cardiorespiratory disorders. Am J Respir Crit Care Med 152:2021–2031

80. Mostert R, Goris A, Weling-Scheepers C, Wouters EF, Schols AM (2000) Tissue depletion and health related quality of life in patients with chronic obstructive pulmonary disease. Respir Med 94:859–867

81. Decramer M, Gosselink R, Troosters T, Verschueren M, Evers G (1997) Muscle weakness is related to utilization of health care resources in COPD patients. Eur Respir J 10:417–423

82. Pitta F, Troosters T, Spruit MA, Decramer M, Gosselink R (2005) Activity monitoring for assessment of physical activities in daily life in patients with chronic obstructive pulmonary disease. Arch Phys Med Rehabil 86:1979–1985

83. Pitta F, Troosters T, Spruit MA, Probst VS, Decramer M, Gosselink R (2005) Characteristics of physical activities in daily life in chronic obstructive pulmonary disease. Am J Respir Crit Care Med 171:972–977

84. Troosters T, Sciurba F, Battaglia S, Langer D, Valluri SR, Martino L, Benzo R, Andre D, Weisman I, Decramer M (2010) Physical inactivity in patients with COPD, a controlled multi-center pilot-study. Respir Med 104:1005–1011

85. Franssen FM, Wouters EF, Schols AM (2002) The contribution of starvation, deconditioning and ageing to the observed alterations in peripheral skeletal muscle in chronic organ diseases. Clin Nutr 21:1–14

86. Bossenbroek L, de Greef MH, Wempe JB, Krijnen WP, Ten Hacken NH (2011) Daily physical activity in patients with chronic obstructive pulmonary disease: a systematic review. COPD 8:306–319

87. Tuder RM, Petrache I (2012) Pathogenesis of chronic obstructive pulmonary disease. J Clin Invest 122:2749–2755

88. Gan WQ, Man SFP, Senthilselvan A, Sin DD (2004) Association between chronic obstructive pulmonary disease and systemic inflammation: a systematic review and a meta-analysis. Thorax 59:574–580

89. Cai D, Frantz JD, Tawa NE Jr, Melendez PA, Oh BC, Lidov HG, Hasselgren PO, Frontera WR, Lee J, Glass DJ, Shoelson SE (2004) IKKbeta/NF-kappaB activation causes severe muscle wasting in mice. Cell 119:285–298

90. Wilcox P, Milliken C, Bressler B (1996) High-dose tumor necrosis factor alpha produces an impairment of hamster diaphragm contractility. Attenuation with a prostaglandin inhibitor. Am J Respir Crit Care Med 153:1611–1615

91. Yende S, Waterer GW, Tolley EA, Newman AB, Bauer DC, Taaffe DR, Jensen R, Crapo R, Rubin S, Nevitt M, Simonsick EM, Satterfield S, Harris T, Kritchevsky SB (2006) Inflammatory markers are associated with ventilatory limitation and muscle dysfunction in obstructive lung disease in well functioning elderly subjects. Thorax 61:10–16

92. Broekhuizen R, Wouters EF, Creutzberg EC, Schols AM (2006) Raised CRP levels mark metabolic and functional impairment in advanced COPD. Thorax 61:17–22

93. Papi A, Luppi F, Franco F, Fabbri LM (2006) Pathophysiology of exacerbations of chronic obstructive pulmonary disease. Proc Am Thorac Soc 3:245–251
94. Agusti A, Morla M, Sauleda J, Saus C, Busquets X (2004) NF-kappaB activation and iNOS upregulation in skeletal muscle of patients with COPD and low body weight. Thorax 59:483–487
95. Crul T, Spruit MA, Gayan-Ramirez G, Quarck R, Gosselink R, Troosters T, Pitta F, Decramer M (2007) Markers of inflammation and disuse in vastus lateralis of chronic obstructive pulmonary disease patients. Eur J Clin Invest 37:897–904
96. Couillard A, Maltais F, Saey D, Debigare R, Michaud A, Koechlin C, LeBlanc P, Prefaut C (2003) Exercise-induced quadriceps oxidative stress and peripheral muscle dysfunction in patients with chronic obstructive pulmonary disease. Am J Respir Crit Care Med 167: 1664–1669
97. Van Helvoort HA, Heijdra YF, Thijs HM, Vina J, Wanten GJ, Dekhuijzen PN (2006) Exercise-induced systemic effects in muscle-wasted patients with COPD. Med Sci Sports Exerc 38:1543–1552
98. Marin-Corral J, Minguella J, Ramirez-Sarmiento AL, Hussain SN, Gea J, Barreiro E (2009) Oxidised proteins and superoxide anion production in the diaphragm of severe COPD patients. Eur Respir J 33:1309–1319
99. Gomes-Marcondes MC, Tisdale MJ (2002) Induction of protein catabolism and the ubiquitin-proteasome pathway by mild oxidative stress. Cancer Lett 180:69–74
100. Dekhuijzen PN, Decramer M (1992) Steroid-induced myopathy and its significance to respiratory disease. a known disease rediscovered. Eur Respir J 5:997–1003
101. Decramer M, de Bock V, Dom R (1996) Functional and histologic picture of steroid-induced myopathy in chronic obstructive pulmonary disease. Am J Respir Crit Care Med 153: 1958–1964
102. Hoppeler H, Vogt M (2001) Muscle tissue adaptations to hypoxia. J Exp Biol 204: 3133–3139
103. Pitsiou G, Kyriazis G, Hatzizisi O, Argyropoulou P, Mavrofridis E, Patakas D (2002) Tumor necrosis factor-alpha serum levels, weight loss and tissue oxygenation in chronic obstructive pulmonary disease. Respir Med 96:594–598
104. Takabatake N, Nakamura H, Abe S, Inoue S, Hino T, Saito H, Yuki H, Kato S, Tomoike H (2000) The relationship between chronic hypoxemia and activation of the tumor necrosis factor-α system in patients with chronic obstructive pulmonary disease. Am J Respir Crit Care Med 161:1179–1184
105. Koechlin C, Maltais F, Saey D, Michaud A, LeBlanc P, Hayot M, Prefaut C (2005) Hypoxaemia enhances peripheral muscle oxidative stress in chronic obstructive pulmonary disease. Thorax 60:834–841
106. Klausen T, Olsen NV, Poulsen TD, Richalet JP, Pedersen BK (1997) Hypoxemia increases serum interleukin-6 in humans. Eur J Appl Physiol Occup Physiol 76:480–482
107. Hartmann G, Tschop M, Fischer R, Bidlingmaier C, Riepl R, Tschop K, Hautmann H, Endres S, Toepfer M (2000) High altitude increases circulating interleukin-6, interleukin-1 receptor antagonist and c-reactive protein. Cytokine 12:246–252
108. Kamischke A, Kemper DE, Castel MA, Lüthke M, Rolf C, Behre HM, Magnussen H, Nieschlag E (1998) Testosterone levels in men with chronic obstructive pulmonary disease with or without glucocorticoid therapy. Eur Respir J 11:41–45
109. Debigaré R, Marquis K, Cote CH, Tremblay RR, Michaud A, LeBlanc P, Maltais F (2003) Catabolic/anabolic balance and muscle wasting in patients with COPD. Chest 124:83–89
110. Laghi F, Langbein WE, Antonescu-Turcu A, Jubran A, Bammert C, Tobin MJ (2005) Respiratory and skeletal muscles in hypogonadal men with chronic obstructive pulmonary disease. Am J Respir Crit Care Med 171:598–605
111. Brodsky IG, Balagopal P, Nair KS (1996) Effects of testosterone replacement on muscle mass and muscle protein synthesis in hypogonadal men – a clinical research center study. J Clin Endocrinol Metab 81:3469–3475

112. Casaburi R, Bhasin S, Cosentino L, Porszasz J, Somfay A, Lewis MI, Fournier M, Storer TW (2004) Effects of testosterone and resistance training in men with chronic obstructive pulmonary disease. Am J Respir Crit Care Med 170:870–878

113. Eisner MD, Anthonisen N, Coultas D, Kuenzli N, Perez-Padilla R, Postma D, Romieu I, Silverman EK, Balmes JR (2010) An official american thoracic society public policy statement: novel risk factors and the global burden of chronic obstructive pulmonary disease. Am J Respir Crit Care Med 182:693–718

114. Montes de Oca M, Loeb E, Torres SH, De Sanctis J, Hernandez N, Talamo C (2008) Peripheral muscle alterations in non-COPD smokers. Chest 133:13–18

115. O'Shea SD, Taylor NF, Paratz JD (2009) Progressive resistance exercise improves muscle strength and may improve elements of performance of daily activities for people with COPD: a systematic review. Chest 136:1269–1283

116. Man WD, Kemp P, Moxham J, Polkey MI (2009) Exercise and muscle dysfunction in COPD: implications for pulmonary rehabilitation. Clin Sci (Lond) 117:281–291

117. Troosters T, Probst VS, Crul T, Pitta F, Gayan-Ramirez G, Decramer M, Gosselink R (2010) Resistance training prevents deterioration in quadriceps muscle function during acute exacerbations of chronic obstructive pulmonary disease. Am J Respir Crit Care Med 181:1072–1077

118. Janaudis-Ferreira T, Hill K, Goldstein RS, Robles-Ribeiro P, Beauchamp MK, Dolmage TE, Wadell K, Brooks D (2011) Resistance arm training in patients with COPD: a randomized controlled trial. Chest 139:151–158

119. McKeough ZJ, Bye PT, Alison JA (2012) Arm exercise training in chronic obstructive pulmonary disease: a randomised controlled trial. Chron Respir Dis 9:153–162

120. Franssen FM, Broekhuizen R, Janssen PP, Wouters EF, Schols AM (2005) Limb muscle dysfunction in COPD: effects of muscle wasting and exercise training. Med Sci Sports Exerc 37:2–9

121. Saey D, Lemire BB, Gagnon P, Bombardier E, Tupling AR, Debigare R, Cote CH, Maltais F (2011) Quadriceps metabolism during constant workrate cycling exercise in chronic obstructive pulmonary disease. J Appl Physiol 110:116–124

122. Lemire BB, Debigare R, Dube A, Theriault ME, Cote CH, Maltais F (2012) MAPK signaling in the quadriceps of patients with chronic obstructive pulmonary disease. J Appl Physiol 113:159–166

123. Constantin D, Menon MK, Houchen-Wolloff L, Morgan MD, Singh SJ, Greenhaff P, Steiner MC (2013) Skeletal muscle molecular responses to resistance training and dietary supplementation in COPD. Thorax 68(7):625–633

124. Theriault ME, Pare ME, Maltais F, Debigare R (2012) Satellite cells senescence in limb muscle of severe patients with COPD. PLoS One 7:e39124

Pathophysiology of Chronic Obstructive Pulmonary Disease

22

Bartolome R. Celli

Chronic obstructive pulmonary disease (COPD) currently ranks as the fourth cause of death in the United States and the world [1, 2]. Its prevalence has increased as overall mortality from myocardial infarction and cerebrovascular accident, the two organ systems (heart and brain) affected by the same risk factor (namely, cigarette smoking), has decreased. Once diagnosed, COPD is progressive and leads to disability usually due to dyspnea, at a relatively early age (sixth or seventh decade). Limitation to airflow occurs as a consequence of the destruction of lung parenchyma or the alterations in the airway itself. This chapter integrates the pathological changes of COPD with the known adaptive and maladaptive consequences of those changes. Knowledge of these factors should help us understand the rationale behind the different therapeutic strategies aimed at decreasing the symptoms and addressing the complications of patients with COPD.

22.1 Definition

COPD is a disease state characterized by the presence of airflow obstruction due to emphysema or intrinsic airway disease. The airflow limitation is associated with an abnormal inflammatory response to inhaled particles or noxious gases (mainly cigarette smoking). The obstruction is generally progressive, may be accompanied by airway hyperactivity, and may be partially reversible. Patients with COPD also suffer from important comorbidities. However, in this monograph, we shall concentrate on the pulmonary consequences of COPD.

Emphysema is defined pathologically as an abnormal permanent enlargement of the air spaces distal to the terminal bronchioles, accompanied by destruction of their

B.R. Celli, MD
Department of Pulmonary and Critical Care Medicine, Brigham
and Women's Hospital, 75 Francis Street, Boston, MA 02115, USA
e-mail: bcelli@partners.org

A. Aliverti, A. Pedotti (eds.), *Mechanics of Breathing*,
DOI 10.1007/978-88-470-5647-3_22, © Springer-Verlag Italia 2014

walls, without fibrosis. Chronic bronchitis is defined clinically as the presence of cough and/or sputum production for at least 3 months in 2 years. Its pathological expression is enlargement of the mucosal glands and inflammatory infiltration of the airways. In most patients both emphysema and airway inflammation coexist simultaneously [1–4]. The disease does not affect all portions of the lung to the same degree. This uneven distribution influences the physiologic behavior of the different parts of the lung.

22.2 Pathophysiology

Biopsy studies from the large airways of patients with COPD reveal the presence of a large number of neutrophils [5]. This neutrophilic predominance is more manifest in smoking patients who develop airflow obstruction compared to smoking patients without airflow limitation [6]. Interestingly, biopsies of smaller bronchi reveal the presence of large number of lymphocytes, especially of the CD8+ type [7]. The same type of cells, as well as macrophages, have been shown to increase in biopsy that include lung parenchyma [7, 8]. Taken together, these findings suggest that cigarette smoking induces an inflammatory process characterized by intense interaction and accumulation of cells, which are capable of releasing many cytokines and enzymes that may cause injury. Indeed, the level of interleukin 8 (IL-8) is increased in the secretions of patients with COPD [9]. This is also true for tumor necrosis factor [10] and markers of oxidative stress [11]. In addition, the release of enzymes known to be capable of destroying the lung parenchyma, such as neutrophilic elastase and metalloproteinases (MMPs) by many of these activated cells, has been documented in patients with COPD [12, 13]. Therefore, an increasing body of evidence indicates that the anatomic alterations of COPD, such as airway inflammation and dysfunction as well as parenchymal destruction, could result from altered cellular interactions triggered by external agents such as cigarette or environmental smoke (Fig. 22.1). Whatever the mechanisms, the disease distribution is not uniform, so in one single patient areas of the lung with severe destruction may coexist with less affected areas.

Functionally, COPD is characterized by a decrease in airflow, which is more prominent on maximal efforts. Like the pathological distribution, the airflow limitation is not uniform in nature. This causes uneven distribution of ventilation and also of blood perfusion [14, 15]. This in turn results in arterial hypoxemia (decreased PaO_2) and, if overall ventilation is decreased, in hypercarbia (increased $PaCO_2$). In those patients with an important component of emphysema or bullous disease, total lung volume increases resulting in hyperinflation. Each of these interrelated elements is important in the adaptive changes observed in patients with COPD and helps explain the clinical manifestations of the disease.

The relationship between structure and function in COPD is not well understood. Whether due to loss of attachments or tethering forces and/or due to inflammation and mucous secretion, patients with COPD have decreased airflow. In spite of this, there is no good correlation between the currently used scoring system of either emphysematous or bronchitic changes and the degree of airflow obstruction.

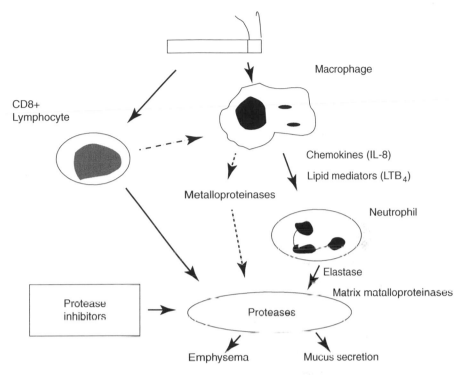

Fig. 22.1 Cigarette smoking induces inflammation. The interaction of different cells results in the release of cytokines that further perpetuate the inflammatory state and cause tissue injury. *IL-8* interleukin-8, *LTB4* leukotriene B4

Therefore, it is practical to describe the patient by the degree of physiologically determined airflow limitation. The severity of airflow limitation expressed by the value of post-bronchodilator forced expiratory volume in 1 s (FEV1) continues to be a good predictor of morbidity and mortality in COPD [16]. However, other variables that can be clinically measured do contribute to better predict the outcome in these patients. Of these, some have been known for a long time such as age and FEV_1 [16, 17]. That data is relatively old and by and large precedes the advent of low flow oxygen, modern long-acting bronchodilators, and mechanical ventilation. Indeed, the presence of hypoxemia and hypercapnia is also important in that they are predictive of mortality, once the patient has moderate to severe airflow limitation [18]. On the other hand, the FEV1 is a better predictor; when its values fall below 50 % of predicted, mortality begins to increase [17].

Over the last two decades, other clinical variables have been explored and found to be better predictors of mortality than the FEV1. The cardinal symptom of COPD is dyspnea [1, 19]. This sensation is the consequence of the interaction between cognitive and non-volitional neural processes and respiratory mechanics including airway obstruction. Dyspnea often limits functional activity and frequently causes the patient to seek medical attention [20, 21] and has been shown to predict mortality in large cohorts [22]. Similarly, the functional capacity measured as either the peak oxygen uptake during an exercise or the capacity [23] to walk over 6 min has also been validated as a predictor of survival [24–26]. Importantly, the combination of several of these variables into single multidimensional index such as the body mass index (B), obstruction (O), dyspnea (D), and exercise capacity (E) or BODE index has been shown to better predict mortality than either variable alone [27], supporting the concept that COPD is a complex disease, difficult to evaluate with a single measurement. With this as a background, we shall concentrate on the respiratory component of COPD because this is the primary locus of the disease and the one more closely related to the perceptive sensations of patients with the disease.

22.3 Airflow Limitation

To move air in and out of the lungs, the bellows must force air through the conducting airways. The resistance to flow is given by the interaction of air molecules with each other and with the internal surface of the airways. Therefore, airflow resistance depends on the physical property of the gas and the length and diameter of the airways. For a constant diameter, flow is proportional to the applied pressure. This relationship holds true in normals for inspiratory flow measured at fixed lung volume. In contrast, expiratory flow is linearly related to the applied pressure only during the early portion of the maneuver. Beyond a certain point, flow does not increase despite further increase in driving pressure. This flow limitation is due to the dynamic compression of airways as force is applied around them during forced expirations. This can be readily understood in the commonly determined flow-volume expression of the vital capacity (Fig. 22.1). As effort increases, expiratory flow increases up to a certain point (outer envelope) beyond which further efforts result in no further increase in airflow. During tidal breathing (inner tracing), only a small fraction of the maximal flow is used, and therefore flow is not limited under these circumstances. In contrast the flow-volume loop of patients with COPD is markedly different. The expiratory portion of the curve is carved out. This shape is due to the smaller diameter of the intrathoracic airways which decreases even more as pressure is applied around them. The flow limitation can be severe enough that maximal flow may be reached even during tidal breathing. A patient with this degree of obstruction (a not uncommon finding in clinical practice) cannot increase flow with increased ventilatory demand. As we shall review later, increased demands can only be met by increasing respiratory rate which in turn is detrimental to the expiratory time and causes dynamic hyperinflation (Fig. 22.2), a significant problem in patients with COPD.

The precise reason for the development of airflow obstruction in COPD is not entirely clear, but it may very likely be multifactorial [28–30]. Because airflow obstruction is physiologically evident during exhalation, COPD has been thought to be a problem of "expiration." Unfortunately, inspiration is also affected because inspiratory resistance is also increased and, importantly, the inability to expel the inhaled air coupled with parenchymal destruction leads to hyperinflation [31, 32].

Fig. 22.2 Patients with severe COPD manifest flow limitation during tidal breathing. Increases in ventilatory demand (i.e., exercise and acute exacerbation) can only be met by increase in breathing frequency. This results in air trapping as expiratory time is shortened. The consequence of these changes is the development of dynamic hyperinflation and associated dyspnea

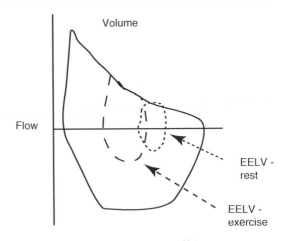

22.4   Hyperinflation

As the parenchymal destruction of many patients with COPD progresses, the distal air spaces enlarge. The loss of the lung elastic recoil resulting from this destruction increases resting lung volume. In a pervasive way, the loss of elastic recoil and airway attachments narrows even more the already constricted airways. The decrease in airway diameter increases resistance to airflow and worsens the obstruction. Decreased lung elastic recoil therefore is a major contributor of airway narrowing in emphysema [30]. Because in most patients the distribution of emphysema is not uniform, portions of the lung with low elastic recoil may coexist with portions with more normal elastic recoil property. It follows that ventilation to each one of those portions will not be uniform. This helps explain some of the differences in gas exchange. It also explains why reduction of the uneven distribution of recoil pressures by procedures that resect more afflicted lung areas results in better ventilation of the remainder of the lung and improved gas exchange.

Increased breathing frequency worsens hyperinflation [31, 32] because the expiratory time decreases, even if patients simultaneously shorten their inspiratory time. The resulting "dynamic" hyperinflation is very detrimental to lung mechanics and helps explain many of the findings associated with higher ventilatory demand, such as exercise or acute exacerbation.

22.5   Alteration in Gas Exchange

The uneven distribution of airway disease and emphysema coupled with the uneven perfusion due to gravitational forces explains the change in blood gases. The lungs of patients with COPD can be considered as consisting of two portions: one more emphysematous and the other one more normal. The pressure-volume curve of the emphysematous portion is displaced up and to the left compared to that of the more normal lung. At low lung volume the emphysematous (more compliant) portion undergoes greater volume changes than the more normal lung. In contrast, at higher lung volume the emphysematous lung is overinflated and accepts less volume change, per unit of pressure change, than the normal lung. Therefore, the distribution of ventilation is nonuniform, and overall, the emphysematous areas of the lung are underventilated compared with the more normal lung. Because perfusion is even more compromised than ventilation in the emphysematous areas, they have a high ventilation/perfusion ratio and behave as dead space. Indeed, this wasted portion of ventilation (VD/VT) corresponding to approximately 0.3–0.4 of the tidal breath of a normal person has been measured to be much higher in patients with severe emphysema [33]. At the same time, narrower bronchi in other areas may not allow appropriate ventilation to reach relatively well-perfused areas of the lung. This low ventilation/perfusion ratio will contribute to venous admixture (V/Q) and hypoxemia [34, 35]. The overall result is the simultaneous coexistence of high VD/VT regions with regions of low V/Q match. Both increase the ventilatory demand, thereby taxing even more the respiratory system of these patients.

As ventilatory demand increases, so does the work of breathing, so the patient with COPD must attempt to increase ventilation in order to maintain an adequate delivery of oxygen. Alveolar ventilation must also be sufficient to eliminate the produced CO_2. If this does not occur, $PaCO_2$ will increase. Indeed, the arterial blood gas changes over time in patients with COPD parallel this sequence. Initially PaO_2 progressively decreases but is compensated by increased ventilation. When the ventilation is insufficient, the $PaCO_2$ rises [36, 37]. This is consistent with the observation that patients with COPD who develop severe hypoxemia and hypercarbia have a very poor prognosis [17].

22.6 Control of Ventilation

For gas exchange to occur, it is necessary to move air in and out of the lung. This is achieved by the respiratory pump which is composed of the respiratory centers, the nerves that carry the signals from those centers, the respiratory muscles which are the pressure-generating structures, and the rib cage and abdomen. These components are linked and ordinarily function in a well-orchestrated manner whereby ventilation goes unnoticed and utilizes very little energy [38, 39].

The central controller or respiratory center is located in the upper medulla and integrates input from the periphery and other parts of the nervous system [40]. The output of this generator is modulated not only by mechanical, cortical, and sensory input but also by the state of oxygenation (PaO_2), CO_2 concentration ($PaCO_2$), and acid–base status (pH). Once generated, the output is distributed by the conducting nerves to the respiratory muscles which shorten and deform the rib cage and abdomen and generate intrathoracic pressures. These pressure changes displace volume and air moves in and out depending on the direction of the pressure change.

The relation between "drive" and inspiratory pressure or volume is referred to as "coupling." Coupling is usually smooth and occurs with minimal effort. That is the reason why breathing is perceived as effortless. Whenever the act of breathing requires effort, this "effort" is perceived as "work" which we define as the unpleasant sensation of dyspnea. The interaction between the central drive (controller output) and the final output (ventilation) is complex and involves many components [41, 42]. This complexity renders it very difficult to ascribe dyspnea to a dysfunction in any individual portion of the system. The ventilatory control can be assessed at different levels. The simplest is the minute ventilation (VE) which reflects the final effectiveness of the ventilatory drive. Further insight can be obtained by measuring the two contributors to VE, the tidal volume (VT) represented by the volume of air inhaled in a breath and the respiratory frequency.

Analysis of these variables in COPD reveals that as the disease progresses, VE increases [42]. This is expected, as the need to keep oxygen uptake and CO_2 removal constant is challenged by the changes in lung mechanics and ventilation-perfusion. The increase in VE is achieved first by an increase in VT; but as the resistive work due to airflow obstruction worsens, tidal volume decreases. The respiratory rate responds in a more linear fashion, increasing as the obstruction progresses [43]. The VE can also be expressed in terms of the mean inspiratory flow rate. This is obtained by relating the VT to the inspiratory time (VT/Ti) and the fractional duration of inspiration or (Ti/Tot). VT/Ti reflects drive and Ti/Ttot reflects timing. In COPD, both are altered by the need to increase VE. The Ti/Ttot, which normally has values of close to 0.38, shortens somewhat while the VT/Ti increases more in order to accommodate the increase in respiratory rate and shortened Ti/Ttot.

A relatively noninvasive way to measure central drive is the mouth occlusion pressure measured 0.1 s after the onset of inspiration (P0.1) [44]. With increased central drive, the increase in P0.1 is higher than that of VT/Ti [45]. This is due to airflow impedance that decreases mean inspiratory flow measured at the mouth while air is moving. The P0.1 is much less affected in COPD, because it is measured in conditions of no airflow, as the airway is temporarily obstructed. Mouth occlusion pressure or P 0.1 has been shown to increase as the degree of obstruction worsens irrespective of the alteration in arterial blood gases. The central drive increases as the degree of airflow obstruction progresses, reaching its maximum in patients with respiratory failure [37, 46]. The drive is effectively "coupled" to increased VT in the early stages of obstruction, but VT actually drops as the work to move air becomes very high. The only alternative is to increase respiratory rate. This also occurs, but as determined by the flow limitation characteristics of these patients, this adaptive phenomenon may result in further hyperinflation. As described earlier, hyperinflation displaces diseased portions of lung higher in their pressure-volume relationship. This effectively turns many portions of the lung into "restrictive" tissue. At this point, respiration is less demanding (in terms of work or pressure changes) when a fast and shallower ventilatory pattern is adopted. Indeed, this is the observed breathing strategy in patients with the most severe COPD [47].

22.7 Respiratory Muscles

As noted before, breathing depends on the coordinated action of different groups of muscles. The respiratory muscles can be divided into those that help inflate the lungs (inspiratory) and those that have an expiratory action. In addition, there are upper airway muscles (tongue and muscles of the palate, of the pharynx, and of the vocal cords), the function of which is to contract at the beginning of inspiration and hold the upper airways open throughout inhalation. Although very important in normal function, they play a limited role in pure COPD and will not be discussed further.

The diaphragm and the other inspiratory muscles are innervated by a wide array of motor neurons that range from cranial nerve 11 (C-11) which provides neuronal input to the sternomastoid to lumbar roots L2–L3 which innervate the abdominal muscles. The respiratory cycle is regulated by a complex series of centrally organized neurons, which maintain rhythmic breathing that goes usually unnoticed, that can be voluntarily overridden by the cortex.

The most important inspiratory muscle is the diaphragm [48]. It is well suited to perform its work due to its anatomic arrangement and histochemical composition. Its long fibers extend from the noncontractile central tendon and are directed down and outward to insert circumferentially in the lower ribs and upper lumbar spine. This concave shape allows the muscle its lifting action as it contracts. The diaphragm can shorten up to 40 % between full expiration and end inspiration [49]. During quiet breathing, it accounts for most of the force needed to displace the rib cage. Other inspiratory muscles are also agonists during quiet breathing and contribute to inspiratory effort. They are the scalene and parasternal intercostal muscles. There are yet other muscles (truly accessory in nature) that are not active during quiet breathing in normals but may contribute to ventilation in situations of increased demand. Muscles such as the sternomastoid, pectoralis minor, latissimus dorsi, and trapezius are some of these truly "accessory" muscles [38, 43]. The abdominal muscles are expiratory in action, since their contractions will decrease lung volume [50]. Inasmuch as that they provide tone to the abdominal wall, they help the diaphragm, because they contribute to the generation of the gastric pressure needed for diaphragmatic contraction to be effective.

It has been postulated that the automatic and voluntary ventilatory pathways are different and that the respiratory and tonic functions of these muscles are driven from different central nervous areas and integrated at the spinal level. In patients in whom some of these muscles are participating in respiration, to perform non-ventilatory work, they must maintain a high degree of coordination. Either because of the load or because of competing central integration, muscle function may become dyscoordinated and result in dysfunction. We have seen this occurring in patients with COPD who perform unsupported arm exercise. This type of exercise leads to early fatigue of the muscles involved in arm positioning and to dyssynchrony between rig cage and diaphragm-abdomen. This could also be caused by competing outputs of the various driving centers that control rhythmic respiratory and tonic activities of the accessory ventilatory muscles and the diaphragm. This dyssynchrony may be perceived as dyspnea. Its occurrence has been observed in normal subjects breathing against resistive loads and in patients with COPD breathing during voluntary hyperventilation [51, 52]. Likewise, it has been observed in patients immediately after disconnection from ventilators but before evidence of contractile fatigue. This suggests that dyssynchrony is a consequence of the load and not an indication of fatigue itself. Whatever the reason, this breathing pattern is ineffective and is associated with respiratory muscle dysfunction [42, 51].

22.8 Dyspnea

Many patients with COPD stop exercising because of dyspnea [53, 54], and dyspnea is the dominant symptom during acute exacerbations of the disease [55]. Several studies have shown that in COPD, dyspnea with exercise correlates better with the degree of dynamic hyperinflation [32, 56] than with changes in airflow indices or blood gas exchange. Dyspnea also correlates better to respiratory muscle function than to airflow obstruction [23, 41]. Studies in normals have shown that dyspnea increases as the ratio between the pressure needed to ventilate and the maximal pressure that the muscles can generate (P breath/Pi max) increases [53]. Dyspnea also worsens in proportion to the duration of the inspiratory contraction (Ti/Ttot) and respiratory frequency. These are also the factors that are associated with EMG evidence of respiratory muscle fatigue [57]. Therefore, it has been suggested that patients with COPD develop dynamic hyperinflation which compromises ventilatory muscle function, and that this is the main determinant of dyspnea in these patients. Although respiratory muscle fatigue has been reasonably well documented in patients with COPD suffering from acute decompensation [58], its presence in stable patients remains in doubt. It is fair to state that the respiratory muscles of patients with severe COPD are functioning at a level closer to the fatigue threshold but are not fatigued. It is possible that restoration of the respiratory muscles to a better contractile state could improve the dyspnea of these patients. Indeed, Martinez et al. observed that the factor that best predicted the improvement in dyspnea reported by COPD patients after lung volume reduction surgery was the lesser dynamic hyperinflation seen during exercise after the procedure [59]. This is consistent with similar reports from other groups [60, 61] and the close association between decreased dynamic hyperinflation and dyspnea in patients treated with bronchodilators [62, 63].

Dyspnea in patients with severe COPD may also be due to the level of resting respiratory drive and the individual's response of the central output to different stimuli. In other words, at similar mechanical load and similar levels of respiratory muscle dysfunction, dyspnea may result from an individual's response of the central motor output. This hypothesis is supported by work from Marin et al. [64] who demonstrated that the most important predictor of dyspnea with exercise was the baseline central drive response to CO_2. The importance of this observation lies in the possibility that there may be a group of patients with COPD who manifest increased central drive and in whom adequate manipulation of this drive may result in decreased dyspnea. Until further studies are completed, this remains just an interesting hypothesis.

22.9 Peripheral Muscle Function

Many patients with COPD will stop exercising because of leg fatigue rather than dyspnea. This observation has prompted renewed interest in the function of limb muscles in these patients. Perhaps the most important of these studies are those

Fig. 22.3 Schematic
model that integrates the
different components of
breathing in patients with
COPD

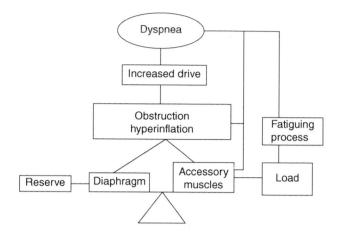

reported by Maltais et al. [65, 66] who performed biopsies of the vastus lateralis, before and after lower extremity exercise training, in patients with severe COPD. At baseline, patients with COPD have lower levels of the oxidative enzymes citric synthase (CS) and 3-hydroxy-acyl-CoA-hydrogenase (HADH) than normal. After exercise, the mitochondrial content of these enzymes increased. This was associated with an improvement in exercise endurance and decreased lactic acid production at peak exercise. These biochemical changes are in line with the observation of several groups that have suggested the presence of a dysfunctional myopathy in patients with COPD. The importance of deconditioning peripheral muscle dysfunction and training in COPD is addressed in a different chapter in this book.

22.10 Integrative Approach

The overall function of the respiratory system in COPD can be represented by the model shown in Fig. 22.3. Central to the model is the problem of airway narrowing and hyperinflation. In order to reverse the model to a normal state, it is necessary to resolve those two problems. Efforts to prevent the disease from developing (smoking cessation) must be associated with methods aimed at reversing airflow obstruction (Fig. 22.4). Indeed, pharmacotherapy including bronchodilators, antibiotics, and corticosteroids is given to improve airflow. If this were effective, hyperinflation should consequently decrease. One alternative is to resect the portion of the lungs which are severely diseased, such as has been done in cases of large bullae [67]. Partial resection of lesser evident emphysematous areas (surgical or bronchoscopic lung volume reduction procedures) seems effective for a minority of patients [68, 69]. Finally, in acute exacerbations or under situations of increased ventilatory demands, the system may fail and respiratory failure with death may occur. Fortunately, the advances in noninvasive and invasive mechanical ventilation have made possible the support required to guarantee the survival of most patients with acute or chronic respiratory failure. After such an event, pulmonary rehabilitation

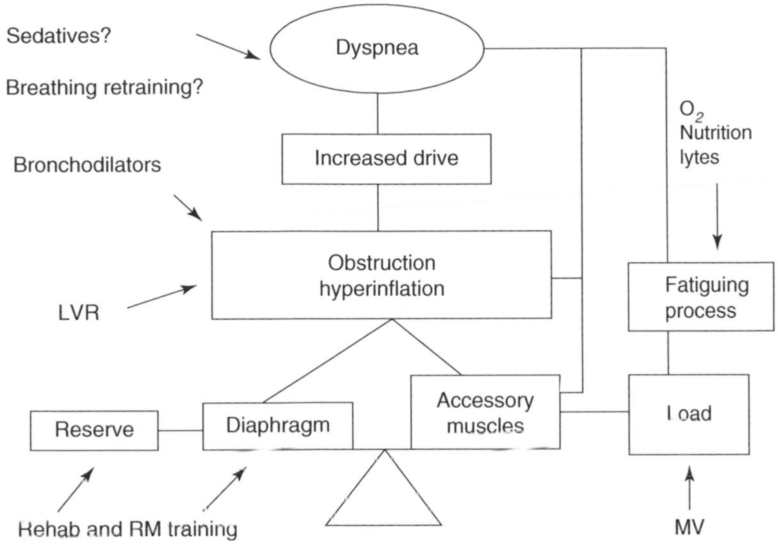

Fig. 22.4 Based on this model, several interventions may be beneficial as shown in this graph

through improvement in peripheral muscle function, nutrition, and implementation of adequate coping mechanisms remains the best available option.

References

1. Celli B, MacNee W (2004) Standards for the diagnosis and care of patients with chronic obstructive pulmonary disease (COPD). Eur Respir J 23:932–46
2. Global obstructive lung disease initiative. www.goldcopd.com. Last accessed 17 June 2013
3. Mitchell RS, Stanford RE, Johnson JM et al (1976) The morphologic features of the bronchi, bronchioles and alveoli in chronic airway obstruction. Am Rev Respir Dis 114:137–145
4. Thurlbeck WM (1990) Pathophysiology of chronic obstructive pulmonary disease. Clin Chest Med 11:389–403
5. Jeffrey PK (1998) Structural and inflammatory changes in COPD: a comparison with asthma. Thorax 53:129–136
6. Keatings VM, Barnes PJ (1997) Granulocyte activation markers in induced sputum: comparison between chronic obstructive pulmonary disease, asthma and normal subjects. Am J Respir Crit Care Med 155:449–453
7. Saetta M, Di Stefano A, Turato G (1998) CD8+ T-lymphocytes in peripheral airways of smokers with chronic obstructive pulmonary disease. Am J Respir Crit Care Med 157:822–826
8. Finkelstein R, Fraser RS, Ghezzo H, Cosio MG (1995) Alveolar inflammation and its relation to emphysema in smokers. Am J Respir Crit Care Med 152:1666–1672
9. Yamamoto C, Yoneda T, Yoshikawa M, Fu A, Tokuyama T, Tsukaguchi K, Narita N (1997) Airway inflammation in COPD assessed by sputum level of interleukin-8. Chest 112:505–510
10. Barnes PJ (2000) Chronic obstructive pulmonary disease. N Engl J Med 343:269–280
11. Pratico D, Basili S, Vieri M et al (1998) Chronic obstructive pulmonary disease is associated with an increase in urinary levels of isoprostane F2a-111, an index of oxidant stress. Am J Respir Crit Care Med 158:1709–1714

12. Finlay GA, O'Driscoll LR, Russell KJ, D'Arcy E, Materson J, Fitzgerald M, O'Connor C (1997) Matrix- metalloproteinase expression and production by alveolar macrophages in emphysema. Am J Respir Crit Care Med 156:240–247

13. Vignola AM, Riccobono L, Mirabella A, Profita M, Chanez P, Bellia V, Mautino G, D'Accardi P, Bousquet J, Bonsignore G (1998) Sputum metalloprotinase-9/tissue inhibitor of metalloprotinase-1 ratio correlates with airflow obstruction in asthma and chronic bronchitis. Am J Respir Crit Care Med 158:1945–1950

14. Berend N, Woolcock AJ, Marlin GE (1979) Correlation between the function and the structure of the lung in smokers. Am Rev Respir Dis 119:695–702

15. Buist AS, Van Fleet DL, Ross BB (1973) A comparison of conventional spirometric tests and the tests of closing volume in one emphysema screening center. Am Rev Respir Dis 107:735–740

16. Fletcher C, Peto R (1977) The natural history of chronic airflow obstruction. Br Med J 1: 1645–1648

17. Anthonisen NR (1989) Prognosis in chronic obstructive pulmonary disease: results from multicenter clinical trials. Am Rev Respir Dis 133:95–99

18. Hodgkin JE (1990) Prognosis in chronic obstructive pulmonary disease. Clin Chest Med 11:555–569

19. Sweer L, Zwillich CW (1990) Dyspnea in the patient with chronic obstructive pulmonary disease. Clin Chest Med 11(3):417–455

20. Mahler DA, Weinburg DH, Wells CK, Feinstein AR (1984) The measurement of dyspnea: contents, interobserver agreement, and physiologic correlates of two new clinical indexes. Chest 85:751–758

21. Ries A, Kaplan R, Limberg T, Prewitt L (1995) Effects of pulmonary rehabilitation on physiologic and psychosocial outcomes in patients with COPD. Ann Int Med 122:823–832

22. Nishimura K, Izumi T, Tsukino M, Oga T (2002) Dyspnea is a better predictor of 5 years survival than airway obstruction in patients with COPD. Chest 121:1434–1440

23. Oga T, Nishimura K, Tsukino M, Sato S, Hajiro T (2003) Analysis of the factors related to mortality in chronic obstructive pulmonary disease: role of exercise capacity and health status. Am J Respir Crit Care Med 167:544–549

24. Gerardi D, Lovett L, Benoit-Connors J, ZuWallack R (1996) Variables related to increased mortality following outpatient pulmonary rehabilitation. Eur Respir J 9:431–435

25. Cote CG, Casanova C, Marín JM, Lopez MV, Pinto-Plata V, de Oca MM, Dordelly LJ, Nekach H, Celli BR (2008) Validation and comparison of reference equations for the 6-min walk distance test. Eur Respir J 31:571–578

26. Polkey MI, Spruit MA, Edwards LD, Watkins ML, Pinto-Plata V, Vestbo J, Calverley PM, Tal-Singer R, Agustí A, Bakke PS, Coxson HO, Lomas DA, MacNee W, Rennard S, Silverman EK, Miller BE, Crim C, Yates J, Wouters EF, Celli B, Evaluation of COPD Longitudinally to Identify Predictive Surrogate Endpoints (ECLIPSE) Study Investigators (2013) Six minute walk test in chronic obstructive pulmonary disease: minimally clinical important difference for death or hospitalization. Am J Respir Crit Care Med 187:382–386

27. Celli BR, Cote CG, Marin JM, Casanova C, Montes de Oca M, Mendez RA, Pinto Plata V, Cabral HJ (2004) The body mass index, airflow obstruction, dyspnea and exercise capacity index in chronic obstructive pulmonary disease. N Engl J Med 350:1005–1012

28. Greaves IA, Colebatch HJ (1980) Elastic behavior and structure of normal and emphysematous lungs postmortem. Am Rev Respir Dis 121:127–128

29. Hogg JC, Macklem PT, Thurlbeck WA (1968) Site and nature of airways obstruction in chronic obstructive lung disease. N Engl J Med 278:1355–1359, 24

30. Nagai A, Yamawaki I, Takizawa T, Thurlbeck WM (1991) Alveolar attachments in emphysema of human lungs. Am Rev Respir Dis 144:888–891, 29

31. O'Donnell SE, Sanil R, Anthonisen NR, Younis M (1987) Effect of dynamic airway compression on breathing pattern and respiratory sensation in severe chronic obstructive pulmonary disease. Am Rev Respir Dis 135:912–918

32. O'Donnell D, Lam M, Webb K (1998) Measurement of symptoms, lung hyperinflation and endurance during exercise in COPD. Am J Respir Crit Care Med 158:1557–1565

33. Javahari S, Blum J, Kazemi H (1981) Pattern of breathing and carbon dioxide retention in chronic obstructive lung disease. Am J Med 71:228–234
34. Rodriguez-Roisin R, Roca J (1995) Pulmonary gas exchange. In: Calverly PM, Pride NB (eds) Chronic obstructive pulmonary disease. Chapman & Hall, London, pp 167–184
35. Parot S, Miara B, Milic-Emili J, Gautier H (1982) Hypoxemia, hypercapnia and breathing patterns in patients with chronic obstructive pulmonary disease. Am Rev Respir Dis 126: 882–886
36. Begin P, Grassino A (1991) Inspiratory muscle dysfunction and chronic hypercapnia in chronic obstructive pulmonary disease. Am Rev Respir Dis 143:905–912
37. Montes de Oca M, Celli BR (1998) Mouth occlusion pressure, CO2 response and hypercapnia in severe obstructive pulmonary disease. Eur Respir J 12:666–671
38. Celli BR (1986) Respiratory muscle function. Clin Chest Med 7:567–584
39. Roussos C, Macklem PT (1982) The respiratory muscles. N Engl J Med 307:786–797
40. VonEuler C (1983) On the central pattern generator for the basic breathing rhythmicity. J Appl Physiol 55:1647–1659
41. Derenne JP, Macklem PT, Roussos CH (1978) The respiratory muscles: mechanics, control and pathophysiology. Am Rev Respir Dis 119:119–133, 373–390
42. Sears TA (1990) Central rhythm and pattern generation. Chest 97:45S–51S
43. Martinez FJ, Couser JI, Celli BR (1990) Factors influencing ventilatory muscle recruitment in patients with chronic airflow obstruction. Am Rev Respir Dis 142:276–282
44. Murciano D, Broczkowski J, Lecocguic M, Milic Emili J, Pariente R, Aubier M (1988) Tracheal occlusion pressure. A simple index to monitor respiratory muscle fatigue during acute respiratory failure in patients with chronic obstructive pulmonary disease. Ann Int Med 108:800–805
45. Milic-Emili J, Grassino AE, Whitelaw WA (1981) Measurement and testing of respiratory drive. In: Horbein TF (ed) Regulation of breathing, Lung biology in health and disease. Marcel Dekker, New York, pp 675–743
46. Sasoon CS, Te TT, Mahutte CR, Light R (1987) Airway occlusion pressure. An important indicator for successful weaning in patients with chronic obstructive pulmonary disease. Am Rev Respir Dis 135:107–113
47. Loveridge B, West P, Anthonisen NR, Krnigger MH (1984) Breathing patterns in patients with chronic obstructive pulmonary disease. Am Rev Respir Dis 130:730–733
48. Rochester DF (1985) The diaphragm contractile properties and fatigue. J Clin Invest 75: 1397–1402
49. Braun NM, Arora NS, Rochester DF (1982) The force-length relationship of the normal human diaphragm. J Appl Physiol 53:405–412
50. DeTroyer A, Estenne M (1988) Functional anatomy of the respiratory muscles. Clin Chest Med 9:175–193
51. Sharp JT (1983) The respiratory muscles in emphysema. Clin Chest Med 4:421–432
52. Tobin MJ, Perez W, Guenther SM, Lodato RF, Dantzker DR (1987) Does rib-cage abdominal paradox signify respiratory muscle fatigue? J Appl Physiol 63:857–860
53. Killian K, Jones N (1988) Respiratory muscle and dyspnea. Clin Chest Med 9:237–248
54. LeBlanc P, Bowie DM, Summers E, Jones NL, Killian KJ (1986) Breathlessness and exercise in patients with cardiorespiratory disease. Am Rev Respir Dis 133:21–25
55. Girish M, Pinto V, Kenney L, Livnat G, Talamo C, Rassulo J, Celli B (1998) Dyspnea in acute exacerbation of COPD is associated with increase in ventilatory demand and not with worsened airflow obstruction. ACCP Chest 114:266S
56. Marin J, Carrizo S, Gallego B, Gascon J, Alonso J, Celli BR (1999) Walk distance and exertional dyspnea is better predicted by dynamic hyperinflation than FEV1 in COPD. Am J Respir Crit Care Med 159:A476
57. Bellemare F, Grassino A (1983) Forces reserve of the diaphragm in patients with chronic obstructive pulmonary disease. J Appl Physiol 55:8–15
58. Cohen C, Zagelbaum G, Gross D, Roussos C, Macklem PT (1982) Clinical manifestations of inspiratory muscle fatigue. Am J Med 73:308–316

59. Martinez F, Montes de Oca M, Whyte R, Stetz J, Gay S, Celli B (1997) Lung-volume Reduction Surgery improves dyspnea, dynamic hyperinflation and respiratory muscle function. Am J Respir Crit Care Med 155:2018–2023

60. Brantigan OC, Mueller E, Kress MB (1959) A surgical approach to pulmonary emphysema. Am Rev Respir Dis 80:194–202

61. Cooper JD, Trulock ER, Triantafillou AN, Patterson GA, Pohl MS, Delaney PA, Sundaresan RS, Roper CL (1995) Bilateral pneumonectomy (Volume reduction) for chronic obstructive pulmonary disease. J Thor Cardiovasc Surg 109:116–119

62. Belman M, Botnick W, Shin W (1996) Inhaled bronchodilators reduce dynamic hyperinflation during exercise in patients with chronic obstructive pulmonary disease. Am J Respir Crit Care Med 53:967–975

63. Celli B, ZuWallack R, Wang S, Kesten S (2003) Improvement of inspiratory capacity and hyperinflation with tiotropium in COPD patients with severe hyperinflation. Chest 124(5): 1743–1748

64. Marin J, Montes De Oca M, Rassulo J, Celli BR (1999) Ventilatory drive at rest and perception of exertional dyspnea in severe COPD. Chest 115:1293–1300

65. Maltais F, Simard A, Simard J, Jobin J, Desgagnes P, LeBlanc P (1995) Oxidative capacity of the skeletal muscle and lactic acid kinetics during exercise in normal subjects and in patients with COPD. Am J Respir Crit Care Med 153:288–293

66. Maltais F, LeBlanc P, Simard C et al (1996) Skeletal muscle adaptation of endurance training in patients with chronic obstructive pulmonary disease. Am J Respir Crit Care Med 154: 442–447

67. Fitzgerald MX, Keelan PJ, Cugel DW, Gaensler EA (1974) Long-term results of surgery for bullous emphysema. J Thor Cardiovasc Surg 68:566–587

68. Criner GJ, Pinto-Plata V, Strange C, Dransfield M, Gotfried M, Leeds W, McLennan G, Refaely Y, Tewari S, Krasna M, Celli B (2009) Biologic lung volume reduction in advanced upper lobe emphysema: phase 2 results. Am J Respir Crit Care Med 179:791–798

69. Naunheim KS, Wood DE, Mohsenifar Z, Sternberg AL, Criner GJ, DeCamp MM et al (2006) Long-term follow-up of patients receiving lung-volume-reduction surgery versus medical therapy for severe emphysema by the National Emphysema Treatment Trial Research Group. Ann Thorac Surg 82(2):431–443

Old and New Trends in Invasive Mechanical Ventilation

23

Maria Vargas, Iole Brunetti, and Paolo Pelosi

The aim of mechanical ventilation is to decrease the work of breathing and to reverse acute hypoxemia and/or respiratory acidosis. Most of critically ill patients require invasive mechanical ventilation [1]. There are three main types of invasive mechanical ventilation: controlled, assist-control, and assisted.

In controlled mechanical ventilation, the ventilator delivers a set tidal volume or pressure independently from the patient respiratory activity. In assist-control ventilation, the ventilator delivers a set tidal volume when triggered by the patient's inspiratory effort or independently, if such an effort does not occur within a preselected time. In assisted ventilation, the ventilator assists the respiratory effort of the patient according to the change of his breathing pattern.

The modality of mechanical ventilation is important to optimize respiratory function according to the patient's characteristics. Studies have shown that optimal setting of mechanical ventilation and its use according to physiopathologic rationale may improve outcome [2].

Different modes of invasive mechanical ventilation have been developed and used in daily clinical practice; in this chapter we discuss the *conventional, nonconventional,* and the most recent modes of invasive mechanical ventilation in critically ill patients.

M. Vargas • I. Brunetti • P. Pelosi (✉)
Department of Anesthesia and Intensive Care Medicine,
IRCCS AOU San Martino – IST, l.go R. Benzi 16, 16132 Genoa, Italy
e-mail: vargas.maria82@gmail.com; ibrunetti@tin.it; ppelosi@hotmail.com

A. Aliverti, A. Pedotti (eds.), *Mechanics of Breathing*,
DOI 10.1007/978-88-470-5647-3_23, © Springer-Verlag Italia 2014

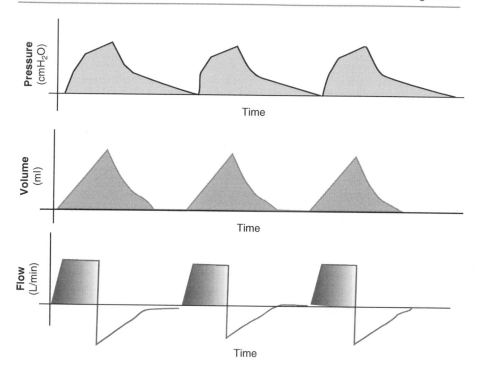

Fig. 23.1 Pressure, volume, and flow curves during volume control ventilation

23.1 Conventional Modes of Invasive Mechanical Ventilation

23.1.1 Volume-Cycled Ventilation Modes

Volume-cycled ventilation is the oldest mode of ventilation used in the operating room or intensive care unit. Volume control, assist-control, intermittent mandatory ventilation, and synchronized intermittent mandatory ventilation are different modes of volume-cycled ventilation.

In *volume control ventilation*, the operator is required to set a fixed tidal volume, respiratory rate, inspired oxygen fraction, inspiratory flow, and the alarm limits for airway pressure. The alarm limits of airway pressure are very important because in this type of ventilation, the variation of airway pressure is determined by the compliance of the patient's respiratory system. In volume control ventilation, the respiratory effort depends completely on the ventilator because the patient is not able to breathe adequately.

Figure 23.1 shows the pressure, volume, and flow curves during volume control ventilation.

Assist-control (AC) is a common mode of mechanical ventilation used in medical intensive care units. A key concept in the AC mode is that the tidal volume of each delivered breath is the same, regardless of whether it was triggered by the

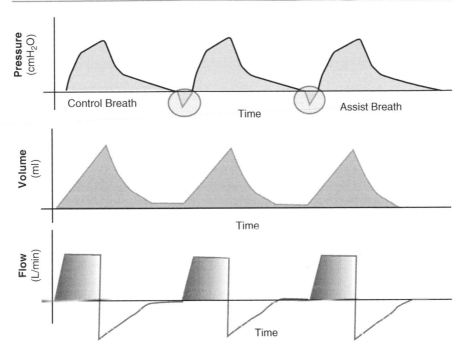

Fig. 23.2 Pressure, volume, and flow curves during assist control ventilation. The ventilator delivers the first breath, while the patient initiates the second and third breaths with a drop in airway pressure

patient or the ventilator. At the start of an inspiratory cycle, the ventilator senses a patient's attempt at inhalation by detecting negative airway pressure or inspiratory flow. The pressure or flow threshold needed to trigger a breath is generally set by the operator and is termed the trigger sensitivity [3]. If the patient does not initiate a breath before a requisite period of time determined by the set respiratory rate (RR), the ventilator will deliver the set tidal volume. However, if the patient starts a breath, the ventilator in AC mode will deliver the set tidal volume; these breaths are patient-triggered rather than time-triggered.

Figure 23.2 shows the pressure, volume, and flow curves for assist-control ventilation.

Synchronized intermittent mandatory ventilation (SIMV) is another commonly used mode of mechanical ventilation [4]. As AC, SIMV delivers a minimum number of fully assisted breaths per minute that are synchronized with the patient's respiratory effort. These breaths are patient- or time-triggered, flow-limited, and volume-cycled. However, any breaths taken between volume-cycled breaths are not assisted; the volumes of these breaths are determined by the patient's strength, effort, and lung mechanics. A key concept is that ventilator-assisted breaths are different than spontaneous breaths.

Figure 23.3 shows the pressure, volume, and flow curves for synchronized intermittent mandatory ventilation.

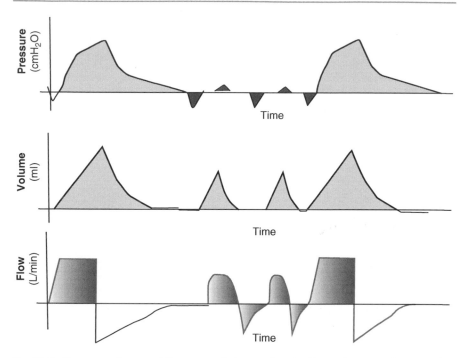

Fig. 23.3 Pressure, volume, and flow curves during synchronized intermittent mandatory ventilation. The first and fourth breaths are mandatory and patient-triggered, while the second and the third unsupported breaths are determined by the patient's inspiratory effort and respiratory compliance

23.1.2   Pressure-Cycled Ventilation Modes

Pressure-cycled ventilation is characterized by the setting of an inspiratory pressure that results in a delivered tidal volume determined by the dynamic compliance of the patient. Pressure control, pressure support, and airway pressure release are different modes of pressure-cycled ventilation.

Pressure control ventilation (PCV) is pressure- and time-cycled ventilation, which produces a tidal volume that varies according to the compliance or impedance of respiratory system [5]. In PCV during the inspiration, gas flows in the ventilator circuit to pressurize the system until the pressure level set by the operator was reached. The gas flow lasts until the alveolar pressure rises at the level of ventilator circuit pressure; after that the flow is stopped. In this way a gradient between the preset pressure, ventilator circuit pressure, and alveolar pressure is established, but if the gap between this three-step gradient is very large, flow is brisk.

Figure 23.4 shows pressure, volume, and flow curves for pressure control ventilation.

Pressure support ventilation (PSV) is patient-triggered, pressure-limited, and flow-cycled [6]. With this strategy, breaths are assisted by a set inspiratory pressure that is delivered until inspiratory flow drops below a set threshold. In this mode of ventilation, the inspiratory pressure facilitates the spontaneous breath triggered by

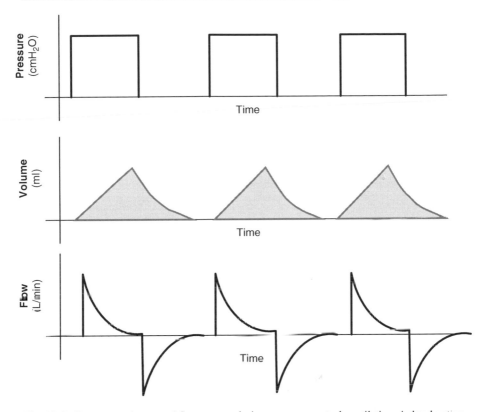

Fig. 23.4 Pressure, volume, and flow curves during pressure control ventilation. A decelerating inspiratory flow pattern is delivered resulting in a fixed pressure throughout the breath

the patient who controls his own respiratory rate and tidal volume. PSV may be used to overcome the resistance of endotracheal tube, to facilitate the respiratory effort of the patient, and to wean critically ill patients.

Figure 23.5 shows pressure, volume, and flow curves for pressure support ventilation.

Airway pressure release ventilation (APRV) may be considered as a partial ventilatory support mode with the possibility to allow spontaneous breathing in each point of ventilation cycle [7]. APRV is a time-cycled ventilation in which the operator sets two levels of pressure (pressure high and pressure low) and the time that the patient spends to maintain each level of pressure (time high and time low) [7]. Theoretically, maximizing the time spent at pressure high allows optimal alveolar recruitment and improved oxygenation; the brief intermittent release of breath to pressure low allows adequate ventilation. Furthermore, the time spent at pressure high may be customized to allow spontaneous breathing and progressive alveolar recruitment at the set level of pressure. Attention should be given in the setting of time low, because if it is too short intrinsic PEEP will result [8]. Spontaneous breaths may be supported or not, according to the patient's clinical needs.

Figure 23.6 shows pressure-time curves during APRV.

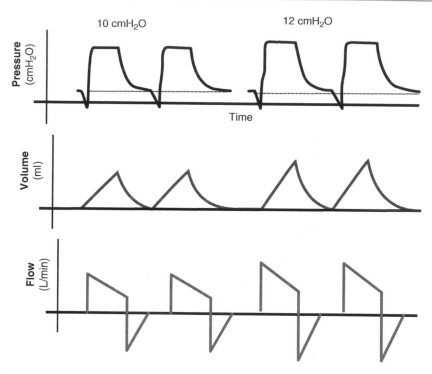

Fig. 23.5 Pressure, volume, and flow curves during pressure support ventilation. Spontaneous breaths are patient-triggered at different levels of pressure support (10 and 12 cmH$_2$O)

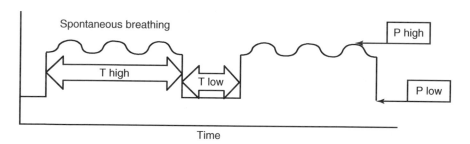

Fig. 23.6 Pressure-time curves during APRV. *P high* pressure high, *P low* pressure low, *T high* time high, *T low* time low

23.2 New Modes of Invasive Mechanical Ventilation

The patient's tailored modes are the new methods developed for invasive mechanical ventilation. These new modes of ventilation may offer several advantages to optimize the patient's respiratory effort and ventilator synchrony. It has been shown that increased patient's ventilator asynchrony might be associated with prolonged weaning and higher morbidity and mortality [2].

23.2.1   Proportional Assist Ventilation

Proportional assist ventilation (PAV) has the ability to provide the best synchronism between the patient's effort and ventilator partial assistance. In this ventilation, the ventilator generates a level of pressure in proportion to the patient's effort, and the ventilator output is under the full control of the patient's respiratory center.

In spontaneous breathing, the pressure generated by the inspiratory muscles (Pmus) is used to overcome the compliance and resistance of the respiratory system. In mechanically ventilated patients, the total pressure applied to the respiratory system (Ptot) equals the Pmus from the patient plus supplied airway pressure (Pappl). In PAV, the support is supplied by a combination of volume assist (VA) and flow assist (FA) based on the percentage of total work of breathing (WOB) that is dialed in for the ventilator to give [9]. The balance of the total WOB is then assumed by the patient. Since his inspiratory muscles have only to cope with the afterload, which has been reduced by the dialed WOB to be done by the ventilator (VA and FA), the ventilator essentially amplifies the patient effort [9]. The new generation of PAV (i.e., PAV +), allowing a better continuous estimation of the respiratory system resistance and compliance, seems to provide more flexible setting of the support according to the patients' need [10].

Figure 23.7 shows pressure, volume, and flow curves for proportional assist ventilation.

23.2.2   Neurally Adjusted Ventilatory Assist

Neurally adjusted ventilatory assist (NAVA) has been developed with the aim to overcome the limitation of PAV. In this ventilation the electrical activity of the inspiratory muscles can be used as an index of the inspiratory neural drive [11]. For this reason NAVA requires the placement of a gastric feeding tube with bipolar electrodes that measure the electrical signal leading to diaphragmatic stimulation by the vagus nerve (Edi). The diaphragmatic bipolar electrodes are not affected by the activity of postural and expiratory muscles. The signal obtained by the active region of the diaphragm is transferred to the ventilator, which regulates the respiratory support needed by the patient [12].

NAVA can be used if the respiratory center, phrenic nerves, and diaphragmatic activity of the neuromuscular junction are intact and the respiratory drive is not affected by sedation [13]. This situation implies that the complex system of feedback needed by NAVA is functional and the signal is not compromised. NAVA may be a promising tool for the future of mechanical ventilation.

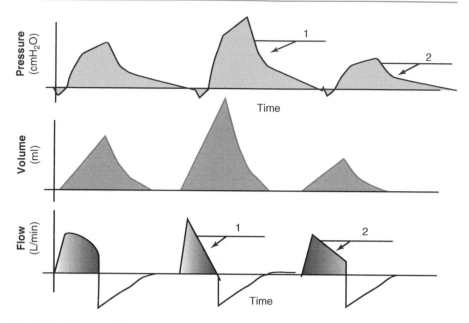

Fig. 23.7 Volume and flow curves for proportional assist ventilation. *1* increased effort of patient associated to an increase in the delivered pressure, *2* decreased effort of patient associated to a decrease in the delivered pressure

23.2.3 Noisy Pressure Support Ventilation

Pressure support ventilation (PSV) is frequently used and mechanical ventilation strategy that permits spontaneous breathing (SB) is investigated. PSV supports every triggered breath with positive pressure, leading to enhanced ventilation or perfusion of dependent zones, with potential improvement of gas exchange, though the work of breathing may increase. Random variation of tidal volume (VT) and respiratory frequency (noisy) may improve lung function during mechanical ventilation [14]. The beneficial effects of noisy ventilation have been demonstrated both in experimental and clinical studies in controlled mechanical ventilation. Basically, noisy PSV differs from other assisted mechanical ventilation modes that may also increase the variability of the respiratory pattern (e.g., proportional assist ventilation) by the fact that the variability does not depend on changes in the patient's inspiratory efforts; rather, it is generated externally by the mechanical ventilator [15]. Thus, *noisy PSV* is able to guarantee a given level of variability by generating different pressure support values, even if the patient is not able to vary the respiratory pattern due to the underlying disease or sedation [16]. In a previous study of a depletion model of acute lung injury, it was reported that the variability level of 30 % seems to represent a reasonable compromise to improve lung functional variables during noisy pressure support ventilation.

Figure 23.8 shows pressure and volume curves for noisy pressure support ventilation.

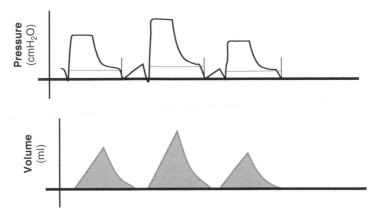

Fig. 23.8 Pressure and volume curves during noisy pressure support ventilation. The variability in the delivered pressure generates a different tidal volume for each breath

23.3   Nonconventional Modes of Invasive Mechanical Ventilation

23.3.1 High-Frequency Ventilation

High-frequency ventilation (HFV) was introduced in the clinical practice in the early 1970s, following the experiences by Oberg and Sjostrand (1969). Many HFV techniques are currently in use, all characterized by breathing frequencies higher than 1Hz (60 breaths/min) where tidal exchanges are less than the combined mechanical and anatomical dead space volume, displaying low peak pressures when compared to conventional mechanical ventilation (CMV). High-frequency ventilation (HFV) operates under two fundamentally different concepts of gas transport: convective gas transport and non-convective flow principles. Thus, gas exchange is at least in part by convection that includes direct alveolar ventilation, pendelluft, and asymmetric flow profiles [17]. HFV techniques, with an associated endobronchial convective displacement, have three essential common elements: a high-pressure flow generator, a valve for flow interruption, and a breathing circuit for connection to the patient [18]. The term high-frequency jet ventilation (HFJV) initially described any cyclic frequency of over a rate of 60 exchanges/min. Variants of this high-frequency definition were further described as flow interruption (HFFI), high-frequency (push-pull) oscillation (HFO), and high-frequency positive-pressure ventilation (HFPPV) based on the specific techniques that discriminate them [19–21].

23.3.2   High-Frequency Percussive Ventilation

High-frequency percussive ventilation (HFPV) was introduced with the intent of overcoming the inconveniences of other variants of HFV (e.g., high-frequency

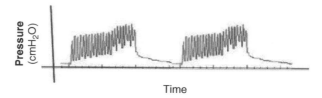

Fig. 23.9 The pressure-time curve for high-frequency percussive ventilation. In the time spent for a single inspiratory phase, HPFV delivers a high percussive pressure with high-frequency set as cycles/min

oscillation, high-frequency jet ventilation) [21]. HFPV associates the positive aspects of conventional mechanical ventilation (CMV) with those of HFV and was initially used for the treatment of acute respiratory diseases caused by burns and smoke inhalation and in the treatment of the newborn affected by hyaline membrane disease or infant respiratory distress syndrome (IRDS). Later on, it was employed in severe gas exchange impairment, where conventional mechanic ventilation (CMV) was useless [21]. Recently HPFV was investigated in a two-compartment heterogeneous mechanical model of the lung whether different mechanical resistive and elastic loads applied to one compartment, while the other is kept constant, would modify gas distribution between the two pathways and air trapping under HFPV [22]. Additionally, these results were compared with those generated in the same model by pressure-controlled ventilation (PCV). In this study the main advantage of HFPV seems to be ventilation at a lower mean airway pressure and lower inspiratory volumes, thus providing a protective effect against volutrauma and barotrauma.

Figure 23.9 shows the pressure-time curve for high-frequency percussive ventilation.

23.3.3 High-Frequency Oscillatory Ventilation

High-frequency oscillatory ventilation keeps the lung open by the application of a constant mean airway pressure. An oscillating piston produces phasic pressure swings around mean airway pressure, which are able to recruit alveolar units and to improve gas exchange, minimizing lung overdistension and atelectasis [23]. Small retrospective studies of HFOV in patients with ARDS and severe hypoxemia and/or elevated plateau airway pressures have revealed significant improvements in oxygenation. For this reason there are increasing evidences to use HFOV in the early phase of ARDS and life-threatening hypoxia [24].

Figure 23.10 shows the pressure-time curve for high-frequency oscillatory ventilation.

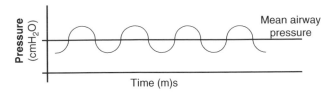

Fig. 23.10 Pressure-time curve for high-frequency oscillatory ventilation. The pressure waveform of HFOV oscillates around mean airway pressure. Time is expressed as ms

---

Conclusions

Invasive mechanical ventilation plays a relevant role in the overall clinical and therapeutic management of critically ill patients, independently from the presence of a specific lung disease. The optimal setting of mechanical ventilation appears to be associated with better outcome. New modes of mechanical ventilation may further improve the beneficial effects of respiratory assistance in critically ill patients.

References

1. Esteban A et al (2008) Evolution of mechanical ventilation in response to clinical research. Am J Respir Crit Care Med 177:170–177
2. Tobin MJ, Jubran A, Laghi F (2001) Patient–ventilator interaction. Am J Respir Crit Care Med 163:1059–1063
3. Singer BS et al (2009) Basic invasive mechanical ventilation. South Med J 102:1238–1245
4. Christopher KL, Neff TA, Bowman JL et al (1985) Intermittent mandatory ventilation systems. Chest 87:625–630
5. Dane N, Sai H (2007) Pressure control ventilation. Crit Care Clin 23:183–199
6. Fiastro JF, Habib MP, Quan SF (1988) Pressure support compensation for inspiratory work due to endotracheal tubes and demand continuous positive airway pressure. Chest 93:499–505
7. Henzeler D (2011) What on earth is APRV? Crit Care 15:115
8. Fan E, Stewart TE (2006) New modalities of mechanical ventilation: high-frequency oscillatory ventilation and airway pressure release ventilation. Clin Chest Med 27:615–625
9. Ambrosino N, Rossi A (2002) Proportional assist ventilation (PAV): a significant advance or a futile struggle between logic and practice? Thorax 57:272–276
10. Georgopoulos D, Plataki M, Prinianakis G et al (2007) Current status of proportional assist ventilation. Int J Intensive Care Med 14:74–80
11. Navalesi P et al (2003) New modes of mechanical ventilation: proportional assist ventilation, neurally adjusted ventilation assist and fractal ventilation. Curr Opin Vrit Care 9:51–58
12. Sinderby C, Navalesi P, Beck J et al (1999) Neural control of mechanical ventilation in respiratory failure. Nat Med 5:1433–1436
13. Verbrugghe W et al (2011) Neurally adjusted ventilatory assist: a ventilation tool or a ventilated toy? Respir Care 56:327–335
14. Suki B, Alencar AM, Sujeer MK et al (1998) Life support system benefits from noise. Nature 393:127–128
15. Gama De Abreu M, Spieth PM, Pelosi P et al (2008) Noisy pressure support ventilation: a pilot study on a new assisted ventilation mode in experimental lung injury. Crit Care Med 36:818–828
16. Spieth PM, Pelosi P, Gama De Abreu M et al (2009) Effects of different levels of pressure support variability in experimental lung injury. Anesthesiology 110:342–350

17. Branson RD (1995) High frequency ventilators. In: Branson RD, Hess DR, Chatburn RL (eds) Respiratory care equipment. J.B. Lippincott Company, Philadelphia, pp 458–469
18. Derdak S, Mehta S, Stewart TE, Smith T, Rogers M, Buchman TG, Carlin B, Lowson S, Granton J, Multicenter Oscillatory Ventilation for Acute Respiratory Distress Syndrome Trial (MOAT) Study Investigators (2002) High-frequency oscillatory ventilation for acute respiratory distress syndrome in adults: a randomized, controlled trial. Am J Respir Crit Care Med 166:801–808
19. Mehta S, Lapinsky SE, Hallet DC, Merker D, Groll RJ, Cooper AB, MacDonald RJ, Stewasrt TE (2001) A prospective trial of high frequency oscillatory ventilation in adults with acute respiratory distress syndrome. Crit Care Med 29:1360–1369
20. Sjöstrand UH (1977) Review of the physiological rationale for and the development of high-frequency positive-pressure ventilation (HFPPV). Acta Anaesthesiol Scand 64(Suppl):7–27
21. Gallagher TJ, Boysen PG, Davidson DD, Miller JR, Leven SB (1989) High frequency percussive ventilation compared with mechanical ventilation. Crit Care Med 17:364–366
22. Lucangelo U, Accardo A et al (2009) Gas distribution in a two compartment model ventilated in high frequency percussive and pressure-controlled modes. Intensive Care Med. doi:10.1007/s00134-010-1993-3
23. Van de Kieft M et al (2005) High-frequency oscillatory ventilation: lessons learned from mechanical test lung models. Crit Care Med 33:s142–s148
24. Diaz JV et al (2010) Therapeutic strategies for severe acute lung injury. Crit Care Med 38:1644–1650

Use of Respiratory Mechanics for Monitoring and Setting of Noninvasive Mechanical Ventilation

24

Luca Fasano, Lara Pisani, and Stefano Nava

Noninvasive ventilation (NIV) is an effective way to supply mechanical ventilation to patients with acute [1] and some forms of chronic respiratory failure [2].

Assisted mechanical ventilation is aimed to support the spontaneous activity of the respiratory system in order to make the insufficient mechanical output of the ventilatory pump adequate to meet the respiratory workload and improve alveolar ventilation. In the meantime, as the patient's ventilatory workload is at least in part performed by the mechanical ventilator, the respiratory muscles are allowed to rest. So the mechanical ventilator is an auxiliary pump which has to work in parallel to the patient's ventilatory pump to manage the workload required by the mechanics of the respiratory system with the dual aim to improve alveolar ventilation and unload respiratory muscles. As stated by Tobin et al., "for the most effective unloading of the inspiratory muscles, the ventilator should cycle in synchrony with the activity of a patient's own respiratory rhythm" [3]. In subjects undergoing invasive mechanical ventilation (IMV) in a controlled mode, patient–ventilator interaction can be enhanced by deep sedation (which reduces the ventilatory drive) up to neuromuscular blockade (which switches off any respiratory muscles activity), so that the patient leans on the ventilator settings up to a completely controlled ventilation. Nevertheless, neuromuscular blocking agents have significant hazards, and the prolonged (>48 h) inactivity of inspiratory muscles rapidly impairs diaphragm function [4–6]. In the

L. Fasano • L. Pisani
Respiratory and Critical Care Unit, Sant'Orsola Malpighi Hospital,
Via Massarenti, 9, Bologna 40138, Italy
e-mail: luca.fasano@aosp.bo.it; larapisani81@gmail.com

S. Nava (✉)
Respiratory and Critical Care Unit, Sant'Orsola Malpighi Hospital,
Via Massarenti, 9, Bologna 40138, Italy

Department of Specialistic, Diagnostic and Experimental Medicine,
Bologna University, Alma Mater Studiorum School of Medicine, Bologna, Italy
e-mail: stefano.nava@aosp.bo.it

A. Aliverti, A. Pedotti (eds.), *Mechanics of Breathing*,
DOI 10.1007/978-88-470-5647-3_24, © Springer-Verlag Italia 2014

case the clinician decides to ventilate noninvasively a patient, a minimal spontaneous activity and an acceptable sensorium are necessary to achieve a successful outcome; that is why sedation is not widely used in this setting [7]. NIV supports spontaneous ventilation instead of replacing or controlling it in collaborative patients, and the respiratory neural activity has to match with the ventilator rather than be abolished. Both the ventilatory pump and the mechanical ventilator are supervised: the ventilator pump is supervised by the patient's central nervous system, and the mechanical ventilator is supervised by the "caregiver" who decides the ventilator settings. As a matter of fact, two different "brains" need to be matched, and since the patient's one is not simple to control, the operator's brain should adapt the ventilator to the patient needs. The real challenge during mechanical ventilation is therefore not only to supply an efficacious support to the ventilatory pump but also to succeed in making the two pumps harmoniously work together, providing the best possible matching between the patient's ventilatory drive and the ventilator settings. Overall, the patient–ventilator interaction depends on how the ventilator responds to patient respiratory effort and, in turn, how the patient responds to the breath delivered by the ventilator [8]. Dealing with patient–ventilator synchrony means to try to improve the agreement between the patient's own neural respiratory cycle and the preset ventilator respiratory cycle so that (1) the patient breath initiation results in ventilator triggering, (2) the assisted-breath delivery matches with patient neural inspiratory time and effort, and (3) the duration of the delivered insufflation ceases when the patient terminates inspiration, avoiding ventilator persistent insufflation during patient exhalation. This is really important as patient–ventilator asynchronies often require a work of respiratory muscles which is necessary to tame the ventilator, but is wasted for ventilation. Furthermore, it has been shown that intubated patients who have a significant asynchrony in triggering the ventilator have worse outcomes; they have longer duration of mechanical ventilation and longer ICU and hospital stays and are less likely to be discharged home [9, 10]. A multiple regression analysis for the risk of intubation found that the SAPS II score and poor toleration of NIV were the two independent predictive factors of the need for mechanical ventilation [11] and tolerance to NIV is correlated with patient ventilator synchrony.

The crucial problem in respiratory mechanics during NIV is to match the two mechanics, the one of the patient and that of the mechanical ventilator, through a semi-open interface which generates air leaks that interfere on both the mechanical output of the two pumps and their interplay. It has been shown that the presence of an inspiratory leak proximal to the airway opening can be accompanied by marked variations in duration of the inspiratory phase and in auto-PEEP. The unstable behavior was observed using the simplest plausible mathematical models and occurred at impedance values and ventilator settings that are clinically realistic [12].

A careful recording of the neural timing is possible only employing sophisticated and invasive measurements such as diaphragmatic electromyography (EMG) with an esophageal electrode which has been shown to precisely reflect the mechanical output of the diaphragm in mechanically ventilated patients during an acute respiratory failure [13]. Indeed the estimation of the onset and duration of neural inspiratory time (Ti), using the flow signal, has been shown to have a poor agreement with

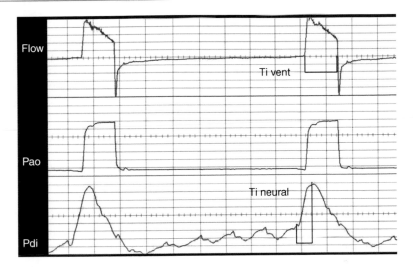

Fig. 24.1 Shows waves of the flow delivered by the ventilator and of airways and transdiaphragmatic pressures: the onset of neural TI was considered the onset of the upward deflection in Pdi and its end the peak transdiaphragmatic pressure

the diaphragmatic EMG-measured neural Ti [14]. In this chapter, indirect estimates of neural Ti were derived, respectively, from the following:

1. Esophageal pressure (Pes) tracing (onset was taken as the point of rapid decline in Pes, and three different points were used to estimate Ti termination: the nadir in Pes, the point of zero flow between inspiration and expiration, and the peak in Pdi)
2. Transdiaphragmatic pressure (Pdi) tracing (onset of neural TI was taken as the onset of the upward deflection in Pdi; the end of neural TI was taken as the return of Pdi to baseline or the point of zero flow between inspiration and expiration)
3. The flow tracing (as the time between the two points of zero flow)

These three different measurements were challenged with EMG-derived neural Ti used as reference measurement. The errors observed in the indirect estimates of neural Ti (from pressure or flow waveforms) had often a time lag from the onset of inspiration with an obvious influence of PEEPi. But sometimes an anticipation of inspiratory onset was observed; in these cases, the muscles involved in the motion of the rib cage may play a major role.

Despite these surrogate estimates of the onset and duration of neural Ti based on flow, esophageal and transdiaphragmatic pressures have proven discrepancies with EMG-measured neural Ti; they are widely used in the clinical practice (Fig. 24.1).

The occurrence of problems in patient–ventilator interaction specifically during the inspiratory triggering phase may be observed as explicit breath mismatching. This type of mismatching can be considered explicit because it may be observed on the flow and pressure tracings on the ventilator screen without requiring the greater precision of EMG measurements to support its evidence. However, this requires expertise by the operator in interpreting the events and close visual monitoring [15].

As stated also by Durbin, ventilator waveforms remain difficult to understand, because of the immense amount of information contained within the wave and the need to understand the context and the clinical conditions in which it is recorded. Indeed, waveforms are more complex than simple measurements or numbers, and therefore, familiarity with them requires frequent exposure and experience. Furthermore, viewing waveforms does not replace the clinical examination [16]. The pressure, flow, and volume waveform eye interpretation may give valuable information without any risk or harm to critically ill and very unstable patients and is a "skill that any practicing intensivist should possess" [17].

Anyway computer-assisted detection of patient–ventilator asynchronies has been attempted:

1. An algorithm embedded in the ventilator able to detect ineffective triggering and double triggering in real time, through the analysis of flow and pressure waves, has been compared with the analysis of transdiaphragmatic pressure waves by two experienced operators used as gold standard for detection of asynchronies with a very good sensitivity (91 %) and specificity (97 %) and a better specificity in patients intubated with respect to the ones undergoing NIV [15].
2. A signal generated noninvasively from flow, volume, and airway pressure using improvised resistance and elastance value and calculating respiratory muscle pressures (PVI monitor, YRT, Winnipeg, Canada) was compared with diaphragmatic pressure and proved to be helpful in monitoring patient–ventilator interaction, to give useful information to optimize the ventilator settings, and to provide breath-by-breath quantitative information of inspiratory muscle pressure [18, 19].
3. Another algorithm analyzing pressure and flow deflection has been shown to be as sensitive and specific in detecting ineffective breaths as the visual diagnosis of three different ICU attendees unaware of the Pes tracing [20].
4. Recently, mathematical algorithms that automatically detect ineffective breaths in a computerized (Better Care®) system that obtains and processes data from ICU ventilators in real time were validated using as control the visual inspection of the traces by five experts and the diaphragm electrical activity [21].

24.1 Putting Mechanics into Clinical Practice

Both in NIV and in IMV, the decision-making process to set the ventilator parameters has two aims:

- To supply an efficacious mechanical support at the ventilator pump
- To allow the best possible patient–ventilator synchrony and therefore patient's comfort

So the monitoring has to take care of the following:

- Ventilatory efficacy: satisfying mechanical output of the two ventilatory pumps working together, that is to say achieving an acceptable alveolar ventilation unloading, at least in part, the respiratory muscles

- Comfort of the patient, which is not only comfort of the patient–ventilator interface but also comfort of the patient–ventilator interplay: that is to say to reduce as far as possible asynchronies

The aims of setting and monitoring of NIV are similar to those of IMV, but the problems to face are different.

Ventilator Settings. Compared with invasive ventilation, NIV has some unique characteristics: First, leaks are unavoidable, even in the most careful settings since the absence of the translaryngeal tube, which directly connects the ventilator with the patient's airways, deeply influences not only airway resistances but also inspiratory flows and volumes owing to the problem of air leaks. Second, the ventilator–lung interaction cannot be considered as a single-compartment model because of the presence of a variable resistance represented by the upper airway.

Both situations may compromise the delivery of an effective tidal volume. As a consequence, increasing the volume delivered by the ventilator or the inspiratory pressure assistance during NIV does not necessarily result in increased effective ventilation. Indeed, it may induce a poor synchrony especially in those patients with high expiratory resistances where the "full exhalation" is almost impossible due to the increased time constants [22].

During IMV, alveolar ventilation is usually better controlled than during NIV and sometimes even reduced to protect the lungs from ventilator-induced lung injury (VILI) and, in patients with COPD, to prevent a further hyperinflation. VILI is not a major problem during NIV as the air leaks around the interface and the resistance of upper airways shields the lungs and the settings of the ventilator are usually adjusted to a level to improve tolerance and reduce air leaks, which means that the level of the inflation pressure at the airways rarely exceeds 25 cmH$_2$O.

Despite these "less aggressive" settings, a poor patient–ventilator interaction is quite frequent during NIV. Typically, the patient may not be able to trigger all the breaths (ineffective efforts) so that the respiratory muscle contraction is not followed by a mechanical support (see Fig. 24.2) and this causes detrimental effects on patient comfort and a variable amount of "wasted work." It may also happen that the patient does not succeed in switching the inspiration off, that is to say that the ventilator goes on insufflating air while the patient's own ventilatory drive is demanding for expiration. So the patient has to recruit his or her expiratory muscles to "fight" the ventilator, switch the inspiratory assistance off, and be allowed to exhale. These conditions are intriguing as the aim of mechanical ventilation is not only to improve alveolar ventilation but also to provide some respiratory muscle rest and not to increase somehow the work of breathing.

Trigger Asynchronies: Triggering is the switching on of the ventilator preset mechanical assistance to inspiration. The mechanical breath begins as the ventilator senses an inspiratory activity (negative pressure or inspiratory flow which attains a preset threshold). Patients reach the set sensitivity by activating their inspiratory muscles, but they cannot switch off respiratory motor output at the point of triggering. As a result, considerable effort is commonly expended over the period of mechanical inflation that follows the trigger phase, and this mainly depends on the patient's drive to breathe [3]. The reduction of respiratory drive is therefore desirable, and sedative could be used, but this indication has to be balanced with the increased risk of

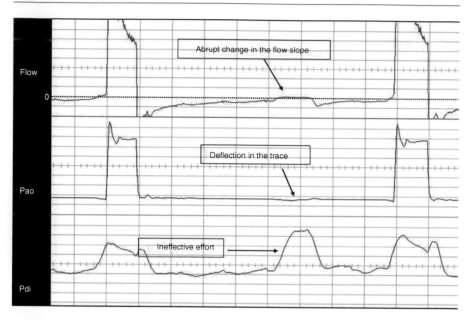

Fig. 24.2 Shows an ineffective inspiratory effort: the "diagnosis" is easier using the Pdi trace, but it can also be detected using only the flow and pressure traces displayed on the ventilator screen

hampering the sensorium and also the capacity of the patient to maintain a spontaneous breathing autonomy; indeed, sedation might be harmful for patient ventilator asynchrony [23]. In this context, remifentanil is a new synthetic opioid that has been proved to provide a good compromise between the reduction of patients' drive and the maintenance of breathing capacity, improving therefore the tolerance to this mode of ventilation. Remifentanil offers several pharmacokinetic advantages such as the steady plasma levels achieved in about 10 min and the half time for equilibration between plasma and its effect compartment of about 1–1.5 min during a constant-rate infusion. A further advantage of remifentanil is its constant and short context-sensitive plasma half time, which allows a prompt recovery after stopping the infusion. In a pilot study performed in an ICU in patients with NIV failure due to intolerance, a remifentanil-based sedation was shown to be safe and effective in improving tolerance and outcome of patients with acute respiratory insufficiency [24].

Asynchronies are both the failure to initiate a mechanical breath and the presence of a mechanical breath which is not demanded by the patient.

Ineffective breathing attempts are patient's inspiratory efforts which fail to trigger the ventilator mechanical breath. It can be detected by close observation of pressure and flow waves on the ventilator monitor, as pressure and expiratory flow sharply decrease without resulting in a ventilator-assisted breath (Fig. 24.2). As discussed earlier, recently different algorithms for a computerized detection of ineffective breaths have been proved to be specific and sensitive [15, 18–21]. Untriggered breaths are wasted respiratory work and may be caused by the patient (respiratory muscle weakness, failing ventilatory drive, or, above all in COPD, dynamic hyperinflation), by the ventilator setting (insensitive trigger, excessive delivered minute ventilation, high levels of pressure support), or by the interface (air leaks which interfere with pressures and flows sensed by the trigger) [25]. The level of sedation is important to blunt the respiratory drive and increase untriggering breaths [23]. Even when the patient is responsible of an ineffective breath, the ventilator setting may play a significant role. An over-assistance of inspiration may lead to the following:

1. Alveolar hyperventilation with respiratory alkalosis which reduces the ventilatory drive. Indeed, a progressive reduction of the respiratory drive has already been shown gradually increasing the inspiratory support [26].

2. High lung volumes which impair the efficiency of the ventilatory pump (unfavorable length/tension ratio of inspiratory muscles) induce alveolar hyperinflation and increase the PEEPi, which is a threshold to overcome before the preset pressure or inspiratory flow is generated.

This last problem is particularly significant in COPD patients and may be offset by applying an extrinsic positive end-expiratory pressure (PEEPe) which is able to reduce the width of the trigger threshold, even if it is not easy to determine in the clinical practice the exact level of PEEPe to set. On the other hand, PEEPe may foster air leaks and discomfort increasing the pressure inside the mask. Nontriggering attempts usually follow breaths with higher tidal volume and shorter expiratory time [26] so that "nontriggering results from premature inspiratory efforts that are not sufficient to overcome the increased elastic recoil associated with dynamic hyperinflation" [3]. The time elapsed between the activation of expiratory muscles and the triggering attempt is important too, above all the expiratory time spent after the mechanical insufflation of the ventilator has ended (see later Asynchronies of Cycling Off Inspiration). Indeed, the longer the expiratory time unopposed by the insufflating ventilator, the lower is the lung volume at which the triggering is attempted. The presence of airflow limitation and the consequent increase of PEEPi are thought to be very important in causing ineffective breaths, which could therefore be more frequent in COPD patients, compared to other patients with acute or chronic respiratory failure. The relationship between a high level of pressure support and rate of ineffective inspiratory efforts was emphasized in COPD patients, due to high lung compliance, which could be responsible for large tidal volumes. It has been shown that in these patients with low elastance, the ventilator continues to inflate the respiratory system long after the inspiratory muscles have ceased to contract and the next inspiratory attempt is likely to occur at a high lung volume, when airway pressure is still markedly positive; the inspiratory effort will not, therefore, always be sufficient to create a pressure gradient capable of being sensed by the ventilator [27, 28]. In a recently published paper, aimed to evaluate the prognostic importance of ineffective efforts in patients with acute respiratory failure undergoing IMV in a medical ICU, the presence of COPD did not discriminate for the presence of ineffective breaths >10 % [9]. Ineffective triggering however was a common problem early in the course of MV and was associated with increased morbidity, including longer MV duration, shorter ventilator-free survival, longer length of ICU stay, and lower likelihood of home discharge. These data were obtained in studies performed in subjects undergoing IMV, but a recently published paper addresses the

Fig. 24.3 Shows a double trigger that can be explicitly seen as a second inspiratory act delivered by the ventilator shortly after the end of the previous inspiration

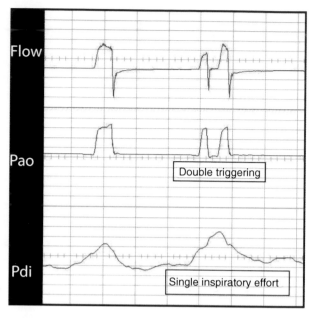

patient ventilator interaction during NIV in an acute setting. Patient–ventilator asynchronies were studied in subjects, admitted in ICU for acute respiratory failure and ventilated noninvasively observing pressure and flow traces on the ventilator screen and surface diaphragm EMG. Ineffective breaths were significantly correlated with air leaks even if the weak correlation suggests that leaks are not the only determinant of untriggering breaths. PEEPi may play a role but was not evaluated in this study; nonetheless, ineffective efforts were not more prevalent or severe in the group of COPD patients [25]. Patients with obstructive disease had a higher PTPdi/min, that is, an estimation of oxygen consumption of the diaphragm, mainly due to a higher R_L and PEEP$_{dyn}$. The level of pressure support was significantly higher in the presence of ineffective efforts >10 % confirming the importance of over-assistance of inspiration in inducing untriggering attempts of breath which has already been shown by other authors [29]. Vitacca et al. have demonstrated that during NIV, using the clinical settings based on the physician's experience, almost half of the patients enrolled for a home ventilatory program had ineffective efforts. The use of a more sophisticated and invasive technique of titration, with the insertion of gastric and esophageal balloons to record the respiratory mechanics, reduced (down to 30 %) the problem of asynchrony during NIV [30].

There are other two forms of triggering asynchronies: double triggering and autotriggering.

Double triggering happens when a second inspiratory act is delivered by the ventilator shortly after the end of the previous inspiration (Fig. 24.3). It happens when the patient respiratory drive is high, the neural Ti is longer than the mechanical Ti, or the ventilatory support is inadequate [8]. Indeed, in a series of acutely ill patients ventilated with NIV, double triggering was associated with a longer patient

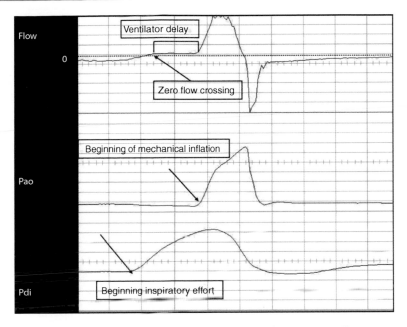

Fig. 24.4 Delayed triggering: the time lag between neural inspiration and ventilator inspiration is uncomfortably widened

inspiratory time, assessed by surface diaphragm EMG, and lower inspiratory pressure support [25]. *Autotriggering* is a ventilator-delivered breath in the absence of triggering attempt. It is more frequent when the patient breathes at low respiratory rate, with no PEEPi, and occurs when the triggering threshold of the ventilator is very low or there is water in the ventilator circuits. In patients ventilated in NIV, autotriggering, assessed by visual inspection of pressure and flow traces and of surface diaphragm EMG, is correlated with air leaks [25].

At last, *delayed triggering* happens when the time lag between neural inspiration and ventilator inspiration is uncomfortably widened (Fig. 24.4) and is more frequent when the respiratory drive is "lazy" or the ventilator trigger "hard."

After triggering, *inspiratory flow asynchrony* may happen. In this case, the flow delivered by the ventilator is insufficient to meet the patient expectations so that patients fight their impedance and that of the ventilator, increasing the inspiratory workload, to get more air. Flow asynchrony can be detected by observation of the inspiratory pressure–time trace which has a downward deflection during volume-controlled breaths in these patients "hungry" for air. The dip in the pressure–time wave is caused by the patient's inspiratory effort that pulls down the pressure during an insufficiently assisted inspiration. Increasing inspiratory flow matches the patient's demand but might increase respiratory rate, as Ti reduction is followed by a Te reduction too owing to a not fully understood nonchemical feedback. Very high flows delivered by the ventilator at the beginning of inspiration decrease the inspiratory neural time, and this induces a reduced tidal volume above all if the support to

Fig. 24.5 Premature cycling off: the ventilator ceases its inspiratory assistance while the patient is still breathing in; neural Ti is longer than the ventilator Ti

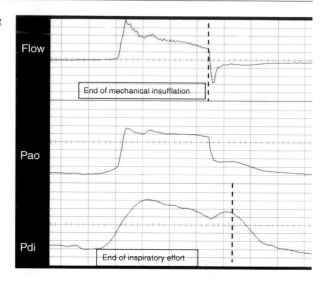

inspiration is low. So high inspiratory flows coupled with low inspiratory support could lead to a rapid shallow breathing pattern that could be misunderstood as persistent weaning failure [31]. Anyway even in COPD patients undergoing volume targeted ventilation, the reduction of the ventilator inspiratory time, notwithstanding the increased respiratory rate, induces a reduction of PEEPi by an increased time for exhalation [32]. Furthermore, it has been shown that in NIV, as pressurization rate increases, there is a reduction of the respiratory workload, assessed by PTPdi, as it happens during IMV; on the other hand, air leaks significantly increase and NIV acceptance decreases. Patient–ventilator interaction, assessed by calculating the ratio between the neural inspiratory time and the mechanical inspiratory time, worsens as this ratio is significantly shorter with the highest flow rate, indicating that, despite the inspiratory effort is reduced, the mechanical breath delivered by the ventilator exceeds what is required by the patient. These two variables seem to determine the tolerance to NIV, on one side the presence of higher leaks and on the other a mismatch between the inspiratory time of the patient and that provided by the ventilator [33].

Cycling Off Asynchronies. Cycling off is the switching from inspiration to expiration: the ventilator stops delivering inspiratory assistance and thereafter does not provide any support until being triggered again. The ventilator Ti may be shorter than neural Ti in controlled mechanical ventilation (CMV); in this case, the ventilator assistance ceases when a neural inspiratory output is still on (Fig. 24.5), and double triggering is expected. Vignaux et al. in their series of acute patients ventilated in NIV found that premature cycling was more prevalent in patients whose acute respiratory failure was caused by community-acquired pneumonia, and this is interesting as one of the main causes of premature cycling is thought to be a restrictive ventilatory defect [25]. On the other hand, the ventilator Ti may be longer than neural Ti; this could happen mainly during pressure support ventilation. In this ventilatory modality, the ventilator duty cycle ends when the inspiratory flow decreases under a preset threshold of maximum inspiratory flow; in COPD patients, the increased resistances to airflow and lung compliance delay the inspiratory flow decay so that the patient begins expiration while the ventilator is still insufflating air. This asynchrony can be seen in the pressure trace of the ventilator monitor as an end inspiratory peak causes an extra respiratory work and discomfort. It can be managed during pressure support ventilation by increasing the threshold of the maximum flow at which the ventilator cycles off. Tassaux et al. showed in intubated patients that increasing the expiratory trigger from 10 to 70 % of the maximum inspiratory flow significantly reduces the time lag between the end of neural and that of mechanical inspiration, PEEPi, the number of ineffective untriggering breaths, and the respiratory work to trigger the ventilator (triggering time product) [34]. While in intubated patients expiratory airflow limitation is the main determinant of delayed cycling, in NIV owing to the semi-open patient ventilator interface, an obstructive respiratory mechanics is only a contributing factor, and air leaks are the major determinant of this very common patient ventilator asynchrony [25]. A form of asynchrony that is a unique feature of PSV used in NIV is when the patient is unable to reach the criteria to switch from inspiration to expiration in the presence of large air leaks, when the inspiratory flow remains higher than the threshold value set for the expiratory trigger, because the ventilator tries to compensate for leaks. In this case, the flow signal reaches a sort of plateau after an initial brisk decay. Since all the ventilators now have a safety feature to avoid what was called the "hangover" phenomenon, inspiratory time cannot be longer usually than 3 s.

24.2   Clinical "Take-Home Messages"

Most of the studies assessing the incidence of asynchronies during NIV were performed during pressure support ventilation. Neurally adjusted ventilatory assist (NAVA) is an assisted ventilatory mode that delivers a pressure proportional to the integral of the electrical activity of the diaphragm (EAdi). Ventilator support begins when the neural drive to the diaphragm begins to increase, and pressure is cycled off when the respiratory centers end the EMG of the diaphragm. Compared with PSV, NAVA significantly reduces severe patient–ventilator asynchrony and results in similar improvements in gas exchange during NIV for acute respiratory failure [35, 36].

As stated before, the close observation of the flow and pressure traces on the ventilator screen may help the clinicians to detect and solve some "major" problems of patient–ventilator interaction. In COPD patients with an acute exacerbation, the visual detection of these waveforms has been shown to lead to a more rapid normalization of pH at 2 h (51 vs. 26 % of patients), to a significant improvement of the patient's tolerance to ventilation at 2 h, and to a higher decrease of PaCO2 at 2 and 6 h, compared to the group of patients ventilated with the parameters chosen by an operator with an "obscured" screen of the respirator [37].

Concerning the problem of chronic respiratory failure and home mechanical ventilation, it has been shown that NIV delivered in pressure support mode was effective in improving arterial blood gases and in unloading inspiratory muscles independent of whether it is set on the basis of patient comfort or tailored to a patient's respiratory muscle effort and mechanics. However, a tailored setting of the ventilator may result in reduction in ineffective inspiratory efforts, but this requires on one side expertise of the team and on the other side a "semi-invasive" measurement using the balloon-catheter techniques [30].

One particular problem in setting the ventilator in order to achieve the best interaction between the patient and the ventilator is that in the large majority of cases in the clinical practice, the ventilator settings are "decided" during the daytime. In patients with severe respiratory muscle weakness, patient–ventilator dyssynchrony may be a cause of suboptimal ventilation, especially at nighttime, when profound modifications in the recruitment of the respiratory muscle may occur during the various stages of sleep. In particular, in elderly patients recovering from an episode of acute hypercapnic respiratory failure in ICU, late NIV failure was associated with early sleep disturbances including an abnormal electroencephalographic pattern, disruption of the circadian sleep cycle, and decreased rapid eye movement sleep [38].

In a physiological study, we have shown, in stable patients with neuromuscular disorders, that the settings of NIV chosen on an empirical basis while the patient is awake do not predict ventilator synchrony while asleep and that an incorrect titration of inspiratory support or PEEPe may interfere with the triggering of the mechanical breath. A physiological setting, based on recording the inspiratory efforts, may minimize the rate of ineffective efforts, resulting in improvement of sleep quality and gas exchange [39]. For this reason, it has been suggested that the patient who is not tolerating, or benefiting from, NIV should be carefully evaluated during wakefulness with respiratory mechanics and then during sleep, and this should include respiratory polygraphy [40].

Last but not least, the choice of the ventilator and interfaces is a critical factor in improving patient–ventilator interaction during NIV. In a very recent in vivo and in vitro study, the authors showed that most dedicated NIV ventilators allowed better patient–ventilator synchronization than ICU and transport ventilators, even when the NIV algorithm was engaged, especially regarding the risk of autotriggering. Interestingly, most of the dedicated NIV ventilators exhibited a synchronization performance in the presence of leaks equivalent to that of the ICU ventilators in the absence of leaks [41].

Concerning the effects of the different interfaces on the incidence of asynchronies, few studies have been performed. Tarabini Fraticelli et al. have tested, among other clinical variables, the effects of four different interfaces (integral, full face, oronasal, and mouthpiece) on patient–ventilator interaction. Leaks were significantly larger with the mouthpiece, and not surprisingly the amount of asynchronies was higher with this kind of interface [42]. The helmet, an interface basically used in Europe, when compared to the full-face mask is equally tolerated and effective in ameliorating gas exchange and decreasing inspiratory effort. The helmet, however, was less efficient in decreasing inspiratory effort and worsened the patient–ventilator interaction [43]. Two physiological studies show that the ventilator settings have to be changed to improve the patient ventilator synchrony and this is achieved by increasing by 50 % the level of inspiratory aid and the amount of external positive pressure [44, 45].

Conclusions

Patient–ventilator asynchrony is underestimated in clinical practice. Particularly in patients with airflow limitation, it may cause increased duration of mechanical ventilation and increased frequency of tracheostomy. Air leaks additionally increase asynchrony during NIV and may interfere with the treatment success.

The clinician should consider how best to correct this harmful interaction between the "two brains" (i.e., the patient and the clinician who is responsible for the ventilator settings). The use of respiratory mechanics and EMG of the diaphragm to assess the problem of synchrony and eventually set the ventilatory parameter is definitively useful, but unfortunately it requires skill of the clinician and it is semi-invasive. The close observation of the physiological traces on the ventilator screen remains difficult to understand, because of the immense amount of information contained within the waves and the need to understand the context and the clinical conditions in which they are recorded but are really useful in clinical practice: they need experience in interpretation to be helpful but are a powerful tool in the hand of any intensive care specialist.

References

1. Nava S, Hill N (2009) Non-invasive ventilation in acute respiratory failure. Lancet 374:250–259
2. Hess DR (2012) The growing role of noninvasive ventilation in patients requiring prolonged mechanical ventilation. Respir Care 57:900–918
3. Tobin MJ, Jubran A, Laghi F (2001) Patient-ventilator interaction. Am J Respir Crit Care Med 163:1059–1063
4. Levine S, Nguyen T, Taylor N, Friscia ME, Budak MT, Rothemberg P, Zhu J, Sachdeva R, Sonnad S, Kaiser LR, Rubinstein NA, Powers SK, Shrager JB (2008) Rapid disuse atrophy of diaphragm fibers in mechanically ventilated humans. N Engl J Med 358:1327–1335
5. Petrof BJ, Jaber S, Matecki S (2010) Ventilator-induced diaphragmatic dysfunction. Curr Opin Crit Care 16:19–25
6. Hudson MB, Smuder AJ, Nelson WB, Bruells CS, Levine S, Powers SK (2012) Both high level pressure support ventilation and controlled mechanical ventilation induce diaphragm dysfunction and atrophy. Crit Care Med 40:1254–1260
7. Devlin JW, Nava S, Fong JJ, Bahhady I, Hill NS (2007) Survey of sedation practices during noninvasive positive-pressure ventilation to treat acute respiratory failure. Crit Care Med 35:2298–2302
8. Epstein SK (2011) How often does patient-ventilator asynchrony occur and what are the consequences? Respir Care 56:25–35
9. De Wit M, Miller KB, Green DA, Ostman HE, Gennings C, Epstein SK (2009) Ineffective triggering predicts increased duration of mechanical ventilation. Crit Care Med 37:2740–2745
10. Thille AW, Rodriguez P, Cabello B, Lellouche F, Brochard L (2006) Patient-ventilator asynchrony during assisted mechanical ventilation. Intensive Care Med 32:1515–1522

11. Carlucci A, Richard JC, Wysocki M, Lepage E, Brochard L (2001) Noninvasive versus conventional mechanical ventilation: an epidemiologic survey. Am J Respir Crit Care Med 163:874–880

12. Hotchkiss JR, Adams AB, Dries DJ, Marini JJ, Crooke PS (2001) Dynamic behaviour during noninvasive ventilation. Chaotic support? Am J Respir Crit Care Med 163:374–378

13. Beck J, Gottfried SB, Navalesi P, Skrobik Y, Comtois N, Rossini M, Sinderby C (2001) Electrical activity of the diaphragm during pressure support ventilation in acute respiratory failure. Am J Respir Crit Care Med 164:419–424

14. Parthasarathy S, Jubran A, Tobin MJ (2000) Assessment of neural inspiratory time in ventilator-supported patients. Am J Respir Crit Care Med 162:546–552

15. Mulqueeny Q, Ceriana P, Carlucci A, Fanfulla F, Delmastro M, Nava S (2007) Automatic detection of ineffective triggering and double triggering during mechanical ventilation. Intensive Care Med 33:2014–2018

16. Durbin CG (2005) Applied respiratory physiology: use of ventilator waveforms and mechanics in the management of critically ill patients. Respir Care 50:287–293

17. Georgopulous D, Prinianakis G, Kondili E (2006) Bedside waveforms interpretation as a tool to identify patient-ventilator asynchronies. Intensive Care Med 32:34–47

18. Younes M, Brochard L, Grasso S, Kun J, Mancebo J, Ranieri M, Richard JC, Younes H (2007) A method for monitoring and improving patient: ventilator interaction. Intensive Care Med 33:1337–1346

19. Kondili E, Alexopoulou C, Xirouchaki N, Vaporidi K, Georgopoulos D (2010) Estimation of inspiratory muscle pressure in critically ill patients. Intensive Care Med 36:648–655

20. Chen CW, Lin WC, Hsu CH, Cheng KS, Lo CS (2008) Detecting ineffective triggering in the expiratory phase in mechanically ventilated patients based on airway flow and pressure deflection: feasibility of using a computer algorithm. Crit Care Med 36:455–461

21. Blanch L, Sales B, Montanya J, Lucangelo U, Garcia-Esquirol O, Villagra A, Chacon E, Estruga A, Borelli M, Burgueño MJ, Oliva JC, Fernandez R, Villar J, Kacmarek R, Murias G (2012) Validation of the Better Care® system to detect ineffective efforts during expiration in mechanically ventilated patients: a pilot study. Intensive Care Med 38:772–780

22. Rabec C, Rodenstein D, Leger P, Rouault S, Perrin C, Gonzalez-Bermejo J, on behalf of the SomnoNIV group (2011) Ventilator modes and settings during non-invasive ventilation: effects on respiratory events and implications for their identification. Thorax 66:170–178

23. De Wit M, Pedram S, Best AM, Epstein SK (2009) Observational study of patient-ventilator asynchrony and relationship to sedation level. J Crit Care 24:74–80

24. Constantin JM, Schneider E, Cayot-Constantin S, Guerin R, Bannier F, Futier E, Bazin JE (2007) Remifentanil-based sedation to treat noninvasive ventilation failure: a preliminary study. Intensive Care Med 33(1):82–87

25. Vignaux L, Vargas F, Roeseler J, Tassaux D, Thille AW, Kossowsky MP, Brochard L, Jolliet P (2009) Patient-ventilator asynchrony during non-invasive ventilation for acute respiratory failure: a multicenter study. Intensive Care Med 35:840–846

26. Leung P, Jubran A, Tobin MJ (1997) Comparison of assisted ventilator modes on triggering, patients' effort, and dyspnea. Am J Respir Crit Care Med 155:1940–1948

27. Nava S, Bruschi C, Rubini F, Palo A, Iotti G, Braschi A (1995) Respiratory response and inspiratory effort during pressure support ventilation in COPD patients. Intensive Care Med 21:871–879

28. Nava S, Bruschi C, Fracchia C, Braschi A, Rubini F (1997) Patient-ventilator interaction and inspiratory effort during pressure support ventilation in patients with different pathologies. Eur Respir J 10:177–183

29. Thille A, Cabello B, Galia F, Lyazidi A, Brochard L (2008) Reduction of patient-ventilator asynchrony by reducing tidal volume during pressure-support ventilation. Intensive Care Med 34:1477–1486

30. Vitacca M, Nava S, Confalonieri M, Bianchi L, Porta R, Clini E et al (2000) The appropriate setting of noninvasive pressure support ventilation in stable COPD patients. Chest 118: 1286–1293

31. Laghi F (2003) Effects of inspiratory time and flow settings during assist control ventilation. Curr Opin Crit Care 9:39–44

32. Laghi F, Segal J, Choe WK, Tobin MJ (2001) Effect of imposed inflation time on respiratory frequency and hyperinflation in patients with chronic obstructive pulmonary disease. Am J Respir Crit Care Med 163:1365–70

33. Prinianakis G, Delmastro M, Carlucci A, Ceriana P, Nava S (2004) Effect of varying the pressurisation rate during noninvasive pressure support ventilation. Eur Respir J 23:314–320

34. Tassaux D, Gainnier M, Battisti A, Joillet P (2005) Impact of expiratory trigger setting on delayed cycling and inspiratory muscles workload. Am J Respir Crit Care Med 172: 1283–1289

35. Bertrand PM, Futier E, Coisel Y, Matecki S, Jaber S, Constantin JM (2013) Neurally adjusted ventilatory assist vs pressure support ventilation for noninvasive ventilation during acute respiratory failure a crossover physiologic study. Chest 143:30–36

36. Piquilloud L, Tassaux D, Bialais E, Lambermont B, Sottiaux T, Roeseler J, Laterre PF, Jolliet P, Revelly JP (2012) Neurally adjusted ventilatory assist (NAVA) improves patient–ventilator interaction during non-invasive ventilation delivered by face mask. Intensive Care Med 38:1624–1631

37. Di Marco F, Centanni S, Bellone A, Messinesi G, Pesci A, Scala R, Perren A, Nava S (2011) Optimization of ventilator setting by flow and pressure waveforms analysis during noninvasive ventilation for acute exacerbations of COPD: a multicentric randomized controlled trial. Crit Care 15:R283

38. Roche Campo F, Drouot X, Thille AW, Galia F, Cabello B, d'Ortho MP, Brochard L (2010) Poor sleep quality is associated with late noninvasive ventilation failure in patients with acute hypercapnic respiratory failure. Crit Care Med 38:477–485

39. Fanfulla F, Delmastro M, Berardinelli A, D'artavilla Lupo N, Nava S (2005) Effects of different ventilator settings on sleep and inspiratory effort in patients with neuromuscular disease. Am J Respir Crit Care Med 172:619–624

40. Elliott MW (2011) Non-invasive ventilation during sleep: time to define new tools in the systematic evaluation of the technique. Thorax 66:82–84

41. Carteaux G, Lyazidi A, Cordoba-Izquierdo A, Vignaux L, Jolliet P, Thille AW, Richard JC, Brochard L (2012) Patient-ventilator asynchrony during noninvasive ventilation. A bench and clinical study. Chest 142:367–376

42. Tarabini Fraticelli A, Lellouche F, L'Her E, Taillé S, Mancebo J, Brochard L (2009) Physiological effects of different interfaces during noninvasive ventilation for acute respiratory failure. Crit Care Med 37:939–945

43. Navalesi P, Costa R, Ceriana P, Carlucci A, Prinianakis G, Antonelli M, Conti G, Nava S (2007) Non-invasive ventilation in chronic obstructive pulmonary disease patients: helmet versus facial mask. Intensive Care Med 32:74–81

44. Vargas F, Thille A, Lyazidi A, Roche Campo F, Brochard L (2009) Helmet with specific settings versus facemask for noninvasive ventilation. Crit Care Med 37:1921–1928

45. Mojoli F, Iotti GA, Currò I, Pozzi M, Via G, Venti A, Braschi A (2013) An optimized set-up for helmet noninvasive ventilation improves pressure support delivery and patient-ventilator interaction. Intensive Care Med 39:38–44

Use of FOT for Optimising Mechanical Ventilation

25

Raffaele L. Dellacà, Pasquale P. Pompilio, Ramon Farré, Daniel Navajas, and Emanuela Zannin

Forced oscillation technique (FOT) is a simple and minimally invasive method used to study the mechanical properties of the respiratory system by measuring its response to an externally applied forcing signal (see Chap. 10).

An interesting feature of FOT, which contrasts with the conventional methods of measuring respiratory mechanics, is that FOT does not interfere with the breathing pattern and with ventilator cycling when combined to mechanical ventilation. The fact that FOT measurements do not require patient cooperation is of interest both in invasive and non-invasive artificial ventilation.

25.1   FOT Setup for Mechanical Ventilation

The application of FOT during mechanical ventilation demands an adaptation of the typical setup [1]. To produce the pressure stimuli, two possible approaches have been used. The first one consists of connecting an additional external oscillatory pressure generator in parallel to the inspiratory ventilator circuit. In this case, specific technical solutions must be implemented to make the generator able to withstand the positive pressure applied by the ventilator, such as enclosing the rear part of the loudspeaker in a sealed chamber [2, 3] or to servocontrol the loudspeaker cone position [6]. The second approach is based on controlling the pressure

R.L. Dellacà (✉) • P.P. Pompilio • E. Zannin
TBMLab, Dipartimento di Elettronica, Informazione e Bioingegneria,
Politecnico di Milano, Piazza Leonardo da Vinci, 32, Milan 20133, Italy
e-mail: raffaele.dellaca@polimi.it; pasquale.pompilio@polimi.it

R. Farré • D. Navajas
Unitat de Biofísica i Bioenginyeria, Facultat de Medicina,
Universitat de Barcelona-IDIBAPS-CIBERES,
Casanova 143, Barcelona 08036, Spain
e-mail: rfarre@ub.edu; dnavajas@ub.edu

A. Aliverti, A. Pedotti (eds.), *Mechanics of Breathing*,
DOI 10.1007/978-88-470-5647-3_25, © Springer-Verlag Italia 2014

generator or valve of the mechanical ventilator to enable them to superimpose forced oscillations onto the ventilation waveform [4–6].

In addition to the generation of an appropriate oscillatory waveform, other methodological issues should be taken into consideration when applying FOT in ventilated patients. In case of invasive ventilation, particular attention should be paid to avoid [7] or to correct for [3] the nonlinear impedance of the endotracheal tube. In case of non-invasive ventilation through a nasal/face mask, the artefacts associated to unintentional air leaks should be minimised [8].

Another FOT methodological issue, which is particularly important during mechanical ventilation, is related to the technical characteristics and frequency response of the sensors [9, 10].

25.2 Data Processing

In most studies, broadband pressure waveforms made by simultaneous multiple sinusoids [11] or small-amplitude random noise [12] are applied at the airway opening of the subject where pressure and flow are also measured. The flow and pressure signals are then decomposed into their individual frequency components using standard Fourier analysis [13–15], and the value of the impedance is determined at each particular frequency.

One drawback of using Fourier analysis for the estimation of respiratory impedance is the assumption of system stationarity during the measurement period. When a discrete sinusoidal forcing is used with a frequency sufficiently faster than breathing rates (i.e. 5–10 Hz), it is possible to compute impedance with a high temporal resolution and track within-breath variations of respiratory mechanical properties. In this case, the impedance can be obtained from algorithms based on cross-correlation [16, 17], fast Fourier transforms [2, 18] or various recursive and nonrecursive least square techniques [14, 19–23]. Within-breath analysis of impedance is potentially valuable for a wide range of clinical applications, such as detection of obstructive sleep apnoea and expiratory flow limitation [21, 24, 25], evaluation of lung mechanics during positive pressure ventilation [3] and examination of the effects of deep inspirations on airway constriction [22, 26, 27].

In this chapter, we will focus on the advantages of using within-breath forced oscillation technique for tailoring mechanical ventilation in two different applications: (1) during non-invasive ventilation (NIV) and (2) during invasive mechanical ventilation in patients with acute lung injury (ALI) or respiratory distress syndrome (RDS).

25.3 Application to Non-invasive Mechanical Ventilation

Monitoring the time course of total respiratory system resistance (R_{rs}) and reactance (X_{rs}) could be useful to assess the mechanical load of the respiratory system and to adapt the settings of the ventilator accordingly. Figure 25.1 shows an example of R_{rs}

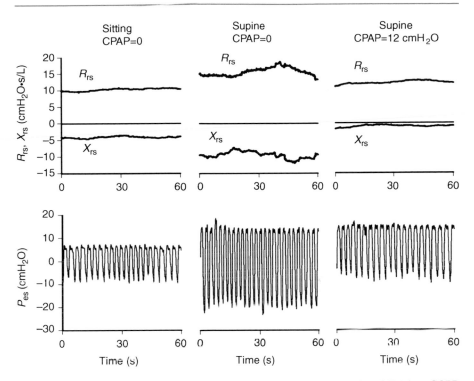

Fig. 25.1 Respiratory resistance (R_{rs}) and reactance (X_{rs}) measured by FOT (5 Hz) in a COPD patient at CPAP=0 in sitting (*left*) and in supine (*centre*) and in supine at CPAP=12 cmH$_2$O (*right*). Inspiratory effort is illustrated by the swings of the oesophageal pressure simultaneously recorded in the patient (P_{es}, *bottom*)

and X_{rs} measured during non-invasive ventilatory support through a nasal mask in a patient with chronic obstructive pulmonary disease (COPD) [22].

When the non-ventilated patient was moved from sitting to supine (at CPAP=0), R_{rs} increased and X_{rs} became more negative, indicating a marked increase in the mechanical load of the patient, which was reflected by an increase of the amplitude of oesophageal pressure swings. This variability of the mechanical load highlights the importance of adjusting the pressure support according to measures of lung mechanics. When the supine patient was subjected to a CPAP of 12 cmH$_2$O, respiratory impedance (and oesophageal pressure effort) considerably improved, probably due to a reduction in expiratory flow limitation (EFL).

In 1993, Peslin et al. reported that during mechanical ventilation, some COPD patients develop large negative swings in X_{rs} measured by FOT [3]. Similar results were also obtained using a simplified mechanical model of the respiratory system which included a flow-limiting resistance [28], as well as in mechanically ventilated rabbits after intravenous methacholine infusion [25]. This behaviour of reactance has been interpreted as follows: under normal conditions, reactance reflects the elastic and inertial properties of the entire respiratory system. When EFL is present, the linear velocity of gas passing through regions of dynamic airway compression (i.e. choke points) equals the local speed of pressure wave propagation (Fig. 25.2) [29]; thus, the

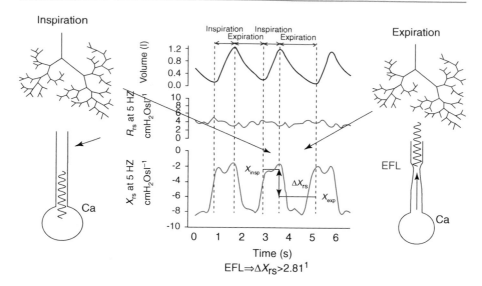

Fig. 25.2 Volume, resistance (R_{rs}) and reactance (X_{rs}) tracings in a representative COPD patient exhibiting expiratory flow limitation. ΔX_{rs} denotes the difference in reactance values measured at the beginning and end of an expiration. *EFL* expiratory flow limitation (Modified from Dellaca et al. [24])

flow becomes independent from the driving pressure with the choke points preventing the propagation of oscillations to the lung periphery. Therefore, when EFL is present, the oscillatory signal cannot pass through these choke points and reach the alveoli. As a consequence, impedance will reflect the mechanical properties of airways proximal to the choke points, which are much stiffer than the periphery. This results in a marked reduction of the respiratory compliance, as well as reactance, when measured by FOT (Fig. 25.2). Intratidal changes in X_{rs} were found to be able to detect EFL with 100 % specificity and sensitivity compared to the gold standard method based on the analysis of flow and transpulmonary pressure signals [24, 30].

Moreover, the measurement of impedance has the advantage of being suitable for the continuous and automatic monitoring of EFL [31] also during continuous positive airway pressure delivered by nasal mask [21], opening new perspectives for the automatic adjustment of positive end-expiratory pressure (PEEP) during non-invasive mechanical ventilation (Fig. 25.3).

Specifically, NIV is often used for the treatment of acute respiratory failure to improve pulmonary gas exchange and to unload the respiratory muscles, supporting the respiratory system while the underlying disease either improves or resolves. Among other ventilatory parameters, the application of PEEP has been widely and successfully used in patients with COPD to counteract the so-called intrinsic PEEP (PEEPi), i.e. the increase of end-expiratory pressure of the total respiratory system at end-expiration compared to the pressure measured in resting condition at the end of an end-expiratory pause. PEEPi is a sign of increased end-expiratory lung volume (EELV) above the mechanical resting volume (the functional residual capacity, FRC), a phenomenon called dynamic hyperinflation (DH).

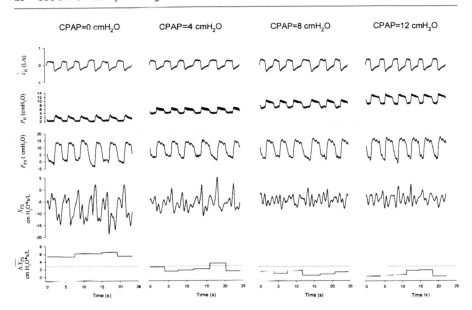

Fig. 25.3 Experimental tracing from a representative COPD patient. From *top* to *bottom*: Flow at the nasal mask (positive when inspiratory), nasal pressure, oesophageal pressure, total respiratory input reactance (X_{rs}) at 5 Hz and ΔX_{rs} for each breath at the four considered CPAP values of 0, 4, 8 and 12 cmH_2O (from *left* to *right*) (From Dellaca et al. [21], with permission)

DH occurs as a result of reduced expiratory flows or time so that inspiration starts before the respiratory system reaches FRC. DH commonly occurs in COPD, where the presence of expiratory flow limitation (EFL) forces the patient to breath at higher lung volumes to produce the necessary expiratory flow. In these patients, PEEPi provides a substantial threshold load that must be counterbalanced by respiratory muscles: the inspiratory flow starts only when the pressure developed by the inspiratory muscles exceeds PEEPi. In these conditions, the inspiratory efforts required by the patient may be excessive. It has been shown both in physiologic and clinical studies that the application of an external PEEP reduces the work of breathing, normalises the breathing pattern, improves blood gases and reduces patient–ventilator asynchrony [32–34].

On the other hand, if the externally applied PEEP is greater than the PEEPi, it results in an increased EELV (and, thus, in an increased work of breathing) and in adverse effects on haemodynamics, as it may severely decrease venous return and cardiac output, depending upon intravascular volume status, myocardial function and other factors [35–37].

For the application of an appropriate support, end-expiratory pressure should be tailored to each individual patient, taking into account that EFL is a condition that may considerably change with time [38], and particularly from night to day, as a consequence of the change in body posture and breathing pattern during sleep.

In a preliminary study, an automatic algorithm based on the continuous monitoring of EFL by FOT has been implemented in a commercial mechanical ventilator (Synchrony, Philips Respironics). Briefly, the ventilator has been modified in order

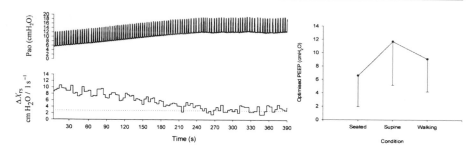

Fig. 25.4 (**a**) Example of automatic PEEP optimisation in a flow-limited COPD patient. PEEP is gradually increased until ΔX_{rs} is reduced to the threshold defining the presence of EFL (*dotted reference line*). (**b**) Optimal PEEP identified by the self-optimising ventilator on a group of COPD patients in three different conditions: seated position, supine and at the end of a 6-min walking test

to provide a 5 Hz sinusoidal pressure oscillation at the nasal mask and to compute in real time the value of ΔX_{rs}. According to the presence of tidal flow limitation, the algorithm adjusted automatically and gradually the PEEP until ΔX_{rs} fell below the threshold for flow limitation (Fig. 25.4a).

This self-optimising PEEP device has been used on COPD patients during three ventilation trials [39]: the first one was performed with the patient resting in the seated position, the second one with the patient in the supine position and the third one during a 6-min walking test (6 MWT). Total respiratory input impedance and breathing pattern parameters for each breath were computed and averaged at the end of each experimental condition.

On average, the optimised PEEP was minimal when the patient was resting in the seated position; it was maximal when patients were supine, likely as a consequence of the reduced lung volumes due to the displacement of the diaphragm in cranial direction; and it was somewhere in between the values identified in seated and supine position during the 6 MWT (Fig. 25.4b).

Even if this trend was highly representative of the behaviour of the patients, the baseline values and the changes with posture and exertion were quite different in each individual patient, leading to the high values of standard deviation. This variability underlines the importance of individual continuous tailoring of PEEP for these patients.

25.4 Applications to Invasive Mechanical Ventilation of Patients with Acute Lung Injury and Acute Respiratory Distress Syndrome

Acute lung injury (ALI) and the acute respiratory distress syndrome (ARDS) are characterised by alveolar flooding, widespread airway closure and disturbed ventilation–perfusion relationship, resulting in increased lung resistance, reduced lung compliance and hypoxaemia [40].

Artificial ventilation associated with various strategies utilising PEEP and lung recruitment manoeuvres (RM) have been shown to improve lung function in ARDS [41–43]. Unfortunately, artificial ventilation itself can worsen the existing injury through two distinct mechanisms: cyclic overdistention of lung units due to high and badly distributed tidal volumes (volutrauma) and shear stress associated with cyclic opening and closing of lung units (or atelectrauma). Both mechanisms can result in the release of inflammatory cytokines (biotrauma) that may worsen the injury. Recently, emphasis has been put on the development of more lung protective ventilation protocols. In particular, there is evidence that PEEP should be adjusted aiming at maximising the fraction of recruited lung [44, 45], while tidal volumes and inspiratory pressures should be set as low as possible in order to minimise overdistention [46]. The ability to quantify mechanical heterogeneities during ventilation may provide insight into the ongoing processes of derecruitment, alveolar flooding and parenchymal overdistention. Such information may therefore be of use for optimising parameters such as PEEP, tidal volume or respiratory rate.

Recent studies in mammalian models of ALI have demonstrated that the frequency-dependent features of impedance can be very sensitive indicators of mechanical heterogeneities in the lungs [4, 47–49]. Moreover, these studies emphasised the importance of monitoring dynamic elastic properties of the lungs or total respiratory system to assess recruitment and overdistention during ventilation. Kaczka et al. measured Z_{rs} in dogs using broadband (0.078 8.1 Hz) oscillations over mean airway pressures from 5 to 20 cmH$_2$O both at baseline and following oleic acid injury [48]. They found that the effective dynamic elastance as well as the heterogeneity of tissue mechanics increased following ALI, consistent with derecruitment. Both of these variables approached pre-injury levels as mean airway pressure increased, consistent with the recruitment of lung units.

An alternative approach consists in within-breath measurements of X_{rs} at a single frequency. In particular, measurements of reactance at 5 Hz have proved to be very sensitive and specific to changes in peripheral lung mechanics [21, 24, 50], and they have been used for the evaluation of lung volume recruitment with the following rationale: in the simplifying hypothesis that the alveolar units can be modelled by compliant elements connected to each other in parallel, the total compliance assessed at the airways opening should measure the sum of the compliance of the single alveolar units which are reached by the oscillations and, therefore, ventilated. Thus, if the distending pressure of the lung is kept constant, changes in compliance should be proportional to the number of alveolar units that are recruited or derecruited.

Dellacà et al. demonstrated that oscillatory compliance, derived from reactance measured at end-expiration at 5 Hz, could be used to monitor recruitment/derecruitment regardless of the model and distribution pattern of lung collapse (Fig. 25.5) [51].

The specificity of C_{X5} in detecting loss of ventilated lung is confirmed by the strong linear relationship between the percentage amount of derecruitment, assessed by CT, and oscillatory compliance ($R^2 = 0.89$).

Compared to the use of dynamic compliance (Cdyn) for monitoring lung volume recruitment and derecruitment, the use of C_{X5} offers three main advantages. First, since FOT requires very small lung volume changes, the measurement can be performed at a specific lung volume, minimising the artefacts due to nonlinearities of the respiratory system. On the contrary, Cdyn is calculated over a whole breath, and this large volume change invalidates the hypothesis of linearity on which the

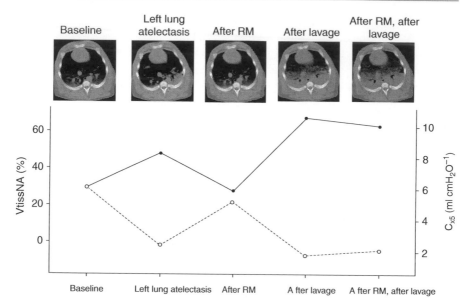

Fig. 25.5 *Upper panel*: CT scans at baseline, during left lung atelectasis, after an RM, post broncho-alveolar lavage and after RM after broncho-alveolar lavage. *Lower panel*: Corresponding non-aerated tissue volume (VtissNA%, *closed symbols*, *solid line*) and C_{X5} (*open symbols*, *dotted line*) (From Dellaca et al. [51] with permission)

calculation of Cdyn is based, especially in diseased lungs. Second, since C_{X5} is not affected by spontaneous breathing, it does not require sedation as Cdyn. Third, since C_{X5} may be measured with a high time resolution, it allows the assessment of within-breath changes of lung mechanics.

The most interesting application of FOT for assessing lung volume recruitment/derecruitment is for supporting the delivery of effective protective ventilation to the patients. In particular, FOT can be an effective tool for tailoring a value of PEEP that maximises recruitment while avoiding overdistention (see Chap. 8). In an experimental model of ALI/ARDS [52], monitoring X_{rs} during a decremental PEEP trial allowed the identification of open lung PEEP (PEEPol), defined as the minimum PEEP level required to prevent lung derecruitment after a recruitment manoeuvre, with high sensitivity and specificity when compared with CT (see Fig. 25.6).

The effects of repeated PEEP optimisation based on X_{rs} on oxygenation, lung mechanics and histologic markers of lung injury have been compared with the results obtained by applying the ARDSNet protocol based on oxygenation alone in a porcine surfactant-depletion lung injury model over a 12-h ventilation period [53]. The FOT-based optimisation strategy resulted in the selection of higher PEEP levels than the ARDSNet protocol. Higher levels of PEEP resulted in higher dynamic compliance in the FOT group leading to lower pressure amplitude and lower or comparable levels of plateaux pressure (Fig. 25.7).

Moreover, the PEEP optimisation strategy based on X_{rs} resulted in a better PaO_2/FiO_2 ratio and in reduced histopathologic evidence of VILI compared to the ARDSNet protocol.

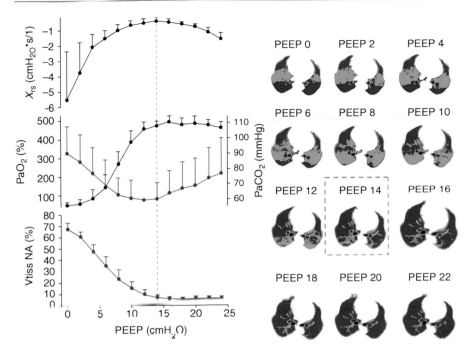

Fig. 25.6 *Left*: X_{rs}, blood gases (PaO$_2$ in *black* and PaCO$_2$ in *blue*) and percentage amount of non-aerated tissue during the deflation limb of the PEEP trial. *Right*: Representative CT slice at the different PEEP levels. *Black* over-aerated, *blue* normally aerated, *green* poorly aerated, *red* non-aerated (Modified from Dellacà et al. [52], with permission)

The same FOT approach can be easily applied during high-frequency oscillatory ventilation (HFOV), an attractive alternative to conventional mechanical ventilation (CMV) that has the potential to reduce ventilator-induced lung injury when optimally applied [54–56]. It has been recently shown that accurate measurements of X_{rs} can be readily obtained from the mechanical response of the respiratory system to the oscillatory waveform being delivered by the high-frequency oscillator [57], and that these measures can be used to tailor mean airway pressure (P_{AW}), the primary variable affecting oxygenation [58] and the most critical determinant of ventilator-induced lung injury.

As FOT can be performed with high temporal resolution and without changing lung volume, during CMV, it can be used to assess lung mechanical properties both at end-inspiration and end-expiration [59] (Fig. 25.8).

The measurement of intratidal changes in X_{rs} has the potentials to be used not only to optimise and individualise PEEP but also to evaluate the tidal recruitment and distention associated to different pressure amplitudes or tidal volumes.

The application of FOT for tailoring mechanical ventilation is particularly interesting for neonatal intensive care. Newborns, especially those born preterm, are more prone to lung damage and VILI because of their immature lung structure and very compliant chest wall. Moreover, the inflammatory process induced by the mechanical stress to lung tissue dramatically increases the mortality and is a major cause of the development of a chronic lung disease called broncho-pulmonary dysplasia (BPD).

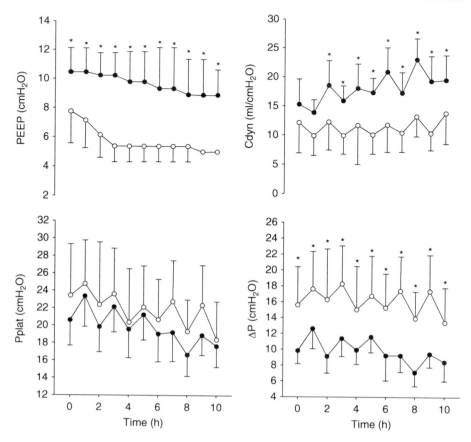

Fig. 25.7 Ventilatory and respiratory mechanics parameters over time. Positive end-expiratory pressure (*PEEP*), plateau pressure (P_{plat}), driving pressure (ΔP) and dynamic compliance (C_{dyn}) for the forced oscillation technique (*FOT*) group (*closed symbols*) and for the ARDSNet group (*open symbols*). Significance of differences between the two: * for $p < 0.01$ (From Kostic et al. [53] with permission)

FOT is an ideal technique to be applied in the neonates as it is less affected by leaks than dynamic compliance, an important feature as in small babies the fragility of tracheal tissues prevents the use of cuffed intratracheal tubes. Moreover, the highly irregular breathing pattern and the high respiratory rate of term and preterm babies make it difficult to use other approaches to assess the mechanical condition of their lungs. Back in 1983, Dorkin et al. described the relationship between impedance and frequency in infants with RDS [60]. Based on the frequency dependency of resistance and reactance, Sullivan et al. [61] distinguished between two classes of patients related to different postnatal age, suggesting that FOT can help in following changes in lung function associated to long-term mechanical ventilation. These interesting results were not transferred to the clinical practice because of the criticalities of the measurement setups used in these first studies. In fact, infants were disconnected from the ventilator and connected to a device that provided a stimulus within a wide range of frequencies. In 1998, Gauthier et al. [62] used single-frequency FOT superimposed to the ventilator waveform to evaluate lung function in ventilated infants affected by bronchiolitis. Infants were evaluated at different levels of PEEP, and two different behaviours were observed: infants with very high resistance and negative reactance at low PEEP were more responsive to changes in PEEP, while in other infants, changes in PEEP produced limited effect on R_{rs} and X_{rs}.

In preterm lambs receiving HFOV, Pillow et al. [63] showed that FOT successfully tracks changes in lung mechanics associated to both recruitment manoeuvres and surfactant administration. The partitioning of lung mechanics into airway and tissue components showed that tissue resistance constitutes the main resistive component of impedance in a structurally immature lung, and that both surfactant prophylaxis and volume recruitment manoeuvres predominantly influence tissue rather than airway impedance, with the reduction in tissue resistance being proportionally greater than the decrease in tissue elastance.

In a recent study, Dellacà et al. [64] evaluated respiratory system impedance during an incremental/decremental PEEP trial in different groups of infants (controls, RDS and infants with evolving BPD) subjected to mechanical ventilation. This study showed that in ventilated preterm newborns, respiratory system impedance is very sensitive to changes in PEEP, and the relationship between impedance and PEEP has specific features in different lung diseases, suggesting that FOT can provide useful information for tailoring the ventilator settings according to the pathophysiological characteristics of these difficult and fragile patients.

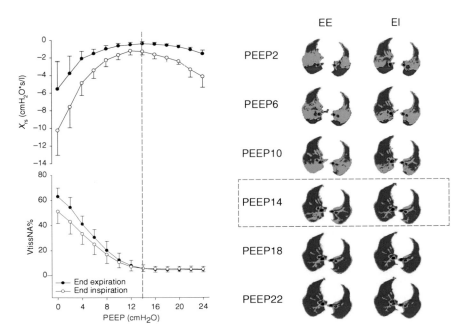

Fig. 25.8 *Left*: Reactance and percentage amount of non-aerated tissue (VtissNA%) at end-expiration (*closed symbols*) and at end-inspiration (*open symbols*) as a function of decreasing PEEP. *Right*: CT images for selected protocol steps. *Red* non-aerated region, *green* poorly aerated, *blue* normally aerated. The *dashed line* indicates open lung PEEP (Modified from Zannin et al. [59] with permission)

Conclusions

FOT allows an easy and accurate assessment of respiratory mechanics during non-invasive and invasive mechanical ventilation. R_{rs} and X_{rs} values reflect the interaction of the elastic, resistive and inertial properties of the whole respiratory system and provide information about the presence of EFL and lung volume heterogeneity and recruitment, variables of a great pathophysiological interest and with direct application in clinical practice. Moreover, FOT may be a useful tool for monitoring the status and evolution of respiratory mechanics in the ventilated patient and could be a complementary tool for optimising the ventilator settings. Although the application of FOT during invasive and non-invasive mechanical ventilation has been so far limited to research studies, the current development of the technique, in particular considering the within-breath approach, facilitates its application in the clinical setting.

References

1. Navajas D, Farrè R (2000) Forced oscillation assessment of respiratory mechanics in ventilated patients. Crit Care 5:3–9
2. Navajas D, Farrè R, Rotger M et al (1998) Assessment of airflow obstruction during CPAP by means of forced oscillation in patients with sleep apnea. Am J Respir Crit Care Med 157:1526–1530
3. Peslin R, Felicio-da SJ, Duvivier C, Chabot F (1993) Respiratory mechancics studied by forced oscillations during artificial ventilation. Eur Respir J 6:772–784
4. Farrè R, Ferrer M, Rotger M, Navajas D (1995) Servocontrolled generator to measure respiratory impedance from 0.25 to 26 Hz in ventilated patients at different PEEP levels. Eur Respir J 8:1222–1227
5. Lutchen KR, Yang K, Kaczka DW, Suki B (1993) Optimal ventilation waveform for estimating low-frequency respiratory impedance. J Appl Physiol 75:478–488
6. Farrè R, Rotger M, Monserrat JM, Navajas D (1997) A system to generate simultaneous forced oscillation and continuous positive airway pressure. Eur Respir J 10:1349–1353
7. Farrè R, Manzini M, Rotger M et al (2001) Oscillatory resistance measured during noninvasive proportional assist ventilation. Am J Respir Crit Care Med 164:790–794
8. Navajas D, Farrè R, Rotger M, Canet J (1989) Recording pressure at the distal end of the endotracheal tube to measure respiratory impedance. Eur Respir J 2:178–184
9. Farrè R, Peslin R, Rotger M et al (1999) Forced oscillation total respiratory resistance and spontaneous breathing lung resistance in COPD patients. Eur Respir J 14:172–178
10. Farrè R, Navajas D, Peslin R et al (1990) A correction procedure for the asymmetry of differential pressure transducers in respiratory impedance measurements. IEEE Trans Biomed Eng 36:1137–1140
11. Daroczy B, Hantos Z (1990) Generation of optimum pseudorandom signals for respiratory impedance measurements. Int J Biomed Comput 25:21–31
12. Michaelson ED, Grassman ED, Peters WR (1975) Pulmonary mechanics by spectral analysis of forced random noise. J Clin Invest 56:1210–1230
13. Cooley JW, Tukey JW (1965) An algorithm for the machine calculation of complex Fourier series. Math Comput 19:297–301
14. Kaczka DW, Barnas GM, Suki B, Lutchen KR (1995) Assessment of time-domain analyses for estimation of low-frequency respiratory mechanical properties and impedance spectra. Ann Biomed Eng 23:135–151

15. Welch PD (1967) The use of fast Fourier transform for the estimation of power spectra: a method based on time averaging over short, modified periodograms. IEEE Trans Audio Electroacoustics 15:70–73

16. Horowitz JG, Siegel SD, Primiano FPJ, Chester EH (1983) Computation of respiratory impedance from forced sinusoidal oscillations during breathing. Comput Biomed Res 16:499–521

17. Peslin R, Ying Y, Gallina C, Duvivier C (1992) Within-breath variations of forced oscillation resistance in healthy subjects. Eur Respir J 5:86–92

18. Cauberghs M, Van de Woestijne KP (1992) Changes of respiratory input impedance during breathing in humans. J Appl Physiol 73:2355–2362

19. Avanzolini G, Barbini P (1985) A comparative evaluation of three on-line identification methods for a respiratory mechanical model. IEEE Trans Biomed Eng 32:957–963

20. Avanzolini G, Barbini P, Cappello A, Cevenini G (1990) Real-time tracking of parameters of lung mechanics: emphasis on algorithm tuning. J Biomed Eng 12:489–495

21. Dellaca RL, Rotger M, Aliverti A, Navajas D, Pedotti A, Farre R (2006) Noninvasive detection of expiratory flow limitation in COPD patients during nasal CPAP. Eur Respir J 27:983–991

22. Jensen A, Atileh H, Suki B, Ingenito EP, Lutchen KR (2001) Selected contribution: airway caliber in healthy and asthmatic subjects: effects of bronchial challenge and deep inspirations. J Appl Physiol 91:506–515

23. Lauzon AM, Bates JH (1991) Estimation of time-varying respiratory mechanical parameters by recursive least squares. J Appl Physiol 71:1159–1165

24. Dellaca RL, Santus P, Aliverti A, Stevenson N, Centanni S, Macklem PT et al (2004) Detection of expiratory flow limitation in COPD using the forced oscillation technique. Eur Respir J 23:232–240

25. Vassiliou M, Peslin R, Saunier C, Duvivier C (1996) Expiratory flow limitation during mechanical ventilation detected by the forced oscillation method. Eur Respir J 9:779–786

26. Baldi S, Dellaca R, Govoni L, Torchio R, Aliverti A, Pompilio P et al (2010) Airway distensibility and volume recruitment with lung inflation in COPD. J Appl Physiol 109:1019–1026

27. Pellegrino R, Pompilio PP, Bruni GI, Scano G, Crimi C, Biasco L et al (2009) Airway hyperresponsiveness with chest strapping: a matter of heterogeneity or reduced lung volume? Respir Physiol Neurobiol 166:47–53

28. West JB (2008) Pulmonary pathophysiology: the essentials, 7th edn. Lippincott Williams & Wilkins, Baltimore

29. Peslin R, Farre R, Rotger M, Navajas D (1996) Effect of expiratory flow limitation on respiratory mechanical impedance: a model study. J Appl Physiol 81:2399–2406

30. Dawson SV, Elliott EA (1977) Wave-speed limitation on expiratory flow-a unifying concept. J Appl Physiol 43:498–515

31. Mead J, Whittenberger JL (1953) Physical properties of human lungs measured during spontaneous breathing. J Appl Physiol 5:779–796

32. Appendini L, Patessio A, Zanaboni S, Carone M, Gukov B, Donner CF et al (1994) Physiologic effects of positive end-expiratory pressure and mask pressure support during exacerbations of chronic obstructive pulmonary disease. Am J Respir Crit Care Med 149:1069–1076

33. Elliott MW, Mulvey DA, Moxham J, Green M, Branthwaite MA (1993) Inspiratory muscle effort during nasal intermittent positive pressure ventilation in patients with chronic obstructive airways disease. Anaesthesia 48:8–13

34. Nava S, Bruschi C, Fracchia C, Braschi A, Rubini F (1997) Patient-ventilator interaction and inspiratory effort during pressure support ventilation in patients with different pathologies. Eur Respir J 10:177–183

35. Ambrosino N, Nava S, Torbicki A, Riccardi G, Fracchia C, Opasich C et al (1993) Haemodynamic effects of pressure support and PEEP ventilation by nasal route in patients with stable chronic obstructive pulmonary disease. Thorax 48:523–528

36. Baigorri F, de Monte A, Blanch L, Fernandez R, Valles J, Mestre J et al (1994) Hemodynamic responses to external counterbalancing of auto-positive end-expiratory pressure in mechanically ventilated patients with chronic obstructive pulmonary disease. Crit Care Med 22:1782–1791

37. Ranieri VM, Giuliani R, Cinnella G, Pesce C, Brienza N, Ippolito EL et al (1993) Physiologic effects of positive end-expiratory pressure in patients with chronic obstructive pulmonary disease during acute ventilatory failure and controlled mechanical ventilation. Am Rev Respir Dis 147:5–13

38. Patel H, Yang KL (1995) Variability of intrinsic positive end-expiratory pressure in patients receiving mechanical ventilation. Crit Care Med 23:1074–1079

39. Bernard GR, Artigas A, Brigham KL, Carlet J, Falke K, Hudson L et al (1994) The American-European Consensus Conference on ARDS. Definitions, mechanisms, relevant outcomes, and clinical trial coordination. Am J Respir Crit Care Med 149:818–824

40. Meade MO, Cook DJ, Guyatt GH, Slutsky AS, Arabi YM, Cooper DJ et al (2008) Ventilation strategy using low tidal volumes, recruitment maneuvers, and high positive end-expiratory pressure for acute lung injury and acute respiratory distress syndrome: a randomized controlled trial. JAMA 299:637–645

41. Mercat A, Richard JC, Vielle B, Jaber S, Osman D, Diehl JL et al (2008) Positive end-expiratory pressure setting in adults with acute lung injury and acute respiratory distress syndrome: a randomized controlled trial. JAMA 299:646–655

42. Villar J, Kacmarek RM, Perez-Mendez L, Aquirre-Jaime A (2006) A high positive end-expiratory pressure, low tidal volume ventilatory strategy improves outcome in persistent acute respiratory distress syndrome: a randomized, controlled trial. Crit Care Med 34:1311–1318

43. Bellardine Black CL, Hoffman AM, Tsai LW, Ingenito EP, Suki B, Kaczka DW et al (2008) Impact of positive end-expiratory pressure during heterogeneous lung injury: insights from computed tomographic image functional modeling. Ann Biomed Eng 36:980–991

44. Ware LB, Matthay MA (2000) The acute respiratory distress syndrome. N Engl J Med 342:1334–1349

45. Brower RG, Lanken PN, MacIntyre N, Matthay MA, Morris A, Ancukiewicz M et al (2004) Higher versus lower positive end-expiratory pressures in patients with the acute respiratory distress syndrome. N Engl J Med 351:327–336

46. Ventilation with lower tidal volumes as compared with traditional tidal volumes for acute lung injury and the acute respiratory distress syndrome. The Acute Respiratory Distress Syndrome Network (2000) N Engl J Med 342:1301–1308

47. Bellardine CL, Ingenito EP, Hoffman A, Lopez F, Sanborn W, Suki B et al (2005) Heterogeneous airway versus tissue mechanics and their relation to gas exchange function during mechanical ventilation. Ann Biomed Eng 33:626–641

48. Kaczka DW, Hager DN, Hawley ML, Simon BA (2005) Quantifying mechanical heterogeneity in canine acute lung injury: impact of mean airway pressure. Anesthesiology 103:306–317

49. Kaczka DW, Brown RH, Mitzner W (2009) Assessment of heterogeneous airway constriction in dogs: a structure-function analysis. J Appl Physiol 106:520–530

50. Johnson MK, Birch M, Carter R, Kinsella J, Stevenson RD (2005) Use of reactance to estimate transpulmonary resistance. Eur Respir J 25:1061–1069

51. Dellaca RL, Andersson OM, Zannin E, Kostic P, Pompilio PP, Hedenstierna G et al (2009) Lung recruitment assessed by total respiratory system input reactance. Intensive Care Med 35(12):2164–2172

52. Dellaca RL, Zannin E, Kostic P, Olerud MA, Pompilio PP, Hedenstierna G et al (2011) Optimisation of positive end-expiratory pressure by forced oscillation technique in a lavage model of acute lung injury. Intensive Care Med 37:1021–1030

53. Kostic P, Zannin E, Andersson OM, Pompilio PP, Hedenstierna G, Pedotti A et al (2011) Positive end-expiratory pressure optimization with forced oscillation technique reduces ventilator induced lung injury: a controlled experimental study in pigs with saline lavage lung injury. Crit Care 35(12):2164–2172

54. McCulloch PR, Forkert PG, Froese AB (1988) Lung volume maintenance prevents lung injury during high frequency oscillatory ventilation in surfactant-deficient rabbits. Am Rev Respir Dis 137:1185–1192

55. Meredith KS, de Lemos RA, Coalson JJ, King RJ, Gerstmann DR, Kumar R et al (1989) Role of lung injury in the pathogenesis of hyaline membrane disease in premature baboons. J Appl Physiol 66:2150–2158

56. Froese AB (1997) High-frequency oscillatory ventilation for adult respiratory distress syndrome: let's get it right this time! Crit Care Med 25:906–908

57. Bond DM, Froese AB (1993) Volume recruitment maneuvers are less deleterious than persistent low lung volumes in the atelectasis-prone rabbit lung during high-frequency oscillation. Crit Care Med 21:402–412

58. Dellacà R, Zannin E, Ventura M, Sancini G, Pedotti A, Tagliabue P et al (2013) Assessment of dynamic mechanical properties of the respiratory system during high frequency oscillatory ventilation. Crit Care Med 41:2502–2511

59. Zannin E, Dellaca RL, Kostic P, Pompilio PP, Larsson A, Pedotti A et al (2012) Optimizing positive end-expiratory pressure by oscillatory mechanics minimizes tidal recruitment and distension: an experimental study in a lavage model of lung injury. Crit Care 16:R217

60. Dorkin HL, Stark AR, Werthammer JW, Strieder DJ, Fredberg JJ, Frantz ID (1983) Respiratory system impedance from 4 to 40 Hz in paralyzed intubated infants with respiratory disease. J Clin Invest 72:903–910

61. Sullivan KJ, Durand M, Chang HK (1991) A forced perturbation method of assessing pulmonary mechanical function in intubated infants. Pediatr Res 29:82–88

62. Gauthier R, Beyaert C, Feillet F, Peslin R, Monin P, Marchal F (1998) Respiratory oscillation mechanics in infants with bronchiolitis during mechanical ventilation. Pediatr Pulmonol 25:18–31

63. Pillow JJ, Sly PD, Hantos Z (2004) Monitoring of lung volume recruitment and derecruitment using oscillatory mechanics during high-frequency oscillatory ventilation in the preterm lamb. Pediatr Crit Care Med 5:172–180

64. Dellaca RL, Veneroni C, Vendettuoli V, Zannin E, Matassa PG, Pedotti A et al (2013) Relationship between respiratory impedance and positive end-expiratory pressure in mechanically ventilated neonates. Intensive Care Med 39:511–519

Index

A. Aliverti, A. Pedotti (eds.), *Mechanics of Breathing*,
DOI 10.1007/978-88-470-5647-3, © Springer-Verlag Italia 2014